DATE DUE			

The First Session in Brief Therapy

The First Session in Brief Therapy

Edited by

Simon H. Budman,
Michael F. Hoyt,
and Steven Friedman

THE GUILFORD PRESS
New York / London

© **1992 The Guilford Press**

A Division of Guilford Publications, Inc.

72 Spring Street, New York, NY 10012

Printed in the United States of America

This book is printed on acid-free paper.

Last digit is print number: 9 8 7 6 5 4 3 2

Library of Congress Cataloging-in-Publication Data

The First session in brief therapy / edited by Simon H. Budman,
    Michael F. Hoyt, and Steven Friedman.
        p.   cm.
    Includes bibliographical references and index.
    ISBN 0-89862-138-0
    1. Brief psychotherapy.   I. Budman, Simon H.
II. Hoyt, Michael   F.   III. Friedman, Steven, 1945–
    [DNLM: 1. Psychotherapy, Brief.   WM 420 F527]
RC480.55.F56   1992
616.89′14—dc20
DNLM/DLC
for Library of Congress   92-1533
                                                              CIP

Contributors

STEVE ANDREAS, MA, NLP Comprehensive, Boulder, Colorado

CONNIRAE ANDREAS, PhD, NLP Comprehensive, Boulder, Colorado

HARRY J. APONTE, ACSW, Family Therapy Training Program of Philadelphia, Philadelphia, Pennsylvania

DONALD H. BAUCOM, PhD, Department of Psychology, University of North Carolina–Chapel Hill, Chapel Hill, North Carolina

JEFFREY L. BINDER, PhD, Georgia School of Professional Psychology, Atlanta, Georgia

SIMON H. BUDMAN, PhD, Harvard Community Health Plan and Department of Psychiatry, Harvard Medical School; and Innovative Training Systems, Boston, Massachusetts

STEPHEN F. BUTLER, PhD, Department of Psychology, Northeast Psychiatric Associates/Brookside Hospital, Nashua, New Hampshire

ROBERT CARELS, Graduate Student, Clinical Psychology, University of North Carolina–Chapel Hill, Chapel Hill, North Carolina

JUDY DAVIDSON, MA, Brattleboro Family Institute, Brattleboro, Vermont

ALBERT ELLIS, PhD, Institute for Rational–Emotive Therapy, New York, New York

NORMAN EPSTEIN, PhD, Department of Family and Community Development, University of Maryland, College Park, Maryland

RICHARD FISCH, MD, Brief Therapy Center of the Mental Research Institute, Palo Alto, California

STEVEN FRIEDMAN, PhD, Harvard Community Health Plan–The Braintree Center and Lesley College Graduate School, Braintree, Massachusetts

LESLIE S. GREENBERG, PhD, Department of Psychology, York University, Toronto, Ontario, Canada

ALAN S. GURMAN, PhD, Department of Psychiatry, University of Wisconsin Medical School, Madison, Wisconsin

MICHAEL F. HOYT, PhD, Department of Psychiatry, Kaiser-Permanente Medical Center, Hayward, California; and Clinical Professor, Langley Porter Institute, University of California, San Francisco

SUSAN M. JOHNSON, PhD, Department of Psychology and Psychiatry, University of Ottawa, Ottawa, Ontario, Canada

ROBERT ROSENBAUM, PhD, California Institute of Integral Studies, San Francisco

HANS H. STRUPP, PhD, Department of Psychology, Vanderbilt University, Nashville, Tennessee

MOSHE TALMON, PhD, P.O. Box 9593, Kfar Shmarione 46910, Israel

RALPH M. TURNER, PhD, Department of Psychiatry, Temple University School of Medicine, Philadelphia, Pennsylvania

MICHAEL D. YAPKO, PhD, Milton Erickson Institute of San Diego, California

JOHN H. WEAKLAND, MD, Brief Therapy Center of the Mental Research Institute, Palo Alto, California

Preface

The First Session in Brief Therapy arose out of our interest in updating *Forms of Brief Therapy* (Budman, 1981). Initially we thought of simply offering a revision of the material covered in *Forms*. It rapidly became apparent to us that over a period of 10 years so much had changed in the realm of brief treatment that such coverage would be insufficient. Instead, we began to think about including in the new volume many of the areas of brief treatment that have gained in prominence since the publication of *Forms*. We also decided on a major revision of the format to allow more "interactive learning" for us and for the reader. Out of a series of cross-country brainstorming conversations grew *The First Session in Brief Therapy*.

The brief therapy landscape has changed tremendously over the past decade. While psychoanalytic brief treatment has been durable and retains many adherents, cognitive behavioral therapies are ever more important; solution-oriented approaches have gained a broad following; and the concept of integrative, "time-effective" psychotherapy is increasingly salient. From our perspectives, however, the greatest change in the past 10 years is that brief therapies, short-term therapies, and time-effective treatments are no longer viewed as peculiar, "specialized" approaches to be tried only with the healthiest patients seeking care. Rather, with the rising prominence and expansion of managed behavioral health care in this country and the escalated interest in brief and time-effective treatments that this expansion has brought, such models of treatment are rapidly becoming a standard component of conventional mental health practice.

Compiling *The First Session in Brief Therapy* was a wonderful opportunity for us to reflect with distinguished, thoughtful clinicians upon the work that they do. We could "sit in" on the session, learn about precisely what was transpiring, and then ask questions about what had occurred. In the process our own views on brief and time-effective treatment were honed and evolved. We hope that the reader will find some of the same types of opportunities to sharpen and develop his or her own thinking in this area as a function of *The First Session*.

As always there are people to be thanked and appreciated. Seymour Weingarten and Bob Matloff at Guilford remain a pleasure to work with. Their never-failing cooperation and support made our task immeasurably easier. The chapter authors required no threats, little pressure, and minimal coaxing to get material to us in a timely and professional manner. We are also grateful to Lori Jacobs for the exceptional and rapid job of text editing she did for this book, and to our families, who loved, tolerated, and supported us during this process.

As this book was moving toward completion, two of the very important and eminent supporters of the brief therapy movement in this country died. Gerald L. Klerman, M.D., and Robert L. Goulding, M.D., contributed much to the study and evolution of brief treatment. They will be greatly missed.

Simon H. Budman, PhD
Michael F. Hoyt, PhD
Steven Friedman, PhD

Contents

INTRODUCTION

CHAPTER 1   **First Words on First Sessions**   3
Simon H. Budman, Michael F. Hoyt,
and Steven Friedman

INDIVIDUAL APPROACHES

Introduction to Individual Brief   9
Therapy Approaches
Michael F. Hoyt, Simon H. Budman,
and Steven Friedman

CHAPTER 2   **Neuro-Linguistic Programming**   14
Steve Andreas and Connirae Andreas

CHAPTER 3   **Brief Therapy: The Rational–**   36
Emotive Approach
Albert Ellis

CHAPTER 4   **Planned Single-Session Therapy**   59
Michael F. Hoyt, Robert Rosenbaum,
and Moshe Talmon

CHAPTER 5   **Time-Limited Dynamic Psychotherapy**   87
Stephen F. Butler, Hans H. Strupp,
and Jeffrey L. Binder

CHAPTER 6   **A Time-Sensitive Model of Brief Therapy:**   111
The I-D-E Approach
Simon H. Budman and Alan S. Gurman

CHAPTER 7   **Launching Cognitive-Behavioral Therapy**   135
             for Adolescent Depression and
             Drug Abuse
             Ralph M. Turner

CHAPTER 8   **Therapy with Direction**   156
             Michael D. Yapko

COUPLE AND FAMILY APPROACHES

             Introduction to Couple and Family   183
             Brief Therapy Approaches
             Steven Friedman, Simon H. Budman,
             and Michael F. Hoyt

CHAPTER 9   **Integrative Marital Therapy: A**   186
             Time-Sensitive Model for Working
             with Couples
             Alan S. Gurman

CHAPTER 10   **Emotionally Focused Therapy:**   204
             Restructuring Attachment
             Susan M. Johnson and Leslie S. Greenberg

CHAPTER 11   **A Cognitive-Behavioral Model of**   225
             Marital Dysfunction and Marital Therapy
             Donald H. Baucom, Norman Epstein,
             and Robert Carels

CHAPTER 12   **Reflecting Conversations in the**   255
             Initial Consultation
             Judy Davidson and William D. Lax

CHAPTER 13   **Constructing Solutions (Stories) in**   282
             Brief Family Therapy
             Steven Friedman

CHAPTER 14   **Brief Therapy—MRI Style**   306
             John H. Weakland and Richard Fisch

CHAPTER 15   **The Black Sheep of the Family: A**   324
             Structural Approach to Brief Therapy
             Harry J. Aponte

CONCLUSION

CHAPTER 16   **Last Words on First Sessions**   345
                Simon H. Budman, Steven Friedman,
                and Michael F. Hoyt

                Index   359

INTRODUCTION

First Words on First Sessions

SIMON H. BUDMAN
MICHAEL F. HOYT
STEVEN FRIEDMAN

BEGINNING AT THE BEGINNING

The therapist waited expectantly in her office, anticipating the arrival of Timothy Simmons, with whom she had a 4:00 P.M. Friday appointment. At precisely 3:59, the receptionist buzzed her to indicate that "Mr. Simmons just arrived."

There was a minimal amount of material to go on. A week before, the therapist had a brief phone conversation in which the client (really a potential client) explained that he felt depressed about "a relationship situation as well as other issues"; a note from Ginny Graham, the internist, indicating that this was a man who "really needs your help."

When she greeted Mr. Simmons in the waiting area, the clinician observed his tense, uncomfortable smile and his wan face. Even as they began to walk down the long hallway to her office, she felt some uncertainty about the possibilities of treating him effectively in less than 12 visits. By the time this constricted, thirtyish gentleman sat down in the smallest, hardest chair in the interview room, the therapist was wondering what she could do for him in less than 12 months.

Should she begin the interview in her usual manner by asking, "What brings you in?" Was it better to start with, "How did you decide that this was the time for you to seek help?" Or, alternatively, the intervention she had learned at a recent workshop seemed like a possibility: "What would you like to get out of today's visit?" Her day had been so difficult and demanding that she even had the fleeting idea—which she quickly dismissed—of asking Mr. Simmons, "Of all the therapists in this area, why (in the world) did you decide to see me?"

Ever since she had started providing brief therapy services for a managed-care company, she began to call many of her old approaches into question. "In what ways

3

can I offer a useful, albeit limited, service to this client?" was a question she found herself facing in most first visits.

Her graduate training had never prepared her for anything like the work she was doing now. Neither Jenson's course on psychoanalytic treatment nor Hilman's behavior therapy practicum had given her a clear sense of what to do at this facility. Even the years of work in her own private practice seemed to be of marginal use.

"Damned insurance companies—all they think about is money," went through her mind more than once on a busy day. Still, there was something engrossing and valuable about attempting to offer services to a wide range of people in a manner that was helpful and effective and still affordable.

She decided to go with her old: "What brings you in?" It was too late in the day and definitely too late in the week for novelty. Next time she would use an alternative opener.

As active staff therapists at two of the largest health maintenance organizations in the country (Harvard Community Health Plan and Kaiser Permanente) we have had to hone our brief therapy skills. Each of us has researched and written about various aspects of brief treatment for many years (Budman, 1981; Budman & Gurman, 1988; Friedman & Fanger, 1991; Friedman & Pettus, 1985; Hoyt, 1985, 1990).

As managed mental health care has increasingly affected the professional lives of psychotherapists throughout this country (Austad & Berman, 1991; Austad & Hoyt, 1992), brief treatment, which at one time was seen as a specialized category of therapeutic intervention, has come to the forefront as the standard model of care. Most insurers cover their subscribers for somewhere between 6 to 20 visits unless the subscriber has a condition that may lead to psychiatric hospitalization. (Only the more enlightened companies put added resources into outpatient care in order avoid a hospitalization.) It is thus becoming increasingly important that most mental health clinicians have a familiarity, comfort, and reasonable level of proficiency in brief treatment (Budman & Armstrong, in press).

In considering the most important aspects of brief therapy, it is clear that in some ways the entire process of brief psychotherapy, or perhaps any therapy, is shaped by the first visit. The first encounter sets the tone, tenor, structure, direction, and foundation of the therapy. Obviously, errors and corrections may be made and directions changed following this visit, as the patient/client* reveals additional information about his or her situation. However, it is often the quality of the initial meeting that has an enormous bearing on what comes later in the treatment.

In reviewing patients' requests during initial interviews, for example, Eisenthal and Lazare (1976) emphasized the importance of specifically eliciting how the patient hopes to be helped; in a later study,

Eisenthal and Lazare (1976) found patients' satisfaction to be significantly correlated with their perception that the clinician assisted them in verbalizing their request. Mohl, Martinez, Ticknor, Huang, and Cordell (1991) found that various psychiatrist intake screeners in an initial visit had significantly different impacts on whether a patient would return for treatment (with a different therapist) or stay for more than five visits if he or she did return. In another interesting recent study, Adams, Piercy, and Jurich (1991) compared families who were given a solution-oriented task at the end of the first session of therapy with families given a problem-oriented task at the end of the initial session. Results indicated significantly higher compliance with assigned tasks, clarity of treatment goals, and rapid improvement for those in the solution-oriented condition. A study by Seeman, Tittler, and Friedman (1985) also found that "early interactional change" during initial sessions of family therapy was predictive of favorable outcome as reflected in improved family functioning. It is quite clear that the opening moves in treatment matter.

There is also the rather large probability (see Hoyt, Rosenbaum, & Talmon, Chapter 4, this volume) that there will *not* be another visit after the first, since about 30% of all therapies cease after a single visit. Thus, the initial session must be viewed as paramount.

The First Session in Brief Therapy is structured in a manner that we hope is both interesting and informative. We asked a variety of experts in the field of brief treatment to present a concise description of their clinical model and method of treatment. Their next task was to demonstrate what they do in a first session through the use of an annotated transcript of an initial visit. Finally, after a chapter was submitted, we, as editors, reviewed the case material and sent the author(s) a series of questions about their methods and/or what they had done in the particular case. We also asked each author how he or she had become a brief therapist. The authors' responses to our questions are thoughtful and enrich each chapter.

We intend for this to be a casebook in which the reader can learn what therapists in fact do in their clinical practices with real patients on a day-to-day basis. As we all recognize, it is far different to read theoretical disquisitions than to see how various clinicians function in their treatment interactions.

NOTES

*We shall use the terms "patient" and "client" interchangeably throughout this volume. For more discussion of the implications of the terms, see Hoyt (1979, 1985).

REFERENCES

Adams, J. F., Piercy, F. P., & Jurich, J. A. (1991). Effects of solution focused therapy's "formula first session task" on compliance and outcome in family therapy. *Journal of Marital and Family Therapy, 17*, 277–290.

Austad, C. S., & Berman, W. H. (Eds.). (1991). *Psychotherapy in managed health care: The optimal use of time and resources*. Washington, DC: American Psychological Association.

Austad, C. S., & Hoyt, M. F. (1992). The managed care movement and the future of psychotherapy. *Psychotherapy, 29*, 109–118.

Budman, S. H. (Ed.). (1981). *Forms of brief therapy*. New York: Guilford Press.

Budman, S. H., & Armstrong, E. (in press). Brief therapy training in managed care settings: Making it happen. *Psychotherapy*.

Budman, S. H., & Gurman, A. S. (1988). *Theory and practice of brief therapy*. New York: Guilford Press.

Eisenthal, S., & Lazare, A. (1976). Specificity of patients' requests in the initial interview. *Psychological Reports, 38*, 739–748.

Eisenthal, S., & Lazare, A. (1976). Evaluation of the initial interview in a walk-in clinic: the patient's perspective on a "customer approach." *Journal of Nervous and Mental Disease, 162*, 169–176.

Friedman, S., & Fanger, M. T. (1991). *Expanding therapeutic possibilities: Getting results in brief therapy*. New York: Lexington/Macmillan.

Friedman, S., & Pettus, S. (1985). Brief strategic interventions with families of adolescents. *Family Therapy, 12*, 197–210.

Hoyt, M. F. (1985). Therapist resistances to short-term dynamic psychotherapy. *Journal of the American Academy of Psychoanalysis, 13*, 93–112.

Hoyt, M. F. (1990). On time in brief therapy. In R. A. Wells & V. J. Giannetti (Eds.), *Handbook of the brief psychotherapies* (pp. 115–143). New York: Plenum Press.

Mohl, P. C., Martinez, D., Ticknor, C. Huang, M., & Cordell, L. (1991). Early dropouts from psychotherapy. *Journal of Nervous and Mental Disease, 179*, 478–481.

Seeman, L., Tittler, B. T., & Friedman, S. (1985). Early interactional change and its relationship to family therapy outcome. *Family Process, 24*, 59–68.

INDIVIDUAL
APPROACHES

Introduction to Individual Brief Therapy Approaches

MICHAEL F. HOYT
SIMON H. BUDMAN
STEVEN FRIEDMAN

Striving for more rapid effect and parsimony, theoreticians and clinicians have developed various brief and time-effective treatment systems that, in different ways, address and attempt to modify how a patient thinks, feels, and behaves (see Budman, 1981; Gustafson, 1986; Wells & Giannetti, 1990; Zeig, 1987; Zeig & Gilligan, 1990). Each system or approach has its own characteristic ways of understanding psychological functioning (and dysfunctioning), and each has its particular methods for bringing about psychological change. These differential methods reveal themselves throughout the course of any psychotherapy. When the treatment is deliberately intended to be brief, "time sensitive," or "time effective" (Budman & Gurman, 1988), however, differences in theory and practice must reveal themselves all the more quickly. Just as the therapist's opening intervention in any session may set the theme for that session (Kaiser, 1965), so does the initial session determine much of the tone and direction of what follows (Hoyt, 1990). If the adage holds truth, "As the twig is bent so grows the tree," we can expect to see differences (and commonalities) in how skillful practitioners of diverse brief therapy approaches begin their work with patients.

The initial stages of brief therapy (or any psychotherapy) involve forming a working relationship and assessing a problem and creating a treatment focus (Margulies & Havens, 1981). The brief therapist also actively begins the initiation or facilitation of change via therapeutic intervention. "Where/how is the patient stuck?" "What is needed to help the patient get unstuck?'' and "How can the therapist facilitate or provide what is needed?'' are three heuristic questions that underlie clinical work (Hoyt, 1990). In the chapters that follow, the reader can study many fascinating answers to these questions.

First, Steve and Connirae Andreas provide a concise theoretical summary of the neurolinguistic programming model followed by their description of two rapid intervention cases (Chapter 2). In both cases, the patients' specific complaints and treatment goals are elicited. The therapist in each case clearly directs the treatment, asking the patient to perform certain mental tasks and to recount, in the session, the resultant experiences. There is a comfortable, positive tone between patient and therapist in each case, as well as an expectation of rapid change or improvement. The focus is clearly on the here and now and on the nuts and bolts of current mental processing. There is an unmistakable expectation on the therapist's part that the desired transformations can and will take place rapidly, and this is precisely what occurs.

Albert Ellis provides us with a fine exposition of his classic rational–emotive therapy model (Chapter 3). Again, the patient's problems are pinpointed, and the therapist then directs the treatment, both within and outside the therapy sessions. The expectation is that the patient can make the desired changes if he applies the lessons of rational–emotive therapy. The therapist–patient tone is again positive, and the focus is on here-and-now thoughts and behaviors. As Ellis makes clear in this case and in the question-and-answer section that follows, the patient knows that responsibility for success ultimately rests with the patient, and that therapy will progress much more quickly if he or she is actively committed to the change process. This is what occurs and the outcome is striking.

Michael F. Hoyt, Robert Rosenbaum, and Moshe Talmon report on their experience attempting to facilitate patients' finding a useful solution in a single therapeutic encounter (Chapter 4). They emphasize that such an ultra-brief approach is not appropriate for everyone and that their goal is patient empowerment and constructive movement rather than "cure." One-session treatment is offered as an option but not required. In the case they present, that of a young man bothered by stress and conflicts at work with his supervisor, the patient's complaints are traced back to "unfinished business" with his father. The treatment focus and expectation of change are cast in terms of current psychological and behavioral options, with role playing a new approach to the father being used as a model. Again, the therapist forms a positive relationship with the patient. On follow-up, the patient is less stressed and feels more in control of himself but has left his old job and has not yet found a new one. Hoyt and his colleagues note that single-session therapy may well be a part of "intermittent therapy" or "serial treatment." They make the interesting point that while single-session therapy is obviously time sensitive, the decision about whether one session has been sufficient is generally left up to the patient and is not forced. Thus, single-session therapy, the briefest treatment contact, is not actually a form of time-limited therapy.

In the next chapter, Stephen F. Butler, Hans H. Strupp, and Jeffrey L. Binder (Chapter 5) present an interpersonal psychodynamic model that emphasizes analysis of the patient–therapist relationship. The therapist functions as a participant–observer, helping the patient both to recognize a cyclical maladaptive pattern and to undergo a corrective emotional experience within the therapeutic relationship. The authors view "time limits" as an attitude that focuses patient activity, but they recommend against any strict or rigid predetermined time frame. Indeed, in the case of the depressed woman they present, which had a favorable outcome, the therapist ceded to the patient's request for 10 additional sessions. This decision was based on the considered awareness of the patient's cyclical maladaptive pattern in which she would characteristically want more from a relationship but would fear abandonment or abuse if she became a burden to others. Butler and his colleagues emphasize that their goal is to enhance the patient's sense of autonomy, and that efforts to encourage success in a brief amount of time need to be considered within the context of the patient's expectations and fantasies of what the therapist wants, lest a pressure for change (in the first session or later, especially during the termination phase) be construed in a manner that maintains the patient's self-defeating patterns. In the case presented, the therapist listens and interacts with great empathy and successfully helps the patient to modify her views of self and others and her subsequent actions.

Simon H. Budman and Alan S. Gurman present their interpersonal–developmental–existential model (Chapter 6). They advocate an approach that is "time sensitive" rather than "brief" per se, meaning that treatment is rationed and allotted in a manner to maximize time/cost-effectiveness. They recognize the possibility and advantages of intermittent or serial contact as the patient deals with various issues throughout the life cycle. A series of pro-brief therapy beliefs and attitudes are presented such as the promotion of improvement or growth rather than "cure," the desire of the therapist to become unnecessary, and the recognition that change is inevitable and will largely occur after formal therapy ends. The key question, "Why now is the patient seeking therapy?" is answered: Because the patient wants to change, doesn't want to change, and/or has changed. Their approach is conceived as broadly useful, with typical foci involving loss, developmental dysynchronies, interpersonal conflicts, symptomatic disorders, and personality disorders. In the case they present, that of a 29-year-old woman complaining of panic attacks, they elaborate on their I–D–E approach with control–mastery theory informing their understanding of the therapeutic relationship and the various "tests" the therapist faced in establishing a working alliance with the patient. These therapeutic "trials" were particularly pertinent as the case developed because of the patient's involvement with alcohol and drug abuse and her history of incest victimization. The therapist is able to "pass" the patient's initial tests and the therapy successfully proceeds (with sessions initially being weekly, then monthly, then occasionally). Of interest in this case is the implication that even in situations of significant early trauma, a time-effective model can still be of great value.

Ralph Turner (Chapter 7) provides a good theoretical overview of the basic premise that cognitive processes causally affect our behavior and emotions. Cognition is viewed as an active process, with attention to the cognitive triad (attributions regarding self, experiences in the world, and the future), cognitive distortions, and underlying schema. Integrative links to more psychodynamic conceptualizations are also traced. The case presented, a 17-year-old woman first seen in the emergency room after an overdose following a dispute with her boyfriend, illustrates the approach in action. The therapist quickly makes good contact with the patient and assesses the genesis of the problems and the types of cognitive schema and distortions involved and devises a treatment approach. He carefully evaluates the psychiatric status of the patient, of course, including her current potential for suicidal behavior. The therapist is active and responsive, engages the patient well, and provides her with a clear cognitive–behavioral understanding of her problems. He enlists her active participation by telling her, "We will not just be talking." He assures her that they will work together to enhance her skills for handling stress and solving problems and to change the ways she thinks about herself and others; that homework will be assigned and she will be asked to try out behaviors and ideas; and that she will be taught to monitor her thoughts and see how they affect her emotionally. The follow-up report indicates that the patient responded well, learning to recognize and refute her cognitive distortions; asserting her needs better with her parents; ending the dysfunctional relationship with her boyfriend; and entering college.

In the final chapter of this section (Chapter 8), Michael D. Yapko begins with his observation that all effective psychotherapies have in common the interruption of existing problematic patterns and the building of new ones that are more adaptive and life enhancing. Strongly influenced by the work of Milton Erickson, Yapko prefers a strategic approach that modifies counterproductive dissociation by hypnosis (direct and indirect) plus directives that send the patient out into the "real world" to experiment with new response patterns. His focus is on the *how* rather than the *why* of clients' experiencing, as he attempts to accept and utilize the client's reality. His approach is nicely illustrated in his work with a young woman unsure of her emotions who is struggling to decide whether to continue within a marriage or to divorce. We see him form a good rapport and working relationship with her, build a positive expectation (hope), meet her within her reality, and negotiate the presented problem into something treatable and changeable. He assists her in ordering therapeutic priorities and initially intervenes using hypnotic communications and directives. In the follow-up report, we learn that the patient had four more therapy sessions. These focused on establishing more realistic expectations for herself and others and interrupting the pattern of putting others' needs above her own while trying to avoid conflict. After these initial sessions, she filed for a divorce. The patient continued to have "occasional" therapy sessions (23 in 2 years), consulting with her therapist to get an "outside" opinion about important life decisions as part of taking better care of herself.

REFERENCES

Budman, S. H. (Ed.). (1981). *Forms of brief therapy.* New York: Guilford Press.

Budman, S. H., & Gurman, A, S. (1988) *Theory and practice of brief therapy.* New York: Guilford Press.

Gustafson, J. P. (1986). *The complex secret of brief psychotherapy.* New York. W. W. Norton.

Hoyt, M. F. (1990). On time in brief therapy. In R. A. Wells & V. J. Giannetti (Eds.), *Handbook of the brief psychotherapies* (pp. 115–143). New York: Plenum Press.

Kaiser, H. (1965). *Effective psychotherapy: The contribution of Hellmuth Kaiser* (L. B. Fierman, Ed.). New York: Free Press.

Margulies, A., & Havens L. L. (1981). The initial encounter: What to do first? *American Journal of Psychiatry, 138,* 421–428.

Wells, R. A., & Giannetti, V. J. (Eds.). (1990). *Handbook of the brief psychotherapies.* New York: Plenum Press.

Zeig, J. K. (Ed.). (1987). *The Evolution of psychotherapy.* New York: Brunner/Mazel.

Zeig, J. K., & Gilligan, S. G. (Eds.). (1990). *Brief therapy: Myths, methods, and metaphors.* New York: Brunner/Mazel.

Neuro-Linguistic Programming

STEVE ANDREAS
CONNIRAE ANDREAS

Neuro-Linguistic programming (NLP) offers the field of brief therapy new ways of determining, understanding, and changing the structure of experience. This in turn opens the door for (1) a wide range of detailed procedures designed for specific limitations or symptoms and (2) clearer and more immediate evidence, both nonverbal and verbal, for when procedures are effective—when our clients have gotten the results they want. This understanding of the process and structure of limitations makes possible more rapid and thorough change processes that respect the whole person and the larger context he or she lives in.

All our experiences—our memories and plans, hopes and fears, values and decisions, etc.—are composed of the building blocks of sensory experience. There are five major modalities of experience: visual (sights), auditory (sounds), kinesthetic (feelings), and to a lesser degree olfactory (smells) and gustatory (tastes). These modalities in turn are made up of smaller components called submodalities. In the visual modality, for instance, we can see an image as bright or dim, large or small, close or far away. It can be in color or black and white, three dimensional or flat, still or movie. Likewise, sounds or words can be loud or soft or near or far, and they can differ in pitch, timbre, etc.

Submodalities are true process variables because they are completely independent of the content of the image or sound. Typically, people respond much more fully to a large, bright, close image than to a small, dim, distant one. By changing submodalities, we can change our responses to any image, whether pleasant or unpleasant. If someone is bothered by an unpleasant memory, when he or she makes the visual image of it small, dimmer, and farther away, he or she will feel less burdened by it. If the individual continues to make it smaller and farther away until it is only a black dot on the distant horizon, it will be so small and invisible that it may not be responded to at all.

Although most people are not consciously aware that these submodality shifts change responses, it is easy to verify by performing simple subjective mind experiments. If you think of a memory that you respond to strongly—either pleasantly or unpleasantly—and alternately make the image large/bright/close and then small/dim/distant, you can notice how the intensity of your feelings changes. By adjusting submodalities, we can selectively intensify or diminish our responses to specific events, memories, and thoughts so as to enhance our lives.

People can recall memories in one of two very different modes, "associated" or "dissociated." In an associated memory, you remember an event as if you are reliving it, reexperiencing every aspect of the original event.

However, you can also recall the same event dissociated by stepping back out of the image until you can see yourself, as if watching a movie on a TV set.

There are two major differences between these two ways of remembering: (1) the associated image elicits the full range of feeling responses from the original event—whether pleasant or unpleasant—while a dissociated image provides only the less intense feelings of an impartial observer, (2) since you can see yourself in the dissociated image, you have more information about how your own behavior elicits responses from others in that situation. This knowledge empowers, since you can see how to adjust your own behavior to get the kinds of responses you want from others. Association–dissociation is a very powerful submodality shift and is essential in the two case examples presented in this chapter.

NLP has also identified observable nonverbal cues that signal dominant modality and submodality changes in internal experience. This makes it possible to assess internal processing even when the client is not subjectively aware of it. For instance, it is usually true that when a client looks up and left, he or she will be using, and responding to, remembered images, while up and right indicate creative imagery. If a client moves his or her head back slightly while visualizing, that usually indicates that the image is becoming dissociated. These same nonverbal cues can be used later as independent evidence for whether an intervention has successfully resolved the presenting problem.

With this solid operational base, an NLP practitioner gathers information about a problem state and/or desired outcome, using specific language patterns to elicit detailed responses while calibrating to nonverbal cues. The next step is to determine the modality/submodality process that underlies the problem state. Treatment consists of directly modifying this underlying internal process in order to reach the desired outcome.

This chapter offers a glimpse of how NLP enables us to identify the underlying process and structure of problems, using as examples two distinct kinds of difficulties that are often confused: phobias and anxieties.

By studying problems with common underlying processes, NLP has developed specific patterns or "recipes" that can be used routinely to remedy certain categories of problems. This vastly reduces the need for extensive information gathering in many cases. In the first example, all we need to know is that the client had a phobia and that her fear response was instantaneous.

CASE ILLUSTRATION

Lori was 31 years old when she agreed to be a demonstration subject in a weekend training workshop in the phobia method. We told participants that we wanted to have several volunteers with phobias so that we could demonstrate the method we were teaching.

When Lori was 11 years old, she fell into a wasp's nest and was stung hundreds of times. Her whole body swelled up so much that her rings had to be cut off. None of her clothes fit, so for several days she had to wear her father's bathrobe. In the 20 years since then, she had had a severe phobia of bees. As she put it, "If a bee is in the house, *I'm not!*" If a bee got in her car, she had to pull over, stop, open the doors, and wait until the bee left. She also avoided flower beds because of the likelihood of bees.

The First Session

Lori, whom we had not met before, had walked into the room only a few minutes before the therapist (SA) asked her to join him at the front of the room. In order to emphasize the method, the therapist did not tell the audience what type of phobia Lori had. In our experience, the method works with most simple phobias as long as the fear response is essentially instantaneous. The transcript that follows is verbatim. The therapist begins with some "small talk" to gain rapport.

Therapist: Lori, I haven't spoken to you at all.
Lori: No.

T: You talked with Michael, I guess. [She had spoken with a friend who had previous experience with our method.]

L: Umhmmm.

T: I don't know what kind of outrageous promises he's made. (*Smiling*)

L: (*Laughing*) I won't tell you. I won't tell you what he promised.

T: Anyway, you have a phobia, which we won't tell them [the group] about, okay?

L: All right.

T: And, it's a very specific thing, right?

L: Uhmmm.

T: Is it just one thing, or is it kind of a class of things?

L: It's one thing.

T: Just one. Okay. And what I'd like you to do first—well, think of it right now. If one of these were flying around right now. . . .

L: Ohhh! (*She rolls her head around in a counterclockwise circle, laughing tensely*)

This pretest accomplished two things. First it allowed the therapist to verify that Lori had the kind of instantaneous response for which the phobia method is appropriate. Second, now that he has seen Lori's phobic response, he will be able to recognize when her response is different later. Now, however, he needs to get her out of the phobic state before proceeding with the technique. This is done with specific instructions, distracting, reassuring, and asking her about her friend Michael.

T: This is what we call a "pretest." That's fine; come back. (*Lori is still laughing nervously*) Look at the people here. . . . Look at me. . . . Hold my hand.

L: Thank you. . . . Okay.

T: We're not going to do stuff like that, right? Okay.

L: Okay. Whew!

T: Now look out at the folks here. How is it just being in front of these folks? (*Lori looks out at the group*) Is that a little nervous making too?

L: (*Breathes out strongly*) Not bad.

T: Is that okay?

L: Yeah, that's fine.

T: Okay. You've got a friend over there, right?

L: Yeah.

T: He's got a nice smile.

L: He sure does. He's a great friend.

T: Yeah, good.

Now Lori is back to a pleasant normal state, so the therapist can begin the method.

T: Okay. Now what I'd like you to do first, before we do anything—the whole procedure by the way is very simple, and you won't have to feel bad and stuff like that. But we need to make a few preparations. What I'd like you to do first, is imagine being in a movie theater.

L: Okay.

T: And this might be easier with your eyes closed.

L: All right. (*She closes her eyes*)

T: And I want you to see a picture up on the screen, of yourself—a black-and-white snapshot. And it could be of the way you're sitting right now, or something you do at home or at work. . . . Can you see a picture of yourself?

L: (*Nodding*) Uhmmm.

T: Is that pretty easy for you?

L: Uhhuh.

T: Good.

Although most people are consciously able to visualize in this way, occasionally a patient cannot. There are basically two ways to deal with this situation. One is to use the auditory or kinesthetic modality in place of the visual: "Can you hear yourself on a tape recorder?" or "Can you reach out and feel a statue of yourself in that situation?" Usually, however, it is simpler and more direct to use some variation of the "as if" frame, by saying, "Pretend that you can see yourself . . ." or "Get the sense of what it would be like if you were able to see yourself . . ."

T: Now I want you to leave that black-and-white picture on the screen, and I want you to float out of your body that's sitting here in the chair, up to the projection booth of the movie theater. Can you do that? Take a little while. . . .

L: Okay.

T: Okay, so from now on I want you to stay up in that projection booth. Can you see yourself down in the audience, there?

L: (*Smiling slightly*) Uhmmm.

T: And you can also see the black-and-white picture up on the screen?

L: Yeah.

T: Okay. Of yourself?

L: Yeah.

T: Pretty interesting.

L: (*Laughing*) It's good.

T: Do you know you could go to a workshop on "Astral Travel" and pay $250 to learn how to do this? (*Lori laughs*)

T: Okay, now I want you to stay up in that projection booth, and see yourself down in the audience, and see that black-and-white picture on the screen of yourself.

L: Umhmm.

T: Got that?

L: Umhmm.

T: Okay, I want you to stay up in that projection booth, until I tell you to do something else.

L: Okay.

T: So you can kind of see through the glass, and there are holes in the glass so you can hear the movie, because we're going to show a movie pretty soon. What I want you to do is run a movie of yourself in one of those bad times when you used to respond to that particular thing. And run it from beginning to end, and you stay back in that projection booth. You might even put your fingers on the glass and feel the glass. Just run a whole movie, clear to the end. See yourself freaking out over there, in response to one of those situations. That's right. Take all the time you need, and just let me know when you get to the end.

The therapist is watching Lori closely for any nonverbal signs that she might be falling back into the phobic response, but she remains relaxed, with no signs of the fear response she had demonstrated earlier.

L: It's hard to get to the end.

T: Okay. What makes it difficult?

L: It just seems to stop. The thing seems to go over and over. (*Gesturing with her right hand in a circle*) The particular incident goes over and over and over and doesn't seem to have an end, although I know it ended.

T: Okay. So it tends to go over and over and over.

L: Umhmm.

T: Okay. Let's speed up the movie. How many times does it have to go over and over before you can get to the end?

L: Um, half a dozen.

T: Okay. So let it flip through half a dozen, so it'll let you get to the end. . . . And when I say "end," I mean after the whole thing happened and you're back normal again.

L: Okay.

T: Okay. Got to the end?

L: Umhmm.

Although the therapist has not seen any sign of her phobic response, he checks this by asking her, "Was that fairly comfortable for you, watching that?"

L: A little uncomfortable, but not bad.

T: A little uncomfortable, but not bad. Not like the real thing.

L: No.

T: Okay. Now in a minute I'm going to ask you to do something, and I don't want you to do it until I tell you to go ahead. What I want you to do is to get out of the projection booth, and out of that chair in the audience, and go into the movie at the very end, when everything's okay and comfortable. Then I want you to run the whole movie backwards, including those six times around. Have you ever seen a movie backwards, in high school or something?

L: Yeah.

T: Okay. I'm going to have you run it backwards in color, and I want you to be inside it, so it's just like you took a real experience, only you ran it backwards in time, and I want you to do it in about a second and a half. So it will go "Bezzzzoooouuuuuurrrrrpppp," about like that.

L: Okay.

T: Okay. Go ahead. Do that. . . .

L: (*Taking a deep breath and shuddering*) Whooof!

T: Okay. Did you come out on the other side all right?

L: Yeah. (*Laughing*)

T: A little weird in the middle there, eh?

L: (*Shaking her head and continuing to laugh*) Ooooh.

T: Okay. Now I'd like you to do that a couple more times, and do it faster. So go into the end, right at the end, jump into it, and then go "Bezourp," real fast, through the whole thing. . . .

Most people only need to run the movie backwards once, but because of Lori's momentary discomfort, the therapist thought it would be helpful to do it several more times. This time Lori responds much less, sighing a little at the end.

T: Now do it a third time, real fast. . . .

L: Okay.

T: Okay. Was it easier the third time?

L: Umhmm.

T: Okay. Now, that's all there is to it.

Lori opens her eyes, looking very skeptical, grabs the chair with both hands, shakes her head, and then starts laughing loudly. After about 8 seconds of laughter, she says, "I'm glad I didn't pay for this one!" and continues to laugh for another 12 seconds. Although Lori has been very willing and cooperative throughout the process, this demonstrates that she certainly has no belief in what we have been doing. Lori's skepticism is very familiar to us. Even though we have guided literally hundreds of people through this process, we are still amazed that such a simple process can have such a profound impact. The therapist's next comments are both to acknowledge her disbelief and to allow a little time to pass before testing her response to bees again.

T: Fine. It's all right. We love to joke. Joking is one of the nicest ways to dissociate. Think about it. When you're joking, when you're having a humorous response to something, there's really no way to do it other than popping out for a while, looking at yourself, and sort of putting a different frame around what's happening, such that it's funny. It's a really valuable way of dissociating. We believe that dissociation is the essence of a lot of humor—not all, there are different kinds of humor, and so on. But we definitely recommend it.

Now, Lori, would you imagine now that one of these little critters—came. (*Gesturing with one finger, like the flight of a bee, toward Lori*) [She pauses, looks momentarily worried, then thoughtful, but does *not* go into the fear response that she demonstrated at the beginning of the session.]

L: Okay.

T: What's it like?

L: Um hay de hay. (*Lori is at a loss for words, and begins laughing*) Um. . . .

T: Do you still have it [the phobia]?

L: (*Looking down, surprised*) No! (*She laughs and puts her hand on her chest*)

T: This is a nice response because it looks like, "What?" Consciously she's expecting to have this [old] response. She's had it for—how long have you had this?

L: Twenty years.

T: She's had the response very, very dependably for 20 years. It's been a very unpleasant and overwhelming response. There's a very strong conscious expectation. And what you saw there, was this conscious expectation, "Ooooh! It's going to be terrible. . . . What?"

L: (*Laughing*) It's true.

T: Now let's make it a real bad one, you know. Have one come in and land on your hand or something. (*Lori looks down at her hand*) Can you imagine that?

L: Umhmm. (*She shakes her head in disbelief*) Whew!

T: What's it like?

L: Umhmm. . . . (*Neutrally, shrugging her shoulders*) It's like having one sitting on my hand.

T: That's a typical answer—is what's so funny [sic] "It's like being in an elevator, you know." Isn't that a mind-boggler?

L: Yeah, it is! Because I had that happen within the first year after the first incident, I had one land on me, woof!

T: And it was different, right?

L: Yeah! (*Looking down at her hand again*)

This January 1984 session, which took less than 7 minutes, is available on videotape (Andreas & Andreas, 1985). Lori's nonverbal response to bees in her imagination was clearly *very* different at the end of the session than it had been at the beginning.

FOLLOW-UP

Several times during the next summer we contacted Lori and asked if she had seen any bees, because we wanted to know her response to a real-world test. Each time she said she hadn't seen any bees. Finally, in

December 1984, we took a jar with about a dozen honeybees to her house. In the videotaped follow-up interview, she comfortably held the jar with the bees and examined them closely. When we let several of them out of the jar, she watched them crawling on her living room window without any reaction. A bee was in her house, and this time, so was she. Now it is over 8 years since the session, and Lori reports that she still hasn't noticed any bees, though she admits, "They must have been around me."

It's actually fairly common that people become completely oblivious to what had been the stimulus for their phobia. What used to terrorize them becomes so normal and ordinary it is not worth noticing. When we called one woman a few weeks after eliminating her elevator phobia, she thought for a while and then realized she had ridden in several elevators without being aware of it.

This method was developed (Bandler, 1985) as an improvement on an earlier method (Bandler & Grinder, 1979). In our clinical experience, it works very consistently for any situation in which the person responds instantaneously as a conditioned response to a specific stimulus: insects, heights, birds, snakes, water, closed spaces, elevators, etc., that is, in circumstances of a simple phobia.

Traditional diagnosis provides a way of categorizing based on behavioral symptoms. Since these categories aren't directly tied to the internal *structure* of experience, they do not inherently suggest how to move toward a solution. Although the DSM-III-R has over 600 pages of diagnosis, not one page is devoted to specifying interventions.

All NLP procedures have one thing in common: Diagnosis is based on the internal process or structure, which always suggests paths to move directly toward a solution. The NLP process definition of a phobia is that a person associates into a traumatic memory with a powerful unpleasant conditioned response. This immediately specifies the solution—dissociating from the experience. This process definition also makes it obvious that the method used for phobias can be used effectively for many problems that are not generally thought of as phobias, provided there is a quick response to an unpleasant associated memory. This includes a wide range of traumatic responses to past events: accidents, sexual and physical abuse, serious illness, drug "flashbacks," and experiences of war or disaster, including many cases of "posttraumatic stress disorder."

The method for specific phobias is not typically effective with agoraphobia, which usually has an inverse pattern. With a specific phobia, the person feels fine except in the presence of the phobic stimulus. In agoraphobia, the client only feels safe in the presence of "home" and is phobic everywhere else. While "secondary gain" is rarely an issue in simple phobias, it is frequently a very powerful aspect of agoraphobia, requiring a larger treatment frame that includes other family members, etc.

ANXIETY RESPONSES

In contrast to phobias, anxiety typically builds more slowly over a period of time that might take minutes or days. Rather than an instantaneous conditioned response to an external stimulus, an anxiety response is built and maintained by more complex internal representations, which are repetitive and often persistent. Some people become anxious by imagining vividly what might occur in the future; others talk to themselves in a rapid, high-pitched voice. Since there is much greater variety in how people generate anxiety, it is necessary to gather more information about exactly how a particular client creates an anxious state, so that the intervention can be carefully tailored to the individual.

Kate, who was 26, had done office work for us for about 2 years when she came in one morning, her eyes bulging and her skin abnormally white. She definitely did not look her best. Kate stopped Steve to ask him: "Did you hear about what happened?" With an unusual urgency in her voice, she recounted the details of an accident the night before. "I saw the whole thing! A car went out of control right in front of me last night. If I hadn't slammed on my brakes, it would have run right into me. Two people were killed, and two are in intensive care."

Kate had watched a car go out of control, veer inches in front of her, crash into a van, flip over, and land on its roof. She stopped her car immediately and got out, both wanting to help and not wanting to face what she might see. Kate apprehensively carried a blanket over to the van, where she saw a man sitting on the ground, obviously hurt, with blood on his face and arm. As she watched, the man slumped back onto the ground, his eyes rolling upward, showing white. Kate panicked, thinking he might have died. "I couldn't handle the possibility that he had just died, so I walked away." Kate only waited long enough to make her accident report, and then left in a state of shock.

The first time Steve listened to her story about the accident he thought, "It's understandable that she's very shaken. She watched the fatal accident and knows it could easily have been her." Seeing something like that usually makes people think about their mortality. However, each time she came in to work over the next few days, she had something new to report about the accident, always with the same urgency in her voice and disturbed look on her face. "Have you heard what they found out now about the person in intensive care?" The accident seemed to be consuming all her waking attention.

Kate, too, became concerned about her response to the accident and wanted to change it. She told Connirae that since the accident, she had been very nervous any time she was in a car. Her nervousness was even worse at night and when others were driving. She kept imagining accidents were going to happen and panicking. Kate had to drive past the scene of the accident every day on her way home from work. Even after arriving safely at her house, she repeatedly went over the details of the accident in her mind.

Although the accident scene had been unpleasant, that wasn't what was bothering her. What deeply concerned her was that she had been unable to help when the man slumped over. She had wanted to help but couldn't. That was when she "lost it."

Kate indicated that the feeling she got when she panicked at the accident reminded her of the feeling she used to get as a child when her mother woke her up in the middle of the night and shook her violently. Kate said she always felt out of control, and mentally "left" when her mother did that. It seemed likely that this abusive history had contributed to her intense reaction to the accident.

CREATING PANIC

Connirae asked Kate to go back and remember the accident just before her panic, in order to find out exactly what made her respond so strongly. They discovered that when she saw the man lying there, she focused on his bloody face and "zoomed in." The more she zoomed in close on his face, the more she felt out of control and frozen. As Kate did this in her imagination, her whole body became tight and immobile. Zooming in clearly worked to produce panic in Kate. When Connirae asked Kate to "unzoom" the face and move it further away, she felt better. Her whole body relaxed and began to move again and breathe normally.

A NEW SELF-IMAGE

Knowing how Kate mentally created her feeling of helplessness and being out of control provided the information needed in order to change it. The first step was to assist Kate in creating what would become literally a new self-image: the Kate who could deal with the same situation resourcefully. The dialogue that follows is reconstructed from detailed case notes by the therapist (CA).

Therapist: Imagine the Kate who could deal with that kind of situation really well. She's probably not ecstatic about accidents, but if one happens, it's not a problem for her. She has the resources to deal with it effectively. You don't need to know what those resources are; you can just tell by looking at that image of Kate that she has lots of choices and abilities. You can know that by the expression on her face, the way she moves, breathes, and gestures, the sound of her voice, etc.

   [Kate tried to develop this image, but it was clear that she wasn't succeeding to her own satisfaction.] Do you see the Kate who can handle this type of situation yet?

Kate: Well, I can see that Kate, but it's not realistic. I'm not her.

T: What makes her not realistic?

Sometimes when someone says this, it is because they are seeing themselves in black and white, and the picture needs to be in color to become real and convincing. Or they may see it as transparent, and it needs to look solid to be real. However, Kate responded with a different concern.

K: That Kate can handle the situation, but I can't because I don't know how to do first aid or CPR, and I really don't know anything medically about what should be done. Maybe I need to take medical classes to feel better.

It seemed unnecessary for Kate to go around feeling panicked and out of control just because she isn't an MD. Many people have little medical knowledge, and yet can function well at accident scenes doing their best without panicking. Kate seemed to be thinking of this as an either/or situation. Either she had to be completely medically competent so that she could feel in control or she had to feel totally out of control.

T: Kate, rather than seeing the you who could do CPR, I want you to see the you who may not know any more about medicine than you do sitting here now, but she has the resources to deal with a difficult situation as best she can, given what she knows. Perhaps this is the Kate who can walk into an emergency and decide on the spot how she can be most helpful. Panic is irrelevant to her, because she knows how to quickly and calmly assess what she can do, and not try to do anything she knows she can't do. What this Kate knows is not medicine, it's how to use whatever information and skills she has to act in the best way possible. She may make mistakes once in a while—as all of us do—but she also has the resources to learn from them, and use these learnings next time. [Kate's face began to relax. She looked more pleased with, and attracted to, the capable Kate of the future that she was now seeing in her mind's eye.]

CHANGING KATE'S AUTOMATIC RESPONSE

Connirae knew what made Kate panic: the memory of zooming in on the man's face. She had also helped Kate create an image of her capable self. However, being able to see herself as resourceful is not enough. This image must automatically flash in her mind compellingly at the right time—whenever she thinks of the accident, or when she actually encounters an accident in the real world.

The next step is to connect these two images in her mind, so that every time Kate thinks of the man's face, it will automatically transform into the image of seeing herself with the resources to deal with this kind of situation. This is what would allow Kate to immediately feel resourceful when she most needed to.

NLP teaches many ways to connect images in our minds, and each of us is unique in what works best for us. Connirae already knew that "zooming in" had an impact on Kate, so she decided to use that to connect the two images.

She first tested her guess, to find out if Kate felt more attracted to the capable Kate of the future if she brought the image closer and zoomed in on it. When she tried this, she smiled and said, "Yes." Then she asked her to clear her visual screen in preparation for linking the two images.

"Now see the unconscious man up close and zoomed in. As soon as you can see that, also see a very small image of the capable Kate, way out on the horizon. . . . Now let the image of the capable Kate zoom in close very rapidly at the same time as the image of the man in the accident quickly "unzooms" and moves off so far away that you can't see it any more."

Here we ran into another minor obstacle. After trying this, Kate frowned slightly. She stopped and said, "I'm not sure I'm really seeing these images," concerned that she might not be doing it right. Connirae decided to try using the "as if" frame.

"What I'd like you to do is just pretend that you are doing it. Many people don't really see these things consciously, they just do it as if it's real. I'm not very conscious of most of my internal pictures, but if I pretend that I really see these things, it works just as well for me as it does for someone who says she actually sees images in her mind. As long as you pretend well, it works fine."

This seemed to satisfy her. Kate closed her eyes and exchanged the images quickly by zooming one out as the other one zoomed in. This time her nonverbal responses indicated that she was really doing it. As she began, her body was motionless and frozen; a moment or two later she relaxed and smiled in the same way she had previously when she was seeing the close image of the capable Kate.

"Now blank your internal screen and do the same thing five more times. Each time begin with the man's face up close and the image of capable Kate far away, exchange the images by zooming, and then blank the screen. You can let these images exchange even faster each time you do it."

FOLLOW-UP

When Kate was done, Connirae carefully tested to find out if her new response was automatic. First she asked Kate to make the image of the man so that she could observe her response. Instead of feeling panic, she felt capable and resourceful and her nonverbal cues were congruent with her self-report. She also found that she felt the same capable feelings if she thought about any other part of the accident scene, or if she imagined driving a car.

However, Kate wasn't convinced that anything would really be different. Connirae pointed out that driving home would be a much better test, since any driving had bothered her since the accident, and she would also have to drive past the accident scene on her way home. She agreed this would be a good test. This work with Kate took almost an hour.

The next day Kate came to work quite pleased. She had been comfortable driving home and going by the scene of the accident, and she hadn't been preoccupied with driving or accidents during the evening. About a month later, she encountered a bike accident in which the rider cut his head with the rim of his sunglasses and was bleeding. Kate immediately responded by helping him resourcefully and calmly. About 2 months later she came on another accident involving a car and a bicyclist, an older man whose face was bleeding. Again Kate was very resourceful and calm in assisting him and the car driver to calm down and handle the situation. It is now over 7 years since our work together, and Kate remains comfortable and resourceful with respect to driving and accidents.

THE METHOD

The procedure used with Kate is called the "swish pattern" because it is often helpful to make a "swishing" sound as the person exchanges the two images. This pattern (Bandler, 1985; Andreas & Andreas, 1987) can be used for a wide variety of habitual responses, both emotional and behavioral. People have been talking for years about the importance of a good self-image in mental health and in the ability to cope and change. However, no one has previously been able to provide a specific and direct way to create a resourceful self-image using submodalities, or to utilize its power to help people change by linking it directly to the stressful situations where it is most needed. This pattern creates a new stimulus–response connection between the cue for the old habitual response and the positive self-image.

We have used this method to help people with a wide range of unwanted behaviors and responses. It has been particularly useful with unwanted habits such as overeating, smoking, and nail-biting. A demonstration with a woman who had a long-standing nail-biting habit is available on videotape (Andreas & Andreas, 1986). This videotape also contains a second demonstration using the swish pattern in the auditory system with a woman who became enraged when her daughter used a certain tone of voice.

THE WIDER FIELD OF NLP

These two examples are based on the submodalities model—one of several models in NLP. Another set of NLP interventions approaches experience in a different way, beginning with the presupposition that every behavior or response, no matter how objectionable, has some positive purpose, an idea borrowed from Virginia Satir (Bandler & Grinder, 1982). This assumption leads to gathering different kinds of information, often working directly with unconscious parts. While it is more content oriented, these NLP procedures have the same precision that allows us to adapt what we do to respect individual differences.

This chapter provides only two examples of the wide range of specific brief interventions that NLP offers the mental health professional. The first is an example of a categorical intervention that requires minimal information gathering. The second is an example of how NLP practitioners can gather more specific information about internal processes in order to select the most useful and efficient change method, and adapt it to the individual.

Both examples are based on a detailed and operationally defined model of how the mind works. Although the ramifications of this model have only begun to be explored, there are already specific patterns or "recipes" for quickly resolving such problems as grief, guilt, shame, internal conflict, abuse, violence, self-assertion, responding to criticism, motivation, decision making, spelling, reading comprehension and many other learning disabilities, changing habits, weight loss, and even some problems that are usually thought of as primarily medical, such as allergies and self-healing. For examples of all these, see *Heart of the Mind* (Andreas & Andreas 1989), from which the examples in this chapter have been adapted.

EDITORS' QUESTIONS

Q: It appears that the two clients you described (especially the second) liked and trusted the therapist from the beginning. They were willing and compliant. What if the patients had been resistant, difficult, and ornery and had significant personality disorders? How would your method and technique vary?

A: The method and techniques would not vary. However, they would be preceded by a short period of gaining rapport, dealing with objections, and creating a positive and acceptable frame for the intervention or interventions that follow. When working toward outcomes selected by the client, there is already at least a certain degree of willingness and motivation. Resistance or reluctance only indicates that some part of the person is afraid (often correctly) that the proposed change would interfere with other positive outcomes that are important to them. Any parts—whether conscious or unconscious—objecting to the proposed changes are asked for their positive outcomes, so that the proposed change can be adjusted to satisfy them as well. When all outcomes of the person are satisfied, change is much easier to accomplish. When all parts are respected, none of them will "sabotage" the change process (Bandler & Grinder, 1982).

Q: What do you usually tell a patient about the course and prognosis of treatment? When and how do you determine and discuss length of treatment? Both of these cases were quick successes. What guides your decisions about length of sessions, frequency, and spacing of sessions? How do you motivate the patient?

A: Initially we usually tell clients that some problems can be resolved very quickly, while others take more time. In either case we expect that within the first three sessions clients should be able to experience significant progress toward the changes they want. If they don't, we advise them to try some other approach. We do not schedule regular sessions. We accomplish what we can in the first session—which may run to 2 or 3 hours if needed—with follow-up sessions as desired or indicated.

The experience of having made some changes quickly is the best way to motivate someone to come back to pursue additional changes. However, NLP has also studied and characterized how people motivate themselves, and how to change this when it doesn't work well, or when it works too well (in the case of a "workaholic," for instance).

In the second case example, the intervention itself included a very powerful motivator: the image of who Kate wanted to become. Most NLP work accomplishes changes that work automatically and effortlessly, without conscious attention, practice, or motivation. In the first case, Lori even consciously actively disbelieved that any change had been made, yet the change still functioned automatically. Although Kate was not quite as skeptical, she too experienced changes in her responses without the need for any "Insight," conviction, practice, or effort.

We have presented two cases that typify the range of simpler NLP interventions. In these cases, no further sessions were necessary for these problems. However, both Lori and Kate could benefit from further sessions regarding other aspects of their lives. Kate chose to do this, while Lori did not.

Q: How would you focus with a client whose problems were more vague or unclear?

A: NLP includes very detailed and specific methods for gathering information about the problem state and how it is generated by external cues and internal processes. These methods consist primarily of carefully phrased questions, with close attention to the nonverbal responses that indicate how the client is processing information, and with attention to the incongruence that indicates the need for additional information about other (often unconscious) parts with outcomes that need to be considered respectfully, etc.

Q: In the cases presented, if the clients had not responded well, what issues might you consider? How might you change your approach?

A: With these kinds of problems, we very rarely fail. In general, when what we have done does not work, we assume that our information gathering was inadequate and/or our intervention was inappropriate. When this occurs, we return to gather more information in order to adjust or reformulate the intervention. Since we make use of detailed nonverbal feedback throughout a session, most of this reformulation occurs during the session itself, making the intervention appropriate and effective. It is more common that an intervention does work, but incompletely, or not in all the desired contexts, etc. Sometimes the intervention works perfectly, and the client discovers "ecological" problems—perhaps a spouse or boss objects to the new behavior and this was not detected in our careful checking for such problems during the outcome specification process.

Q: What might be contraindications or dangers with the NLP approach? What information would you want before proceeding?

A: Although NLP as a field is still in its infancy, it claims to provide the foundation for a comprehensive practical science of human thinking, behavior, and change. There are still certain problems and certain clients with whom we have been unsuccessful; we consider that to be a statement about where the field needs to be further developed. A few years ago, we had no systematic ways to resolve grief and resentment, but now these two issues can also typically be resolved in one session. Research continues to characterize and provide solutions for other human problems. Whereas most psychotherapies advocate that a general approach be used for all problems, NLP is able to specify, in considerable detail, what approach will work with what kind of problem. If someone were to attempt to use the phobia method for grief resolution, it would only make it worse (and vice versa), because the fundamental structure of these two problems is opposite. In a phobia, the problem is association into an intensely unpleasant memory. In grief, the problem is dissociation from a pleasant memory, yielding the feeling of emptiness. Because of the specificity of NLP, contraindications for specific methods are obvious, but not for the overall NLP approach as a whole.

Obviously, some clients are more of a danger to themselves or others, and each therapist has to make his own decisions about working with such people. However, there is a range of specific NLP methods for helping clients become more resourceful and less impulsive or violent, etc. We would use the same kind of verbal and nonverbal information gathering as with any other client.

Q: What are your thoughts with regard to working with clients while they are on drugs?

A: There are two fundamental issues with regard to working with clients on psychoactive or psychotropic drugs—whether legal or illegal. The first is the problem of state-specific learning. Whatever changes you succeed in helping a client make in the drug state may—or may not—

transfer to the nondrug state. If—as is often the case—the changes don't transfer, then you have to do the same work all over again in the nondrug state.

The second, and more important, issue is that your ability to work with the person on drugs is impaired because there isn't as much of him or her to work with. This occurs in two closely related ways: (1) the person's overall state of mind is often very different. He or she may be uncooperative, as is often the case with alcohol for instance, or simply may not be able to concentrate, follow directions, etc.; (2) many drugs essentially eliminate an aspect of the person's problem or conflict—that's often why people take drugs—so you don't have the opportunity to deal with them and engage them as part of the solution. These parts typically return, untouched, in the nondrug state. For example, a schizophrenic's voices are often silenced by medication, yet these voices are one of the essential parts of the client that need to be reintegrated in order to reach conflict-free congruence.

For these reasons we are very reluctant to work with clients who are on drugs, and when we do, our work is tempered by knowledge of these constraints.

Q: What else is distinctly different about the NLP approach?

A: In addition to the ability to gather detailed information about the process in a client to be changed, the specificity of interventions, and moment-to-moment feedback, there is one other very essential aspect of NLP. The therapist him- or herself is the instrument of change. Study after study has shown that the bulk of communication is nonverbal. Like a good actor, an effective therapist must learn to utilize his or her own nonverbal behavior to elicit powerful responses in the listener. A large portion of NLP training is devoted to practicing flexibility in nonverbal behavior, so that interventions can have maximum impact. Without this nonverbal support, the most carefully designed and appropriate intervention will fall as flat as a poorly told joke.

Although NLP attains deep therapeutic outcomes, we think of most of our work as education—teaching people how to use their minds so that they can have more satisfying responses and behaviors.

NLP flatly refutes the alleged need to build a long-term relationship with a client. And since NLP interventions are typically rapid, there is no chance to develop the dependence that often disempowers clients and burdens therapists in more traditional approaches.

One other aspect of NLP work deserves mention. We do not care if the client achieves "understanding" or "insight" or comprehends the method we are using. After her session, Lori couldn't even remember what we had done, and she certainly did not believe that we had made a change. Kate was also dubious and became convinced that she was different only when she found that her response was different in the real-world situations that had been a problem for her. This kind of behavioral evidence of change should be the only test of good therapy.

Q: How did you become a brief therapist?

S. ANDREAS: Coming from a background in chemistry, in which changes occur very quickly with the right conditions and catalyst, I've always assumed that people could change quickly. However, graduate school with Abraham Maslow in the late 1950s did not teach me how to do it. Carl Rogers was sweet and gentle, but much too slow to hold my interest, so I continued to explore different therapeutic methods while teaching psychology in junior college. Fritz Perls was not sweet, but he often made things happen fast, and I did gestalt therapy for 10 years, until I first experienced the precision and effectiveness of NLP in 1977. Since then, NLP has provided a wonderful, varied, and detailed set of methods for rapid and respectful personal change, as well as a solid pragmatic foundation from which we have gone on to develop additional methods. As Wilson Van Dusen writes in his comment on our recent book, *Heart of the Mind*, "Speed is not the real issue. We must be closing in on the actual design of people."

C. ANDREAS: My long-standing interest in brief therapy became a commitment after my second visit to Milton Erickson. I went with about 12 other therapists to spend a week with Dr. Erickson, who told stories each day about his work with clients. I will always remember the moment, on the last day of our visit, when I suddenly felt like a different person. I had an inner knowing that some pressing personal issues would be taken care of; I knew I would be fine, although I didn't know what I would do. At that exact moment, Dr. Erickson turned to me and said, "Your unconscious mind has just made a very important decision. . . . And you don't know what it is, do you?"

Other people had their stories of dramatic personal change with Erickson, but I had always thought they must be exaggerating. This time I had felt it, and the results in my life were powerful.

Knowing rapid change is possible, I've found NLP to most fully open the possibilities for achieving it. This new field offers ways to tap the structure of deep and lasting changes, such as my experience with Dr. Erickson.

NLP also satisfied one of my ongoing concerns about being a therapist. During my early training, I frequently wondered, "How can I be sure I am doing something of value?" Through NLP, I learned many precise ways of "testing" in the moment, to find out if a particular change was complete or if more needed to be done.

Along with my growing understanding of rapid change, I have increasing respect for the continual nature of change. We human beings always seem to have more progress that we can make, and I doubt that I will ever consider myself "done" with my own evolution.

REFERENCES

Andreas, C., & Andreas, S. (1989). *Heart of the mind*. Moab, UT: Real People Press.

Andreas, S., & Andreas, C. (1987). *Change your mind—and keep the change.* Moab, UT: Real People Press.

Andreas, C., & Andreas, S. (1986). *The swish pattern* [Videotape]. Boulder, CO: NLP Comprehensive.

Andreas, S., & Andreas, C. (1985). *The fast phobia cure* [Videotape]. Boulder, CO: NLP Comprehensive.

Bandler, R. (1985). *Using your brain—for a change.* Moab, UT: Real People Press.

Bandler, R., & Grinder, J. (1979). *Frogs into princes*. Moab, UT: Real People Press.

Bandler, R., & Grinder, J. (1982). *Reframing*. Moab, UT: Real People Press.

Brief Therapy: The Rational– Emotive Method

ALBERT ELLIS

I originated rational–emotive therapy (RET) as a pioneering cognitive–behavior therapy (CBT) in 1955 because I discovered, from working as a psychoanalyst from 1947 to 1953, that just about all forms of psychoanalysis are long-winded and inefficient (Ellis, 1957, 1958, 1962). RET was specifically designed, from the start, to be brief but effective for a sizable number of (not *all*) clients. It assumes that borderline, psychotic, and some other clients are severely disturbed, for biological as well as environmental reasons, and usually require somewhat prolonged therapy, but that a large number of neurotic individuals can be significantly helped in 5 to 12 sessions and can therefore appreciably help themselves by continuing to practice the main RET principles they learned during these sessions.

Although RET brief therapy uses a number of relationship and experiential methods, it stresses self-help and homework. It actively *teaches* clients how to understand and help themselves in between sessions and after formal therapy has ended or has been temporarily suspended (Bernard, 1986, 1991; Dryden & DiGiuseppe, 1990: Ellis, 1962, 1973, 1985, 1988; Ellis & Abrams, 1978; Ellis & Dryden, 1987, 1990, 1991; Ellis & Grieger, 1977, 1986; Ellis & Harper, 1975; Grieger & Boyd, 1980; Walen, DiGiuseppe, & Wessler, 1980; Wessler & Wessler, 1980; Yankura & Dryden, 1990).

RET has a definite, and now somewhat famous, ABC theory of human disturbance and its alleviation, a theory that is also held by most of the other CBTs that, since 1963, have followed RET (Beck, 1967; Glasser, 1965; Goldfried & Davison, 1976; Lazarus, 1971; Mahoney,

1974; Maultsby, 1975; Meichenbaum, 1977; Seligman, 1990). This theory states that when people's goals, views, and desires (G) are blocked or thwarted by negative activating events or adversities (A), they can consciously and/or unconsciously adopt a belief system (B) that largely creates their emotional and behavioral consequences (C). If they choose to have only rational beliefs (rBs), which consist of wishes and preferences, they will almost always have appropriate, self-helping feelings and behaviors at point C, while if they choose to hold mainly irrational beliefs (iBs), which consist of strong, dogmatic *demands, commands*, and *musts*, they will usually have inappropriate self-defeating feelings and behaviors at point C.

Thus, if clients only believe (at B), "I'd *like* to do well and be approved by significant others, but I never *have to*, too bad if I don't," they will normally feel appropriately sorry and disappointed (at C), when they fail and are disapproved. But when they strongly believe (at B), "I *absolutely must* do well and be approved by significant others, and it's *awful* and I'm *no good* when I don't," they usually feel inappropriately dysfunctional, panicked, depressed, and self-hating (at C) when they fail and get rejected.

RET hypothesizes that people partly get (or *accept*) their irrational dysfunctional beliefs from their parents and culture, but, more important, they also *construct* and *create* their iBs from their own innate, biological tendencies to think unrealistically, illogically, and absolutistically. They are also born, RET holds, with powerful innate tendencies to construct and create self-changing, self-actualizing thoughts, feelings, and actions and therefore have the ability to *reconstruct* their self- and social-defeating behaviors.

Moreover, as RET has posited since its beginnings in 1955, human (disturbed and nondisturbed) thoughts, feelings, and actions are probably never pure but include and interact with each other (Ellis, 1956, 1958, 1962, 1992). Clients perceive the As of their lives with cognitive–emotive–behavioral biases. They have Bs that are strongly influenced by emotional and behavioral (motoric) factors. And they experience Cs that involve thinking, feeling, and action elements. Therefore, RET theorizes, therapists and their clients had better not only understand how people largely create their own disturbances, but also steadily—and vigorously—employ a number of cognitive, emotive, and behavioral methods to change their disturbed symptoms and to (ideally) make themselves less disturb*able*.

RET assumes that because the human condition is both self-actualizing and self-disturbing, people had better work *all their lives* to use their self-helping to minimize their self-sabotaging (and social-sabotaging) tendencies. In this sense, good psychotherapy is a lifelong process. However, by far most of this ongoing process can be taught and activated for hard-working neurotics in a brief period of time and then steadily reactivated by clients themselves until the end of their days.

The main therapeutic aspect of RET is the disputing (D) of iBs. Disputing is first done with a number of cognitive techniques, including discovering clients' dysfunctional attitudes; logically, empirically, and philosophically discussing and debating them; using rational coping self-statements; reframing the As of one's life; bibliotherapy and audiotherapy; and reviewing the disadvantages of self-defeating thoughts and behaviors. Emotively, RET teaches clients a number of forceful affective methods of changing their feelings, including shame-attacking exercises, rational–emotive imagery, role playing, the use of rational humorous songs, and strongly reiterated self-statements. Behaviorally, clients regularly work homework assignments with the therapist, do *in vivo* desensitization, use reinforcements and penalties to help change their thoughts and actions, and often engage in skill-training activities.

CASE ILLUSTRATION

The client was a 38-year-old black male, Ted, a high school graduate, manager of a retail store, married 10 years, with two young children. He was referred by his physician, an ex-client, because of his pseudo heart attacks, which were really panic attacks, for which he had been given nitroglycerin for reassurance. Two years before coming to therapy, after worrying about the death of a boyhood friend from a heart attack, he was on a PATH train, returning from Manhattan to Jersey City, when he started having chest pains and immediately hospitalized himself for 2 days, only to find that he was in perfect physical condition with no heart problems. Despite medical reassurance, he then became panicked whenever he took the train to work or back to his office, and whenever he even thought about taking a train. In addition, whenever he thought about having intercourse with his wife he became panicked and lost his erection. He borrowed some Xanax from his mother, and it calmed him down temporarily, but he hated taking medication and only used it infrequently.

With clients like this, who I quickly diagnose as severely neurotic, in the first session I get a brief family and personal history (partly from the 4-page questionnaire we have all clients at our Institute for Rational–Emotive Therapy fill out just before the session). I especially want to know when the presenting symptom (panic) started, how intense it is, if other close members of the family have it or other symptoms, how anxious and self-downing the client is about having it, and what he or she is doing to cope with and change it. I usually focus the first session on explaining some of the ABCs of disturbance creation to the client, showing him how he mainly constructs and maintains his symptoms and what he can quickly start doing to ameliorate them. I assume that most of the treatment, if the client is not borderline or psychotic, can be done in 10 or 20 sessions, and that significant improvement may be affected in perhaps a few weeks.

I feel that the most important things to accomplish in the first session include:

1. Finding the core dysfunctional philosophies the client is strongly believing to create and maintain his or her symptoms.
2. Showing the client what these self-defeating Bs are.
3. Showing the client that, in all probability, he or she constructed his or her own irrational shoulds, oughts, and musts and did not merely learn them from his or her parents and culture.
4. Showing the client that he or she can find these core irrationalities and work cognitively, emotively, and behaviorally to change them and ameliorate their influence.
5. Working out the client's suitable, practical thinking, feeling, and action-oriented homework assignments to perform before the next session.
6. Giving the client some reading material on RET to start perusing at home.
7. Summarizing the first session by emphasizing that the client is to make a note of any dysfunctional Cs during the week, observe what As preceded these Cs, and look for his or her rBs and iBs with which he or she largely created these disturbed feelings and behaviors.

The First Session

After I spent less than 10 minutes determining the client's symptoms, when and how they started and are being perpetuated, and a little background about his family (especially his mother's proneness to anxiety), he says that he borrowed some of his mother's Xanax and took 3 or 4 of them.

Therapist: And does it help you when you take it?

Client: Yes. But the one thing I don't like is to take pills. I know that sometimes you need medication, but I hate it.

T: Well, if we can help you to change your ideas and attitudes about taking trains and about having a heart attack, that will really help you and you won't need medication. You see, you said you were a perfectionist. So you're first making yourself anxious about doing things perfectly well. "I *must do* well! I *must do* well!" Instead of telling yourself, "I'd *like* to do well, but if I don't, I don't. Fuck it! It's not the end of the world." You see, you're rarely saying that. You're saying, "I've *got* to! I've *got* to!" And that will *make* you anxious—about your work, about sex, about having a heart attack, or about almost anything else. Then, once you make yourself anxious, you often tell yourself, "I *must* not be anxious! I *must* not be anxious!" That will make you *more* anxious—anxious about your anxiety. Now, if I can help you to accept *yourself* with your anxiety, first, and stop horrifying yourself about it; if we can help you, second, to give up your perfectionism—your demandingness—then you would not keep making yourself anxious. But you're in the habit of demanding that things *have* to go well and that, when they don't, you *must* not be anxious about them. "I must not be anxious! I must be sensible and sane!" That's exactly how people make themselves anxious—with rigid, forceful shoulds, oughts, and musts.

C: Like yesterday. Yesterday was my worst day in a long time.

T: Yes, because?

C: What I did is when I was going to the train, I said: "I need to put something in my mind."

T: To distract yourself from your anxiety that you expected to have when you got on the train?

C: Yes. I said, "I am going to buy some sports things for the children." So I went to one of the stores and I bought some things, and as soon as I got on the train I started deliberately reading. Ten minutes after I was on the train, I still didn't have any anxiety. I was okay. But then I remembered and I said, "Jesus, I feel okay." At that moment, I started feeling panicked again.

T: That's right. What you probably said to yourself was, "Jesus, I feel okay. But maybe I'll have another attack! Maybe I'll get an attack!" You will if you think that way! For you're really thinking, again, "I *must* not get another attack! What an idiot I am if I get another attack!" Right?

C: Yes.

After briefly showing the client that whenever he has a panic attack he really upsets himself and does not really get upset by the train or anything else, I jump right in and try to teach him that it is not his preferences or wishes for good behavior and good health that upset him but his powerful conscious, and unconscious, demands, and that if he gives them up, changes them back to preferences, he will lose his anxiety about having a heart attack—and also his anxiety about his anxiety. In RET, whenever a client like this one has anxiety, and especially panic, I assume that there is a good chance that he also has panic about his panic, and that that exacerbates the original panic mightily. So I try to make him aware of this immediately, and I find that very often as soon as he or she sees that this is so, the panic about the panic subsides—and, often, so does the original panic.

T: Well let me explain to you in a little more detail how humans disturb themselves—what they think and do to make themselves anxious and panicked. They don't *get* disturbed because of the happenings in their early childhood. That's largely psychoanalytic hogwash. They almost always needlessly disturb *themselves*—by first listening to their nutty parents and, more importantly, taking the goals and standards they are taught and insisting that they absolutely have to live up to them, that they completely must do well. They are born with the tendency to "*must*urbate"; that's their nature. But they can teach themselves not to do so and mainly remain with their preferences. Let me give you a model of most neurotic disturbance, and I know you'll understand it. Suppose you go out of this building at the end of this session into the streets of New York, and you don't know how much money you have in your pocket. It could be a dollar or it could be fifty thousand. You're ignorant of how much you have. And the one and *only* thing you think to yourself is, "I *wish*, I'd *like*, I'd *prefer* to have in my pocket a minimum of ten dollars. Not one hundred, not two hundred, just ten. I'd like to have ten dollars in my pocket, because I might eat, take a cab, or go to a movie." Then you actually look in your pocket and you find nine dollars, one less than ten. Now, how would you feel if you preferred ten and had nine, one less? What would your feeling be?

C: That I don't have enough of what I want.

T: Yes, but how would you *feel* about not having enough of what you want? You'd like to have ten dollars, but then you have nine, one less than ten.

C: Slightly disappointed.

T: Fine. That's a very appropriate feeling, because we wouldn't want you to feel good about not having what you want.

C: Yeah.

T: Okay. Now the second time you're going out, this time you're saying foolishly to yourself—you know it's foolish but you still say and believe it—"*I must, I must, I must*, at all times, at all times have a minimum guarantee of ten dollars. *I have to! I've got to! I must!*" That's what you believe in your head. Then again, you look in your pocket and you find only nine dollars and you can't get the tenth. Now how would you feel?

C: I would feel very upset.

T: Yes, because of your *must*. It's the same nine dollars, but this time you're insisting that you absolutely *must* have it—and, of course, you don't. You see, we humans don't get upset by a bad condition that occurs in our lives. We only get upset—or upset ourselves—because of our *musts*. We take our preferences, our wishes, our desires and we often make them into absolute demands, musts, shoulds, oughts. That—your *must*—would be what's upsetting you.

C: I see. My musts.

T: Now finally, the third time, you go out again and you're still saying to yourself the same thing as the second time: "I *must*, at all times, have a minimum guarantee of ten dollars in my pocket!" And you look in your pocket and this time you find eleven dollars—more than enough. Now how would you feel?

C: I'd feel okay.

T: That's right. But a minute later, something would occur to you to make you anxious. Now, why would you be anxious a minute later? First you say to yourself, "Great! I've got eleven dollars—more than enough!" Then something would occur to make you anxious. Now, why would you become anxious a little later? You've still got the eleven dollars. You haven't lost it and you haven't said, "I must have twelve or I must have thirteen." You're still saying, "I must have a minimum of ten. Great, I've got eleven!" Now what would make you anxious?

C: Well, I—. I don't really know.

T: Well, don't forget: You're saying to yourself: "I must have a minimum of ten dollars *at all times*. I now have eleven. But suppose I spend two. Suppose I lose two. Suppose I get robbed!" All of which could happen, you see, because there *are* no guarantees in the goddamned universe! They don't exist, and you're demanding one.

C: Yes, I see. So I'm still anxious.

T: Right! Now this model shows that anybody in the whole universe—and it doesn't matter what they're status is, black or white, young or old, male or female, rich or poor. Anybody who takes any desire, any goal, any preference for anything and makes it into a *must*, a *got to*, first is miserable when they don't have what they must and, second, they're anxious when they do have it—because they could always lose it. Now do you see how that applies to you?

C: Yes, I do. Any must, any real demands.

T: Yes, and you've got two main musts that make and keep making you anxious: (1) "I *must* do well; I *must* be perfect. I *must* do the right thing and not bring on a heart attack!" And (2) "I *must* not be anxious! I *must* not be panicked! I *must* not be panicked!" With these two musts, you're really going to be off the wall. You see?

C: I never thought of that before.

T: But can you see it now?

C: Yes, I think I can.

T: Fine. Now if we can just help you to think, "I don't *like* being anxious, but if I am, too damned bad, it won't kill me," you'll then get rid of your anxiety about your anxiety, your panic about your panic. If you can convince yourself, "Anxiety is uncomfortable but it won't kill me. It won't lead to a heart attack. And it won't make me an idiot for bringing on my anxiety. It's just uncomfortable. It's not *awful*." Then you'll get rid of most of your problem. Then, as you rid yourself of your anxiety about your anxiety, you can much more easily go back to your original perfectionism—your demand that you always do well and not make serious errors. Then you'll work on being less perfectionistic. You'll still very much *want* to do well, *prefer* to do well, but you'll give up the idea that you *have to*. There's no necessity, you see in doing well; no necessity for you to be unanxious.

During the first session, I often use this model of someone wanting something and not being anxious about its loss and needing the same thing and being very anxious, and often self-hating, first when they do not have what they think they need and, second, even when they do have it—for then they could always lose it. Most of my clients understand this model of neurosis and many of them begin right away to use it in their own lives, and keep mentioning to me how useful it is to them.

C: What is the best way to react—when you feel that stress is too strong? How can you overcome it?

T: When you're anxious?

C: Yes.

T: You say to yourself very strongly, until you really mean it: "Fuck it! So I'm anxious! It'll pass; it'll pass in a few minutes. It won't kill me.

It won't turn my hair gray. It won't send me to the loony bin. Nothing will happen if I just go with the anxiety and relax." So you relax. You sit down and you relax. And you strongly tell yourself, "Too damned bad—so I'm anxious. But it's not the end of the world." Anxiety won't kill you.

C: Well, I know that. But—

T: Well, you don't know that well enough. You're probably saying to yourself, "Yeah, it won't kill me. But maybe it will! Maybe it will! Maybe it will!" Then you'll be *more* anxious!

C: Yeah, I think that I need to be anxious to keep living, to stay alive.

T: Well, you don't! You'd better accept the fact that at times we're all anxious, depressed, or upset. Too bad; tough; that's the way it is. That's the human condition—humans often make themselves anxious. But all you have to do is relax—do some deep breathing or other relaxation exercises. Do you know any relaxation exercises?

C: Yes, I bought a tape the other day. I think I have it here. It shows you how to breathe freely.

T: What's it called? *How To Turn Stress Into Energy.* That may be all right. If you really follow this tape, or one of our own relaxation tapes that you can get downstairs, then you'll learn to immediately relax, and your anxiety will temporarily go away. But if you go back to being a perfectionist and insist that you *must* do well, you *must* not be anxious, your anxiety will come back.

C: Someone told me that when you have great stress, if you do a lot of exercise, you can drain it out.

T: You can distract yourself and feel better. That will temporarily work. But you'd better also change your philosophy—that will work much better. You'd better do two things: (1) distract yourself with some exercise, then your anxiety will go away temporarily. But it will come back because you're still telling yourself, "I *must* do perfectly well. I *must* not be anxious! I *must* not be upset!" (2) you therefore had better change your attitude, as well as relax. Show yourself that you don't have to do that well and that your anxiety won't kill you. Relaxation alone will help, but it will not cure you. Changing your basic musturbatory philosophy will help you permanently.

C: So you have to do it physically and mentally?

T: Exactly! You have to do it physically and mentally. And you really have to tell yourself—and *believe*—"Fuck it! If I'm anxious, I'm anxious. Too damned bad! This too will pass. And if I work on it and change my philosophy, I can make it rarely come back.''

C: You see, that's what I'm trying to do in regard to the train. I think that my problem is that I think that if I have an attack on the train it will be awful.

T: So suppose you do have an attack on the train? What's going to happen to you then?

C: Something will happen to me.

T: What?

C: Most of the time I've said to myself, "Okay, nothing will happen. Because I know that whatever I have is not a heart problem—it's a mental problem, and I create it myself." So I then relax. But what's getting to me is that I have to deal with the same thing every day. Everyday I have to deal with it.

T: I know. Because you're saying, "I *must* not be anxious! I *must* not be anxious!" Instead of, "I don't *like* being anxious, but if I am, I am!" You see, you're terrified of your own anxiety.

C: That's exactly what it is!

T: Okay. But anxiety is only a pain in the ass. That's all it is. It doesn't kill you. It's only a pain. Everybody gets anxious, including you. And they live with it!

C: It's a big pain in the ass!

T: I know. But that's all it is. Just like—well, suppose you lost all the money you had with you. That would be a real pain, but you wouldn't worry about it too much, because you know you'd get some more money. But you're making yourself terrified. "Something awful will happen. Suppose people *see* I'm so anxious! How terrible!" Well, suppose they do.

C: I don't care about that.

T: Well, that's good. Most people are afraid of that and it's good that you're not.

C: When I walk to the train, I know that I am going to start feeling anxious.

T: You know it because you're afraid of it happening. If you said to yourself strongly and really believed, "Fuck it! If it happens, it happens!" Then it won't even happen. Every time you say, "I must not be anxious! I must not be anxious!"—then you'll be anxious.

C: I'm getting—not in the train, I mean—yesterday I was like that in the office all day.

T: It doesn't matter where you are. Anytime you say to yourself, "Suppose I'm anxious," you'll be anxious. Sexually, for example, instead of saying to yourself, "What a great piece of ass my wife is! I'm going to enjoy this!" you say, "Suppose I'm anxious and my goddamned cock goes down!" Then you'll be anxious, not be thinking of sexual enjoyment, and it won't work. Anxiety will take over. But if you didn't give that much of a shit about your anxiety, and went back to thinking, "Look: I'd better focus on her body and on sexual enjoyment. That's how I can get and stay erect," then you'll maintain your erection. But, you see, you're not doing that.

C: A couple of months ago when I was anxious, I did what you're saying. I put a picture in my head, about my wife or about some other sexy woman, and then my anxiety would leave and I'd be all right sexually.

T: Yes, as soon as you focus on anything else, your anxiety will temporarily go. Let me tell you a famous fable. A king didn't want to marry his daughter to a favorite prince, who passed all the tests he was given, so that it looked like he would marry the daughter. But the king was horrified at that, so he said to his wise men, "Look! You find a test this son-of-a-bitch can't pass, or I'll cut your balls off!" The wise men were very horrified about this. So they thought and finally came up with a test that the prince couldn't pass. Do you know what it was?

C: No, I can't think of one.

T: "Don't think of a pink elephant for 20 minutes!" You see, if you say to yourself, as the prince did, "I must not think of a pink elephant! I must not think of a pink elephant!—"

C: Then you're going to think about just that.

T: Right! and that, you see, is exactly what you're doing, You're saying, "I must not be anxious!" Then you'll be anxious. Or, "I must be good sexually." Then you'll make yourself so anxious that you won't be able to concentrate on sexual enjoyment. Because to do well at sex, you have to focus on sexual thoughts—on your wife or on some other desirable woman. You have to have sexy thoughts. But if you say to yourself, "Oh, my God! Suppose I get anxious! Suppose my cock won't go up and stay up!" Then it won't! So that's what you're doing. You're demanding that you have to do well; and you're also insisting that you must not be anxious. So if we can get you to say to

yourself, and really believe, "I'd *like* to do well, but I never *have* to,"
And, "I'd very much prefer to be unanxious, but fuck it, if I'm
anxious, I'm anxious!" then you'll get over this nonsense that you're
now telling yourself. Whenever you take a preference, a goal, a
desire, and you say, "I have to achieve it! I must perform well!"
you're making yourself immediately anxious. That's where your
anxiety comes from. And that's what people do: They take their
strong desires and say, "I absolutely must achieve them! I have to;
I've got to!" Instead of, "I'd like to achieve them, but if I don't,
tough! The earth won't stop spinning!"

C: Okay. So the best way is for me to think, if I am anxious?

T: "Too damned bad! It's only uncomfortable! It won't kill me!" For
nothing terrible does happen if you're anxious. You see? Just like my
diabetes. It's a pain in the ass, and I have to take care of it. But it's
only uncomfortable, and I don't whine and scream about having it.
"I must not have diabetes! I must be perfectly healthy!" If I did that,
I'd be in trouble. So I have diabetes! So?

C: And there's nothing that you can do about it?

T: I take care of it. I stick to my diet and take my insulin regularly. Too
fucking bad! I don't like it, but I don't whine and scream and make
myself miserable by intoning, "I must not have diabetes! I must not,
I must not!"

C: There's nothing you can do. So you just accept it.

T: Yes, we *invent* the horrors. They really don't exist in the world. Many
hassles, many problems do exist. But as a store manager, you know
how to take care of problems. That's your business.

C: Yes, I do that pretty well.

T: So you don't get yourself too excited when there's a problem. You
don't say to yourself, "Oh, my God! I absolutely must solve it!"
Then you'd make yourself anxious and wouldn't be able to solve it
very well.

C: That's right.

T: So if we could get you to take the same attitude toward your anxiety
that you take toward your work, you would do very well and rid
yourself of most of your neurotic problems.

C: See, I never thought of that.

T: Yes, but that's what you'd better think of. That's the thing. Life is a
series of hassles, and you've had a number of them in your life. So
when your children get sick, you don't like it, but you take care of

it. Or if you have problems with your wife, you cope with them. Now, we want you to cope with your anxiety, and also give up some of your perfectionism. For when you say, "I have to do well! I have to do well!" you're going to make yourself upset. There are no absolute necessities in the universe—just things we would like, prefer, desire. There are many of those, but we don't *have* to get them. When people like you change these preferences into musts they upset themselves needlessly. The three main musts are: (1) "I *must* do well and be approved by significant others, or else I'm no good!" (2) "*You* have to treat me well, or you're a shit!" And then people become angry, enraged, homicidal. (3) "Conditions *must* be arranged so that they give me exactly what I want when I want it, and never, no, never give me what I don't want!" Then people have low frustration tolerance and, when conditions are pretty bad, depress themselves. Those three musts really upset people. But, of course, there is no reason whay you have to do well, or why other people must treat you nicely, or that conditions must be easy. So whenever you feel upset, or behave foolishly against your interest, about anything, look for your shoulds, look for your musts. You can easily find them, but it takes a good deal of work and effort to give them up. But you can do it!

C: I see what you're saying. It looks like I can do it.

T: Fine, I am sure that you can. Now what I want you to do is take all these forms home with you [the Millon Clinical Multiaxial Inventory], fill them all out and bring them back together and we'll give you some interesting personality scores. Then, for your homework—for we always give homework in RET—make a note of anything that really bothers you during the week—of any feelings of anxiety, panic, depression, self-hatred, or rage against others. Just a little note to yourself, so that you'll remember these feelings next time you come here. Then note exactly what's happening at point A, your activating event, just before each of these feelings happens. Then look for B, your rational and irrational beliefs, about A. Rationally, you have preferences and wishes, that unfortunate As (or adversities) not occur, and these lead to appropriate feelings at C, your emotional and behavioral consequences, such as sorrow, regret, frustration, and disappointment. But we are particularly interested in your *in*appropriate consequences at C—as I said before, your really upset feelings. So bring me some of these ABCs—and you can take one of our self-help report forms, down at the desk downstairs—to remind you what they are and to help you remember them.

C: Down at the desk?

T: Yes, we always have free forms for you to take and fill out as homework, during the week, down at the desk. Bring me in a few filled out, and especially try to find your irrational Beliefs (iBs)—at point B—your shoulds, oughts, and musts by which you disturb yourself. But if you don't find them, just bring me in a few As and a few Cs and I'll show you how to figure out your iBs at point B.

C: Is that all I have to do during the week?

T: Yes, that's all for this week. Except that we gave you a group of pamphlets, so start reading these RET pamphlets. And, preferably, get a copy downstairs of two paperback books: *A New Guide to Rational Living* and *How to Stubbornly Refuse to Make Yourself Miserable About Anything—Yes, Anything*! And start reading those books. You don't have to finish all the reading, but let's see if you can at least start it. The more RET reading you do and the more you listen to some of our tape cassettes, the quicker and better you will see how to help yourself.

C: Oh, I like reading. I find it helpful.

T: Fine. And, as noted in the instructions for therapy, which we gave you in that envelope, we find it desirable for our clients to record their sessions and then listen to them later. So next time you come, if you wish to do so, you can bring a blank cassette, or get one at the desk downstairs, and record your session and listen to it a few times in between sessions. I think you'll find that helpful. Anything else you want to bring up in the last minute or two of this session?

C: No, I don't think so. I got quite a lot out of the session. I've had some therapy before, but nothing like this! Thank you for helping me. I got a lot.

T: Fine. I am glad you enjoyed the session. Just make another appointment downstairs to see me in a week or so, and I'll look forward to continuing to see you.

C: Fine. Thank you.

Notice how I go over some of the essentials of RET, and particularly the point that the client upsets himself with his musts and then makes himself anxious about his anxiety with more musts, several times. I directly, forcefully, and briefly keep repeating this message, especially during the first session, to achieve several results: (1) explain some of the basic principles of human disturbance and of RET to the client; (2)

try to get quickly to a central problem, so that he or she can see right away how it is largely created by him- or herself and that he or she can immediately start to do something about it; (3) try to get over the idea that the client can quickly start changing him- or herself but that to do so permanently will require a longer period of time; (4) try to show the client that the RET sessions themselves can be relatively brief (usually, half-hour sessions) and infrequent (from 5 to 30 sessions for most clients), but only because the client does most of the therapeutic work himself, in between sessions; and (5) give bibliotherapy homework as well as some kind of cognitive, emotive, or behavioral homework.

The second session with this client took place one week after the first session and showed fair progress as:

> He said, "I feel okay, this week only a couple of times have I had some anxiety."

> On a fairly crowded train, he forced himself to read my book (Ellis, 1988) and distracted himself from his feelings of panic.

> He kept strongly convincing himself that he was creating his panic and that he was not going to have a heart attack and felt uncomfortable rather than anxious.

> In his office, he began to tell himself that he did not have to do everything fast or perfectly well. "And two minutes later, I feel like I can face myself. My anxiety—it is gone. . . .

> "Last week when I got to the train, I started getting anxiety. This week I got anxious only one time. I got to the train and I said to myself, 'There's nothing to worry about. Nothing will happen. So you're creating your anxiety, just like you put wood on a fire. So you can go the other way.' So five minutes later I forgot about it and I didn't have that problem. . . .

> "Before last session, I didn't understand what was going on with me. Now I know my anxiety is a problem that I am creating. I can live with that, and one of these days, I won't have that problem. I think I can really convince myself. I don't feel the way that I felt a week ago. Then I was getting crazy. Now I know that anxiety doesn't matter that much. Any time I can take the train and maybe the first couple of minutes I have to deal with myself, and I say, 'You don't have to feel panicked. You can feel the other way.'"

> For the first time, he confessed to some of his friends that he had an anxiety problem and was seeking help. "I no longer care that much what they think. Because I don't think I'm that crazy. I just have a minor problem. You don't have to be crazy to see a psychologist."

He kept repeating that he was creating his anxiety himself and that he didn't have to do so.

Two weeks later, during the third session, the client showed that he had several real breakthroughs as he kept working on his anxiety and kept reading. Here are some excerpts from the session:

"I'm feeling better. Whatever I'm feeling, like anxiety, is not it. I'm creating it. Whatever I'm feeling I can make it go away in a couple of minutes and if I get upset about my anxiety, I can talk to myself about that."

"When I get to the train I'm not that anxious. . . . Like this morning, I completely forgot about it until I was on the train. Then I remembered and started saying to myself, 'It's nice to be feeling the way I'm feeling now.' It doesn't bother me anymore. . . . And last week, a couple of days, I'm going home, I fall asleep on the train, and I wake up at my station and I said to myself, 'Whatever happened a couple of months ago is gone.'"

"And even in my work I don't feel anxious. I am working better than before without getting that, uh, anxiety to make everything fast and quick. I can pace myself better than before. . . . Another thing I learned to do: not to upset myself about the others in my office who act badly. If I got upset, they're going to act the same way."

"Before I thought my anxiety meant something was physically wrong. Now I see that I'm creating it. It's not that I am sick. . . . I used to say, while going to the train, 'I'm sure I'm gonna get sick.' Now I see that I'm creating that sick feeling. Two or three minutes later, I am okay. Two weeks ago it would have taken me fifteen minutes to be less anxious. Now it takes me two or three minutes and there are days when I don't feel panic."

"The other day I got to the train when it was almost full, and I couldn't sit down and read and distract myself. But it didn't bother me and I didn't wait for another train as I used to have to do. . . . I can talk to myself and say, 'Look, whatever anxiety you feel, you created it. And you can uncreate it.'"

"Your book is not only helping me with this anxiety problem, but it's also helping me to deal with other people. If they didn't do things the way I wanted it, I just would get upset. Now if they don't, it's not like before, I don't upset myself. I can deal with people better and I can deal with myself—not making myself crazy. . . . I used to get angry with them and feel enraged for a long time. But now I tell

myself, 'If I'm getting angry it's because I'm creating the anger'. . . . It doesn't pay for me to do that and feel like that.''

"I still try to do things better in the office but when I think that I have to do it perfectly, I say to myself, 'Please! That is impossible. I will do as best I can—and that's it.' "

"Sexually, I am better now than before. Less anxious. I was having problems with erections because I started thinking, 'I won't have it. Suppose I don't have it!' Now, I'm doing what you say in the book: 'Maybe I can make it, maybe I cannot. Okay, if I don't tomorrow maybe it will be better.' And things like that, I am enjoying it more. . . . The whole thing is changing because if I start thinking, 'I can't,' then I won't be able to. But if I don't think like that, then it will be fine. That's what's helping me a great deal.''

"Since I was feeling better this two weeks, I thought that I don't have to be here every week. I would like every two weeks or every three weeks, to see how I can do by myself. . . . I know that I am not 100% better, but I feel I am getting there.''

"I think the book helped me a lot. The way you described in it how to overcome your—to deal with just about any problem you have. . . . The chapters that I read, I read them intensely, like trying to absorb a hundred percent of it, you know. It's not that I have the will to practice everything I read over a month. But I was feeling so awful that I said that the only way for me to get better is to really confront my problem and then to follow through on it in whatever way I can.''

[Therapist asks, ''Anything else that's been bothering you at all recently?''] ''Not really. What was bothering me was worrying about when I get to the train. And then I was feeling anxious in the office. But now with that and in the home and in the office, I said I couldn't control my anxiety and that I had to do so. . . . But now I think that it's better to see what the problem is and use my thinking to make the problem go. Work it out, no matter how bad it is.''

FOLLOW-UP

I expected to have several more sessions with Ted, because I usually see people like him from 5 to 10 times, but actually this was his last individual therapy session. He and his wife started to attend my regular

Friday night workshops at the Institute for Rational–Emotive Therapy in New York, where I interview volunteer clients each week before an audience of 100 or more people. After working with the clients for about a half hour, I throw the discussion over to the audience and let them question and advise the volunteers under my direction. Ted has participated in these workshops quite actively, as well as in several of our 4-hour workshops for the public, such as one on low frustration tolerance. He has continued to read RET books and to listen to Institute cassettes, especially my tapes *Solving Emotional Problems* and *Unconditionally Accepting Yourself and Others*.

I have spoken with him several times and also with his wife, Myra, who agrees that he is continuing the gains that he indicated during his third session and that he is making still further progress. He has almost completely lost his panic about trains and has also begun to take plane trips, which he was previously afraid to do but had never spoken about it in his sessions with me. He is rarely anxious or angry at the office, and sex with his wife is "by far the best I have ever had." His wife corroborates his progress, and almost every time I see her she loudly tells me, in the presence of my other workshop participants, what an "absolute miracle on Ted" I performed. Both Ted and Myra keep sending their friends and relatives to me for therapy, and some of these referrals also comment on "what a new man" Ted is.

At the present writing, 3 months have passed since I saw Ted for therapy, and he continues to hold his ground. I expect that I will see him occasionally again, as new crises may arise in his life, but that he will generally hold the gains he has already made. My guesses about why he was able to make such good gains in the course of three half-hour sessions in one month's time include these: (1) he was a classic neurotic, unlike many borderline personalities I often see. On the Millon Clinical Multiaxial inventory II, his only really high score was on the anxiety scale, with his compulsive and somatoform scores somewhat above average; (2) he was highly motivated to reduce his anxiety and from the first session worked hard to do so; (3) he was competent and hard working in his business and social life; (4) he took well to my highly active–directive RET approach and kept echoing my insistence that he was responsible for his own anxiety and anger and that he had the ability to work at reducing these disturbances; (5) he read and listened to our RET self-help materials most intently and frequently used *How to Stubbornly Refuse to Make Yourself Miserable About Anything—Yes, Anything!*; (6) after therapy ended, he continued assiduously to attend RET workshops and to work with RET materials.

I look forward to further contacts with Ted, to see whether my expectations of his continued progress are fulfilled.

EDITOR'S QUESTIONS

Q: It appears that the client was a man who liked the therapist from the beginning. His personality seems to fit well with the RET model. He was enthusiastic and willing to comply with your requests. What if the patient had been resistant, difficult, and ornery and had a significant personality disorder? How would your method and technique vary?

A: If the client had been resistant, difficult, ornery, and had a significant personality disorder I probably would have tried to show him that he was going to have a difficult time changing and that therefore he had better work harder and longer at doing so. I would often let him know that he very likely had a strong innate tendency to be the way he was, exacerbated by his life experiences and reinforced by his own creating and practicing dysfunctional thoughts, feelings, and behaviors, and that only very hard work and practice—yes, work and practice—to overcome this tendency would probably be effective in his case. I would stress the pain he was in and how disadvantageous it would be for him to prolong it, and I would vigorously show him that, in all probability, he could significantly change if he *chose* to keep working at doing so. I would try to get him to learn RET and to keep using it to help others, and would encourage him to spend a good part of the rest of his life helping himself be much less miserable than he presently was.

Q: What do you usually tell a patient about the course and prognosis of treatment? When and how do you determine and discuss length of treatment? How do you motivate the patient?

A: I usually tell clients that the treatment will be relatively brief—a matter of months rather than years—*if* they work very hard in between sessions at using the RET methods we go over during the sessions. I motivate them in several ways: (1) by emphasizing their present emotional–behavioral misery and showing them that they definitely can reduce or eliminate it; (2) by strongly showing them that they largely create their *own* disturbances and that therefore they can almost invariably alleviate or undo them; and (3) by pointing them toward the greater pleasures they can have if they work at reducing their disturbances *and* at enhancing hedonic pursuits and at personal self-actualization (Ellis, 1991).

Q: There was a flexible use of time in this case. You advised having the next appointment in a week or so, but later the patient indicated spacing out sessions. What guides about length of sessions, frequence, and spacing do you use?

A: I usually suggest fewer or more-spaced-out sessions after several weeks of therapy, providing that the client is improving. If clients want fewer sessions than I suggest, I say, "Let's try it your way and see how it goes. If you will work hard in between sessions, and keep reading our material and doing your homework, you will probably do a good therapeutic job on yourself and therefore require fewer sessions. If not, we'll soon see a lack of progress and you can arrange for more sessions again."

Q: Did you screen for alcohol abuse? Suppose the patient were alcoholic—would you approach the problem in the same way?

A: Yes, I asked the client about alcohol abuse and he indicated that he only did mild social drinking, and I accepted this answer. If there had been alcohol abuse, I would have worked on his problem drinking from the start, ferreted out the dysfunctional beliefs leading to it—including his self-denigration, his low frustration tolerance, and his squelching of other emotional problems by his drinking—and I would have helped him to stop denigrating himself for his drinking, to work on his low frustration tolerance, and to use a number of cognitive, emotive, and behavioral techniques that are commonly used in RET with problem drinkers (Ellis, McInerney, DiGiuseppe, & Yeager, 1988; Ellis & Velten, 1992).

Q: If the patient had come to you on medication for panic disorder, how would you proceed?

A: I would proceed in much the same way that I did in this case, but I would talk to his psychopharmacologist to see what medication he was taking, what dosage, how long he was expected to take it, what side effects he might have, etc. Depending on the information received from the psychopharmacologist, I might possibly modify some of my treatment methods and the homework assignment worked out with the client.

Q: How would you focus with a client whose problems were more vague or unclear?

A: I would get him to clarify his problems by asking him questions about when and where the problems occurred, why they troubled him, what his goal was in regard to them, what he was thinking when the problems occurred, etc. Usually, after a few sessions, I would wind up with a pretty clear idea of his central problems and I would almost always discover at least one specific issue that was clear to both of us and that he or she wanted to work at.

Q: In the case presented, if the patient had not responded well, what are some of the issues you might consider? How might you change your approach?

A: I would consider: (1) how well the client understood the ABCs of RET and knew what he could do about disputing his dysfunctional Bs; (2) how he was acutally working to use the ABCs of RET and how he was doing the homework that we had agreed on; (3) what he was specifically telling himself when he did not do his cognitive, emotive, and behavioral homework; (4) whether he was really willing to change and to work at changing himself; (5) what, if anything, were his "neurotic" gains from remaining the way he was and from not changing; (6) what unexpressed problems he had that may have been blocking him from working on the expressed ones; and (7) how he was reacting to me, and if his positive or negative attitudes toward me were interfering with his working at changing himself.

Q: If the client said that he saw what he was telling himself, was doing his RET disputing of his irrational and dysfunctional beliefs, and was still not changing, what would you then do?

A: I would tell him that it is quite probable that he was seeing his dysfunctional beliefs and disputing them, but mainly doing it lightly, unvigorously, and not often enough. I would show him, if I had not already done so, that practically all disturbed people have *two* simultaneous sets of beliefs: one rational and self-helping and the other irrational and self-defeating, and that one is usually held lightly and mildly and the other is held strongly and powerfully. In his case, the irrational beliefs were probably *still* being held much more powerfully than the rational beliefs, and therefore he had better see that this was so and keep vigorously and powerfully disputing the former and replacing them with the latter. At the same time, he had better work very strongly to change his feelings and work powerfully and repetitively to change his behaviors, so that these, also, interacted with his crooked thinking and significantly helped him change that thinking. I would show him that RET always has highly emotive and behavioral components, and not merely important cognitive elements, and that he had therefore better keep working and practicing—yes, keep working and practicing—the RET methods and do so very strongly and committedly until he truly believed, felt, and acted on the rational philosophies that he was now (at times) presumably telling himself.

Q: How did you become a brief therapist?

A: I became a brief therapist in the early 1940s, when I started to do a great deal of sex and marital therapy and found that most clients only wanted to come for a few sessions and had no intention of making basic personality changes. To help some of them who wanted depth therapy, I was analyzed, was trained as an analyst, and practiced psychoanalysis for

6 years. Doing so, I found that psychoanalysis intensively goes into every irrelevancy under the sun and, alas, misses just about all the philosophic relevancies by which people mainly disturb themselves. Like many therapies that stem from it, psychoanalysis is obsessed with people's past history, which influenced their goals and values but did not really *make them* disturbed. It largely ignores how they mainly constructed their dysfunctional behavior and what they are now actively doing to keep constructing it. So, in 1955, I founded and started using rational–emotive therapy and specifically designed it to be an efficient and brief therapy for most neurotic clients, although it is often more prolonged and intensive for borderline and other seriously disturbed individuals.

REFERENCES

Beck, A. T. (1976). *Cognitive therapy and the emotional disorders.* New York: International Universities Press.

Bernard, M. E. (1986). *Staying alive in an irrational world: Albert Ellis and rational–emotive therapy.* South Melbourne, Australia: Carlson/Macmillan.

Bernard, M. E. (1991). Using rational–emotive therapy effectively: A practitioner's guide. New York: Plenum Press.

Dryden, W., & DiGiuseppe, R. (1990). A primer on rational–emotive therapy. Champaign, IL: Research Press.

Ellis, A. (1956). An operational reformulation of some of the basic principles of psychoanalysis. *Psychoanalytic Review, 43,* 163–180.

Ellis, A. (1958). Rational psychotherapy. *Journal of General Psychology, 59,* 35–49 (reprinted by Institute for Rational Emotive Therapy).

Ellis, A. (1962). *Reason and emotion in psychotherapy.* Secaucus, NJ: Citadel.

Ellis, A. (1973). *Humanistic psychotherapy: The rational–emotive approach.* New York: McGraw-Hill.

Ellis, A. (1975). *How to live with a neurotic: At home and at work* (rev. ed). Hollywood, CA: Wilshire Books.

Ellis A. (1985). *Overcoming resistance: Rational–emotive therapy with difficult clients.* New York: Springer.

Ellis, A. (1988). *How to stubbornly refuse to make yourself miserable about anything—Yes, anything!* Secaucus, NJ: Lyle Stuart.

Ellis, A. (1991). Achieving self-actualization: The rational–emotive approach. In A. Jones & R. Crancall (Eds.), *Handbook of self-actualization* (pp. 1–18). Corte Madera, CA: Select Press.

Ellis, A. (1992). The revised ABCs of rational–emotive therapy. In J. Zeig (Ed.), *Evolution of psychotherapy: II* (pp. 138–150). New York: Brunner/Mazel.

Ellis, A., & Abrahms, E. (1978). *Brief psychotherapy in medical and health practice.* New York: Springer.

Ellis, A., & Dryden, W. (1987). *The practice of rational–emotive therapy.* New York: Springer.

Ellis, A., & Dryden, W. (1990). *The essential Albert Ellis*. New York: Springer.

Ellis, A., & Dryden, W. (1991). *A dialogue with Albert Ellis*. Stony Stratford, Milton Keynes, England: Open University Press.

Ellis, A., & Grieger, R. (Eds.). (1977). *Handbook of rational–emotive therapy* (Vol. 1). New York: Springer.

Ellis, A., & Grieger, R. (Eds.). (1986). *Handbook of rational–emotive therapy* (Vol. 2). New York: Springer.

Ellis, A., & Harper, R. A. (1975). *A new guide to rational living*. North Hollywood, CA: Wilshire Books.

Ellis, A., McInerney, J. F., DiGiuseppe, R., & Yeager, R. J. (1988). *Rational–emotive therapy with alcoholics and substance abusers*. Englewood Cliffs, NJ: Prentice-Hall.

Ellis, A., & Velten, E. (1992). *When AA doesn't work for you: Rational steps to quitting alcohol*. New York: Barricade Books.

Glasser, W. (1965). *Reality therapy*. New York: Harper and Row.

Goldfried, M. R., & Davison, G. C. (1976). *Clinical behavior therapy*. New York: Holt, Rinehart & Winston.

Grieger, R., & Boyd, J. (1980). *Rational–emotive therapy: A skills-based approach*. New York: Van Nostrand Reinhold.

Lazarus, A. A. (1971). *Behavior therapy and beyond*. New York: McGraw Hill.

Mahoney, M. J. (1974). *Cognition and behavior modification*. Cambridge, MA: Ballinger.

Maultsby, M. C., Jr. (1975). *Help yourself to happiness: Through rational self-counseling*. New York: Institute for Rational–Emotive Therapy.

Meichenbaum, D. (1977). *Cognitive–behavior modification*. New York: Plenum Press.

Seligman, M. E. P. (1991). *Learned optimism*. New York: Knopf.

Walen, S. R., DiGiuseppe, R., & Wessler, R. L. (1980). *A practitioner's guide to rational–emotive therapy*. New York: Oxford.

Wessler, R. A., & Wessler, R. L. (1980). *The principles and practice of rational–emotive therapy*. San Francisco: Jossey-Bass.

Yankura, J., & Dryden, W. (1990). *Doing RET: Albert Ellis in action*. New York: Springer.

Planned Single-Session Psychotherapy

MICHAEL F. HOYT
ROBERT ROSENBAUM
MOSHE TALMON

"The readiness is all."
—HAMLET (Act V, Scene II)

Since Freud's one-session successful treatment of Katarina (Breuer & Freud, 1955), there have been anecdotal reports scattered throughout the psychotherapy literature (cf. Bloom, 1981; Rockwell & Pinkerton, 1982; Rosenbaum, Hoyt, & Talmon, 1990) regarding single-session therapy (SST). Running counter to the conventional belief that long-term treatment is the best psychotherapy and that a one-visit contact must represent a "dropout" or "premature termination," a number of authorities have recognized and advocated the possibilities of brief and single-session treatments. The following quotations, based on the experience of leading practitioners of varying theoretical perspectives, suggest the utility of SST with selected patients:

> Human warmth and feelings, experienced by a patient in one session with an empathic therapist, may achieve more profound alterations than years with a probing, detached therapist intent on wearing out resistance. (Wolberg, 1965, p. 138)

> Before each group session I pause and ask myself, "How can I cure everyone in this room *today*?" (Berne, quoted by Goulding & Goulding, 1979, p. 4)

Clearly, psychiatrists who undertake consultations should not automatically assign patients to long-term therapy or even to brief psychotherapy, but should be aware of the possibility that a single dynamic interview may be all that is needed. (Malan, Heath, Bacal, & Balfour, 1975, p. 126)

The idea behind playing as communication is that if we know about regression in the analytic hour, we can meet it immediately and in this way enable certain patients. . . . to make the necessary regressions in short phases, perhaps even almost momentarily. (Winnicott, 1958, p. 261)

In a surprising number of cases, people may require no more than an initial interview to precipitate lasting change and achieve profound behavioral readjustment. (Lazarus, 1971, p. 50)

In summary, for the average problem in the majority of families who seek therapy, a first interview can be conducted in a way that provides maximum information and begins a change. . . . Some families would like an estimate of the length of therapy; it is best to respond that therapy will be as brief as possible to solve the problems. (Haley, 1977, pp. 44–45)

I've always felt my most successful cases were those that lasted only one session. The family came together, something powerful happened that compelled them to make changes. Longer therapies meant that it took longer to reach this "critical mass" or that we were missing some important aspect. (Whitaker, 1990)

There have been a few encouraging systematic investigations of successful SST. Malan et al. (1975) found that 51% of "untreated" patients who had only an intake interview (which served to increase their insight and sense of personal responsibility) showed significant symptom improvement years later, and that half of those patients could also be judged to have made important personality modifications. Follette and Cummings (1967), working within the Kaiser-Permanente Health Plan setting, found medical utilization to be reduced 60% over 5-year follow-up after a single session of psychotherapy. A second study (Cummings & Follette, 1976) found the benefits of SST still in effect after 8 years and concluded that decreased medical utilization was due to a reduction in physical symptoms related to emotional distress. In our own prospective study (reported in Talmon, 1990), the present authors found that, on 3- to 12-month follow-ups, 34 of 58 (58.6%) nonemergency outpatient patients reported that a single session had been sufficient. Of these SST-only patients, 88% reported either "much improvement" or "improvement" since their session, and 65% also reported other positive "ripple" effects.

Rockwell and Pinkerton (1982) suggested that success in SST depends on the therapist's confidence in his or her ability, believing in the value of brief therapy, and being able to rapidly assess motivation and capacity for change. Spoerl (1975) reported examples of successful SST involving reassurance, catharsis, and problem solving. Bloom (1981) reviewed the history of SST as well as his own experiences, offered some tentative technical principles, and concluded: "We can all accomplish far more in brief therapy than we realize, if we are deliberate and plan well" (p. 181). In a similar vein, Sifneos (1987) has written:

> What is needed is a systematic study which tries to identify these individuals [who have successful SST], which describes clearly their psychodynamics, and which specifies how they manage to utilize the psychiatric interview to set in motion the mechanisms which help them rapidly solve psychological problems that have existed over a long period of time. (p. 87)

Intrigued by these suggestions and challenged by the *de facto* evidence that in outpatient psychiatric clinics 20–60% of patients do not return after the first visit (Baekeland & Lundwall, 1975), we have conducted a series of outpatient studies to learn more about the SST phenomenon. Elsewhere we have presented a broad overview of many issues involved in SST (Rosenbaum, Hoyt, & Talmon, 1990) as well as a discussion of attitudes, indications, and guidelines for enhancing the likelihood of therapeutic success in SST (Talmon, 1990; Talmon, Hoyt, & Rosenbaum, 1990). In this chapter, we briefly highlight some of the findings of our clinical research and then present excerpts from a case illustrating some aspects of planned SST.[1]

ATTITUDES AND INDICATIONS FOR SST

A constructive, solution-oriented perspective is apparent in this list of attitudes that help make SST productive, based on our clinical research (Rosenbaum et al., 1990; Talmon, 1990):

1. View each session as a whole, potentially complete in itself. Expect change.
2. The power is in the patient. Never underestimate your patient's strength.
3. This is it. All you have is now.
4. The therapeutic process starts before the first session and will continue long after it.
5. The natural process of life is the main force of change.
6. You don't have to know everything in order to be effective.

7. You don't have to rush or reinvent the wheel.
8. More is not necessarily better. Better is better. A small step can make a big difference.
9. Helping people as quickly as possible is practical and ethical. It will encourage patients to return for help if they have other problems and will also allow therapists to spend more time with patients who require longer treatments.

Those most likely to benefit from SST include the following:

1. Patients who come to solve a specific problem for which a solution is in their control.
2. Patients who essentially need reassurance that their reaction to a troubling situation is normal.
3. Patients seen with significant others or family members who can serve as natural supports and "cotherapists."
4. Patients who can identify (perhaps with the therapist's assistance) helpful solutions, past successes, and exceptions to the problem.
5. Patients who have a particularly "stuck" feeling (e.g., anger, guilt, grief) toward a past event.
6. Patients who come for evaluation and need referral for medical examinations or other nonpsychotherapeutic services (e.g., legal, vocational, financial, or religious counseling).
7. Patients who are likely to be better off without any treatment, such as "spontaneous improvers," nonresponders, and those likely to have a "negative therapeutic reaction" (Frances & Clarkin, 1981).
8. Patients faced with a truly insoluble situation, such as trying to "fix" or "cure" an aged parent's Alzheimer disease. Since a problem may be defined as something that has a solution, it will help to recast goals in terms that can be productively addressed.

Those for whom SST is contraindicated include the following:

1. Patients who might require inpatient psychiatric care, such as suicidal or psychotic persons.
2. Patients suffering from conditions that suggest strong biological or chemical components, such as schizophrenia, manic–depression, alcohol or drug addiction, or panic disorder.
3. Patients who request long-term therapy up front, including those who are anticipating and have prepared for prolonged self-exploration.

4. Patients who need ongoing support to work through (and escape) the effects of childhood and/or adult abuse.
5. Patients with long-standing eating disorders or severe obsessive–compulsive problems.
6. Patients with chronic pain syndromes and somatoform disorders.

FUNDAMENTAL ECLECTICISM AND THREE IMPORTANT FACTORS

There is no single theory, method, or goal for successful SST. Rather, therapeutic work is guided by the nature of the problem the patient presents for solution, along with three metatheoretical questions (Hoyt, 1990): (1) how is the patient stuck (what is maintaining the problem); (2) what does the patient need to get unstuck; and (3) how can the therapist facilitate or provide what is needed? Answers to these heuristics might lead toward focusing in the realm of the intrapsychic, characterological, interpersonal, or systemic (Gustafson, 1986), with the search being for a conceptualization that would allow a viable and parsimonious solution. The therapist needs to be versatile, innovative, and pragmatic, asking: "What would help this patient today?" Patients may need to begin a process or complete a process; they may need to take hold or to let go; they may need reassurance or confrontation; they may need to look at something deeply or to shift perspective. Ideally, techniques might include an integrated combination of appropriate support, psychoeducational and behavioral skill instruction, interpretation to enhance psychodynamic insight, hypnotherapy, Gestalt-type role playing, and/or systemic realignment via strategic intervention. Nothing works all the time, but what might work this time?

Rather than assuming that therapy is a treatment done *to* a patient, often it is better to assume that what is most needed is to not block or stand in the way of the patient's own capacity for self-healing and problem solving. The idea of "cure" becomes less useful than that of facilitating growth, enhancing coping skills, and seeking solutions (de Shazer, 1985; O'Hanlon & Weiner-Davis, 1988; Talmon, 1990). Encouragement to use what one already knows can be very empowering. Most people have had the experience of a single conversation—sometimes with a friend or loved one, sometimes with a stranger—resulting in a shift, a new perspective, an "aha," an idea that later bears fruit. In planned SST, we try to help the patient find/create an answer that works for him or her.

Therapist–Patient Relationship

Judging from our clinical–research experience, success in SST comes much easier if there is a positive feeling tone between patient and therapist. This may be some combination of a realistic person-to-person reaction and a positive transference–countertransference response that permits rapid patient restabilization via identification and object substitution. Viewed differently, the positive relationship paves the way for the patient to accept without undue resistance suggestions, advice, and guidance that may have salutary effects; as well as for the therapist to trust in the patient's strengths. For some people, as the Rogerians have told us, simply being listened to and heard respectfully may be what is necessary and sufficient to produce personal change.

Patient Power or Autonomy

Patients who make beneficial changes as a result of an SST are often those who recognize, perhaps with the therapist's assistance, that they have the power within themselves to be different or to remain the same (Goulding & Goulding, 1979). It is our working assumption that the power is in the patient and that the therapist's ultimate responsibility is to get the patient to assume responsibility for his or her own thoughts, feelings, and actions. Whether through insight and intentional behavior change or more indirectly or paradoxically, we endeavor to help people by getting them to access their own strengths and resources. We assist them to self-empowerment by helping them recognize ways they hinder or defeat themselves and by helping them utilize healthier options.

Readiness

This somewhat vague concept, which refers to immediate preparedness and willingness, should not be evoked teleologically; that is, one should not assume the cause from the conclusion, reasoning that since someone has changed he or she must have been ready to change. Rather, we conceptualize readiness as a state of *potential imminence* (not inevitability) in which various conditions are near a threshold that can, with recognition and skillful facilitation, be assisted and potentiated into actuality. Clinical sensitivity to this phenomenon is what Rockwell and Pinkerton (1982) were referring to when they wrote: "The therapist must be alert to the possibility [of SST occurring], must assess quickly when s/he has a [potential SST] case in hand, set the process in motion, and determine a satisfactory stopping point" (p. 39).

Readiness may occur when old mental constructs have either decayed "spontaneously," through disuse or maturation (Rosenbaum, 1989), or been actively proved untenable or unworkable—resulting in a crisis with its attendant combination of emotional pain and growth opportunity. This underscores the importance of clarifying "Why now?" has the patient come to therapy (Budman & Gurman, 1988, pp. 72–73). Psychotherapy readiness may also obtain when a patient has already made movement in one sector of the triangle of thinking–feeling–acting but has not yet made the other changes necessary to restore congruence. Of course, some patients may simply decide one day, "This is it." The act of electing psychotherapy involves defining something as a "problem" that can be "helped" or "solved," a major step in readiness for intentional change.[2]

CLINICAL GUIDELINES FOR SST

Although each case involves its own idiosyncrasies and therapeutic subtleties, there are a number of general hints or suggestions for conducting a successful SST. Their creative application with particular patients is part of what makes psychotherapy an interesting and innovative endeavor.

1. *Induction and preparation: Seeding change.* The process of change is already under way when a patient calls for an initial appointment, since he or she has already identified some aspect of experience as changeworthy and has started the steps (getting a therapist) that he or she feels will promote that goal. Therapists can potentiate this movement in a pretherapy phone conversation, setting the stage for a constructive SST by asking patients to collect information about the desired change. Saying to a caller, "I am willing to meet with you. You may be able to resolve your problem quickly, perhaps even in the first visit, if you are willing to start doing something different or whatever is necessary," can be both hope inspiring and self-fulfilling. In planned SST, we welcome "spontaneous improvement" and "waiting-list cures."

2. *Getting started.* Establishing a therapeutic alliance (Margulies & Havens, 1981) and finding a focus are joint tasks in the initial portion of SST (or any therapy). Collecting useful and essential information and helping the patient to define the problem to be solved (Haley, 1976) and the treatment contract (Goulding & Goulding, 1979) are primary. When a new potential SST patient comes to see us, we often open the session by saying: "We have recently learned that many people who come to

therapy do so for only one session and find it to be helpful and sufficient. If we need more sessions, we can schedule them, but what we'll do today is try to get to the bottom of your problem, and look for a helpful solution. I'm willing to work hard on this if you are. Now, what is it that you would like to accomplish today?"[3]

Many patients will work well with such a start, but not all. Clearly, patients who are seeking long-term therapy or at least wanting to build a "substitute relationship" with a therapist will not have their needs satisfied in SST. Other patients may have vague complaints or not be able initially to identify what they wish to change. In all cases, it will be important to explore with the patient his or her needs and motivations before proceeding with any treatment.

3. *Allow enough time.* Too often therapists just get to the "heart" of a session only to realize that there is not enough time to do the work that is now possible. Sometimes this is unavoidable, while other times it is some combination of therapist mismanagement and patient resistance (Hoyt, 1985, 1990). In SST, we try to block out 60–90 minutes for an individual, and 90–120 minutes for a couple or family. All of this time may not be needed, but it is useful to not feel prematurely "jammed." One "long" session may be cost-effective if it obviates two or three (or more) "conventional" (usually 50-minute) sessions.

4. *Focus on pivot chords.* In music, the pivot chord is an ambiguous chord that contains notes common to more than one key, and so can imply several "directions" to the music and facilitate the transition from one key to another (Rosenbaum, 1989; Rosenbaum et al., 1990). An important option for the SST therapist is to construe the client's difficulty in such a way that it can function as a pivot chord for change. The therapist simultaneously meets the patient in his or her view of the world, so that he or she feels understood and validated, while at the same time offering a new perspective. "Reframing" allows the therapist to join with the client while introducing the possibility of viewing things differently.

5. *Open up, go slowly, and look for patients' strengths.* We find that it does not help to rush an SST session. The effective SST therapist is usually prudently active, presenting ideas and possible solutions in a respectfully "what if" manner. We do not try to reinvent the wheel or stir up fire and brimstone. The spectacular is seldom necessary or productive; better to be a "constructive minimalist" (Talmon, 1990). Rather than being brilliant "uncommon therapy" (Haley, 1973), most of the successful SSTs we have studied have been "common therapy" involving an unrushed emphasis on abilities and strengths rather than pathology, the expectation of change, and recognition of the potentially salubrious influence of life's vicissitudes. These are also factors that

Barber (1990) cites as conducive to the success he observes in many workshop demonstrations.

6. *Practice solutions experientially.* A powerful experience in which the patient thinks, feels, and acts differently is undeniable. It moves him or her past the stuck point, it makes real and immediate the desired change, it creates a sense of freedom and increases hope, and helps prove to the patient the uncompelling nature of whatever considerations he or she were using to hold him- or herself back and stay stuck. Therapeutic experience can be generated via imagery, role playing, rituals and ceremonies, Gestalt-type exercises, well-timed transference interpretations, family sculpting and guided transactions, etc. The chance to practice the desired outcome in session allows patient and therapist to experience success directly or recognize and correct any impediments during a "dry run" rehearsal.

7. *Take a time-out.* It is often helpful to take a break either during the session or right before its conclusion. This time can be used to think and consult, or just to take a breather. Restating the focal concern or question before the break makes sure that therapist and patient are on the same wavelength. The time-out also heightens the dramatic impact of whatever message is given after the break.

8. *Before concluding the session, allow time for last-minute issues.* Rather than waiting for concerns to be brought up when there is not time enough to address them adequately in the SST, it is useful to elicit important information late in the session by asking, "Are there any questions or concerns you would like to ask me before we finish?" Asked with enough time in reserve, this "extra" questioning may reveal issues that need to be attended to if the SST is to be complete and satisfactory.

9. *Giving final feedback.* Patient satisfaction and sense of self-mastery are usually enhanced by presentation of an understandable, nonpejorative explanation. We find it helpful to underline what we have learned about the patient's thinking, feelings, and behavior that is useful in the direction of solving his or her problem. We emphasize the connection between existing strengths and resources and what appears as a small and rather natural next step toward a desired goal. We avoid "accusatory" interpretations and labels (Wile, 1984). Positive terms are used "to capture the ear of the listener" (Gustafson, 1986) and cast in an autonomous action language that helps patients to see their ability to respond differently (Goulding & Goulding, 1979). When tasks or "homework" are assigned, we look for simple activities that will appeal to the patient's idiosyncrasies and worldview.

10. *Ending the session and leaving an open door for future change.* At the end of an SST, we pause and ask if the patient would like to make another appointment or would prefer to leave an open door to come

back whenever necessary. If therapist and patient conclude that one session is enough, it is helpful to set a brief follow-up phone call for several months hence.[4] This way, time is allowed for changes to materialize, as well as to avoid feelings of separation anxiety or abandonment on either side. Just knowing that the door is open, so to speak, often relieves the need to knock. If no additional appointment is made at the end of the session, it is good to remind patients that they can still choose to seek services at some time in the future if they so desire and that returning to treatment might simply mean that more help is wanted rather than suggesting that something is wrong with what has already been done. In this way, SST can be a useful part of "brief intermittent psychotherapy throughout the life cycle" (Cummings, 1990), a common characteristic of "HMO therapy" (Austad & Berman, 1991; Austad & Hoyt, 1992; Hoyt & Austad, 1992).

CASE ILLUSTRATION

The following case presentation illustrates many of the guidelines described previously. While no one case can adequately depict a therapeutic approach (perhaps especially one that is fundamentally eclectic and has no single unifying theory, method, or goal), this case may be useful because of its very "commonness," involving a young man complaining of unhappiness and job stress. The therapist's activity in the creation of a focus and utilization of a pivot chord, his nurturing tone and insightful interpretation reinforced with experiential work and suggestions for postsession patient "homework," and the invitation to return as needed and to have a follow-up phone call are all features of a planned SST approach.

The First Session

The patient was a 23-year-old man, Jeff Johnson,[5] who had no psychiatric history. He had contacted our health maintenance organization (HMO) clinic complaining of "stress and problems at work." In this case, the therapist (Rosenbaum) had no contact (such as a preparatory phone call) with the patient prior to their meeting. After a short walk from the waiting room to the therapist's office, getting seated, and introductions, the therapist paused and gazed kindly at the patient with a look of "Shall we begin? Take it."

Jeff: I've never talked to anyone like a doctor about my problems and I'm not sure it'll help me. But my wife, she really thought I should speak to you. I'm under a lot of pressure and feel ready to explode.

Therapist: Well, sometimes talking about things can help. Many people who come here and talk about their problems find that just one time can help a lot. Anyway, I'm willing to work hard today to help you get a better handle on things. Does that sound like something you'd like to do?

J: Sure, okay, I guess.

Notice that in this initial exchange, even before addressing the content of the patient's concerns, the therapist already has introduced four important elements: (1) the idea that talking can help; (2) the idea that for many people just one time can help a lot; (3) his willingness to work hard to help the patient "get a better handle on things"; and (4) the patient's partnership in the endeavor. Having a working alliance and a preliminary definition of roles and purpose, the therapist then proceeds:

T: So, what seems to be the problem?

J: I don't know. It just seems like everything is building up. There's just lots of pressure on me and nobody understands.

T: Could you give me an example?

J: Well, it's mostly work, I guess. My supervisor at work just won't get off my back. It all started about a year ago when he wanted to make me a foreman at the warehouse. That meant I'd have to do things to the other guys at work and I wasn't willing to do that. When the other guys saw my supervisor trying to make me a foreman, they all started getting on my case. I told my supervisor I didn't want any part of it. Ever since then he's been giving me a hard time. He tells me I should be more of a man and he gives me all kinds of advice.

T: He gives you advice?

J: Yeah, he tells me that because I've got a new baby, I have to support him and all. My boss makes me so mad, sometimes I just want to hit him.

T: Do you have a new baby?

J: Yeah, a son. He's about 5 months old.

T: Your first?

J: Yeah.

T: What's it feel like to be a father?

J: I really love the kid, but there's lots to worry about. My brothers, they all tell me to lighten up, but they don't understand how when you have a kid you can't fool around anymore.

T: It sounds like you feel you have to be extra responsible now.

J: Yeah. Everything has changed.

The therapist then checked for any contraindications for SST. Jeff was tense, anxious, and mildly depressed. Since he was not suicidal, psychotic, or on drugs, the therapist attempted to help Jeff solve his problem in this one visit. Although Jeff referred to his problems as being work related, the therapist thought that something in the birth of Jeff's son had contributed to his feelings of not having power in his work situation. (The "Why now?" question.) The therapist noted Jeff's sense of responsibility as a strength and then began to explore the possible linkage between work pressures and fatherhood:

T: Well, let's talk a bit about these feelings of pressure and responsibility. There's a lot of that that goes with the birth of a kid, of course . . . but hopefully there can be some joy, too. Have you had any of that?

J: Oh yeah, I mean, when the kid smiles and all, that really makes you feel something tremendous.

T: Yeah.

J: It means I really gotta take care of him. My brothers kid me about it. They don't understand what it means to take care of a family.

T: Can you talk to anybody else about it? Your wife, or your parents, or friends?

J: No, not really. I mean, I don't want to worry my wife. My mother kind of understands, but I don't have any time to hang out around her. I have too much to do.

T: Look, it's clear you're very responsible. But do you ever take any time to just relax and enjoy yourself?

J: Oh, sometimes, just being around my boy. I don't go out much or do much of anything now.

T: It's clear you're able to shoulder responsibility. It's also important, sometimes, to not take on too much responsibility. Of course, it's clear you already know how to say "No" to responsibility which isn't right for you, like when you told your boss you didn't want to be foreman.

J: Yeah, but ever since that time he's been on my case. He puts me in lousy jobs. . . .

As will be seen in the next passage, the therapist continues to focus on Jeff's feeling pressured by responsibilities and makes the connection to Jeff's own experience of being abandoned by his father and subsequent feelings of hurt and anger. A pivot chord is created as Jeff sees that he is both a father to his son and a son to his father. When he changes how he feels and acts as a son, he changes how he feels and acts as a father and a man. Note in what follows how the therapist strives to empower Jeff, reminding him, "What the hell, you can walk out" on the boss. While encouraging Jeff to confront his feelings about his father, the therapist also asks Jeff (rather than telling him), "How do you want to go about that?" Unlike the boss and the father, the therapist's tone is supportive and respectful.

T: Where does your boss come off saying things like that? Is he your father or something?

J: Jesus, he acts like it.

T: What about your real father? Where's he in the picture?

J: My mom left him when I was pretty small. He never took time with me. Now, though, it's funny. Just a little while ago, since I had my son, he looked me up. He was friendly and acted like nothing had happened.

T: What did you do?

J: I didn't do anything. I mean, I felt it was weird for him to be coming around now, and all, but I didn't want to say anything. I just let it be.

T: But it sounds like you had lots of feelings about his not being around before now.

J: Yeah, well, I was about 11 when my parents split up, and it's not like we moved hundreds of miles away. We stayed in the same area. But he just never visited. My brothers, they were pretty well grown up by then. But I mean, I was just getting older. He could have come around sometime.

T: Sounds like you felt pretty mad at him for just dropping you.

J: Yeah . . . I think I was.

T: Maybe you still are.

J: Yeah, I kind of am.

T: Kind of makes it hard knowing how to be a responsible father when your father wasn't responsible at all.

J: Yeah . . . that's right.

T: Cause you're a father now, and you really want to be responsible to your son, and consistent, and be there for him, not like your father was for you.

J: Darn right.

T: You sound pretty hurt and mad.

J: Yeah, I didn't realize that I was. But I think that's really been bothering me, about my father.

T: You know, it's interesting, I wonder whether some of the anger you're feeling at your supervisor has to do with his acting kind of like a bad father to you.

J: You know, I thought about that. I mean, I didn't really think about it that way before. But I did think, "Where does he come off, acting like he's my father or something?" And I think I get mad at him cause I'm still mad at my dad.

T: Of course he's not your father. In fact, you're a father yourself, now. And you know, whatever happened in the past, you can be the kind of father you decide you want to be. And one way of doing that is to just remind yourself that your supervisor isn't your father. And what the hell, you can walk out of his life every day at 5:00 or whenever. But to be a good father to your boy, it sounds like you need to settle some things about your own father.

J: You know, I think that may be a good idea. Yeah, I really think that makes sense.

T: So, how do you want to go about that?

J: Well, maybe I should sit down and tell my father about some of the things I've been feeling.

At this juncture, the therapist suggested using role playing, an experiential technique, to practice the solution Jeff wanted. Jeff quickly brought up his concern that such things aren't "supposed" to be said to fathers and that his father might get angry. Rehearsing with the therapist gave Jeff a chance to "try on" his desired behavior. Jeff played his ostensibly fearsome father, and the therapist modeled a "Jeff" empowered with the truth of his convictions. Again, the therapist focused on validating Jeff's feelings and conveying control for the work and the outcome to Jeff.

J: I mean, this isn't the kind of thing guys are supposed to say to their fathers. Or, maybe he'll get pissed off.

T: Well, let's try that ourselves and see what would happen. You be your father, I'll play you. You try to make fun of me, or get mad, or whatever you feel he'd do. I'll play you, okay?

J: Okay

T: Listen, Dad, I want to say something to you.

J: Yeah?

T: Look, you want to spend time with my son, but you never spent any time with me after the divorce. I was really upset you just left and never visited.

J: Oh, come off it.

T: What do you mean, come off it? This is important to me. I don't think it was real cool of you to just disappear.

J: Well, I . . . I don't know. I didn't know what else to do.

T: (*Breaking role*) Is that what your father would say there?

J: (*Breaking role*) I don't know, I . . .

T: You were worried he'd get mad at you or make fun of you.

J: Yeah, but when I was playing him and thinking of how he's been acting since he came and visited my son, somehow it didn't seem like he would.

T: I don't know. Maybe he would, maybe he wouldn't. But let's see how you'd feel about it or practice how you'd handle it if he does act difficult. You've had a lot of feelings about this. Let's practice just what you really want to tell him and think about what you really want to accomplish.

After a few minutes more of role playing, in which Jeff successfully practiced and experienced the way of being he desired, it was time to conclude the session. Again, the therapist encouraged and supported Jeff's movement toward autonomy. Unlike Jeff's boss, the therapist didn't tell Jeff what to do.

T: So, let me just mention that there's a couple of ways to go from here. I mean, you could talk to your father. You might want to go over the conversation first in your mind, or you might want to think about it for awhile. You may find our talk has helped you think or feel differently. If you want, I'd be glad to meet with you again after you've had a chance to sort out some of these things, if you want.

The therapist also kept the door open for future contact. This is particularly important since Jeff felt abandoned by his father.

T: Do you want to set up another meeting with me? Or would you like to work on it on your own? Of course, if you decide to work on it on your own, you can always call me and I'd be glad to meet with you. So, what are you going to do when you leave?

J: I think, right now, I'll think about it and probably talk to my dad in a little bit. If it doesn't work out, I can always call.

T: That's fine. But let me just check it with you. . . . How are you feeling now? You originally came in feeling real pressured and upset about your work situation.

J: Yeah, but I think that is what's really been bothering me. I feel a lot better now.

T: So, is this enough for now? Have you accomplished what you wanted today?

J: Yeah, I really feel much better. Thanks a lot.

FOLLOW-UP

The patient sought no further treatment. Twelve months later, Jeff was contacted by phone for follow-up.[6] He was doing fairly well. He was enjoying being a parent without feeling overly burdened, and he was no longer so depressed and tense. He reported that he had finally left the job and was doing temporary jobs while looking for a more permanent position—an unsettled reality that had him feeling only "fairly well" instead of "very well." He remarked about the therapist and the SST: "He helped me a lot. . . . He helped me realize I had to cope. He pressured me to think about what I needed to do." Asked about what might have been more helpful, he said: "There was really no way at the time to know how bad things were going to get with my boss, but I wish he had advised me to confront the situation more and get out of there quicker. But when things got tough, it really helped that I remembered that the doctor had told me that no matter what people say, you have a chance to do things in a good way. That helped me deal with it without really losing it." He indicated no need or desire for further therapy at that time. He was invited to recontact the therapist or clinic if and when he so desired. At the end of the phone interview, when thanked for his time, Jeff replied: "I really appreciate the effort and you guys following up. It feels better just to talk about it now. It makes me feel like a person."

CONCLUSION

Since approximately one third of all psychotherapy patients do not return for a second session, it is important for therapists to approach each session with the idea that it could be the last. Undertreatment or overtreatment is not justified, regardless of whether the patient is seen in fee-for-service private practice or in a public clinic or managed health care program. The SST approach is not indicated and will not work in all situations, but utilization of its attitudes and techniques may make many therapy sessions more effective, regardless of the setting or length of treatment. The possibility of a single therapeutic meeting's being sufficient is an option for therapist and patient to be aware of; the decision whether to meet again is usually best left to the patient.

The following SST steps have been described: screening and preparation; suggestion of possible one-session treatment and cultivation of motivation; expectation of change and creation of a solution-oriented focus; reinforcement of positive strengths; reframing and creation of a pivot chord; practicing solutions experientially; concluding with an open door; and following up with a phone call or office visit. SST is not a panacea or "quick fix" but, rather, a way of helping patients to access inner strengths to make constructive steps.

EDITORS' QUESTIONS

Q: SST appears not to be an approach to therapy as much as it is "doing a single session of very good eclectic therapy." Is this true? Do you believe that there is something inherently different regarding SST other than that it takes place in one session?

HOYT and TALMON: We hope that the therapy is very good and eclectic. What is most distinctive about our SST approach is the explicit belief that one session may be enough and the intentional effort to make the most of the first meeting. While it is true that "there is only one first time," as Jung said, and that this first meeting may provide unique opportunities because of its freshness and "surprise," our main purpose and interests are not in single-session or brief therapy per se but, rather, in empowering patients and having them use their resources to move forward in their lives. It is very important to recognize that the patient is not required to have only one session. SST is actually an open-ended form of treatment—we suggest that one session may be enough to provide structure and promote change, but it is the patient who decides if one visit is sufficient. In this way, SST is *not* time-limited therapy!

ROSENBAUM: There is nothing at all unique to SST. I approach *each* session—even of long-term psychotherapies—as if it could be the only session. After this session, the patient or I might die. To be effective, we must both die—give up our old selves—during the course of the session. The apparent length of the session—whether we meet one or more times—is a conventional description. Perhaps we meet once, and the client thinks about it for the rest of her life. Perhaps we meet once, the client forgets me, and I think about her the rest of my life. Single-session therapy is marked not by clock time but by psychological time.

Q: How strictly do you hold to the SST format? How often does your push for one session trigger oppositional reactions in your clients? I find that by offering more (by indicating my availability by phone and in person and by making a second appointment), my clients act very prudently and judiciously in how they access my services. If, however, I try to offer less, they will inevitably demand more. What are your thoughts on this in light of the fact that you set the expectation, up front, for the initial visit to be the only visit?

HOYT, ROSENBAUM and TALMON: You are referring to what Brehm (1966) called "psychological reactance," the interesting response of valuing something more if you cannot have it. You are certainly right that patients might become oppositional (iatrogenic resistance) if they felt forced or pushed into one session. This is a fine line. We try to convey the idea that one session may be enough, that therapist and patient together may be able to find a good solution in a single meeting. We also emphasize that more sessions are available as needed, and make a point of leaving an "open door" and recommend a follow-up contact by phone or in person. What is key is that the patient feel the length of treatment is under his or her control. The one-session model is offered as a possible choice, not forced; and under such conditions, many patients choose it.

Q: What signs, signals, or criteria do you use to determine when it makes sense to offer a second session to a client? How does the SST therapist avoid feeling like a "failure" if he or she does not complete the work in one session?

HOYT: There is no such thing as an "SST therapist." We hope that our approach will encourage therapists to work efficiently and respectfully, and to be alert to the potential for a single session being sufficient and satisfying. Our "goal" is to help the patient use his or her powers to find a parsimonious solution—this might take a single session, a series of sessions, or a long series of sessions. The length of treatment is usually determined by the patient, although we would suggest another meeting if we felt a patient had not found a viable solution and would insistently recommend continuing therapy if it became apparent that the patient would otherwise be at risk for life-threatening behavior or other severe negative consequences.

ROSENBAUM: I always offer additional sessions to clients, and leave the decision to them. There is no success or failure in SST, just as there is no success or failure in manifesting your true self: therapy, and lives, are always works in progress, and being so, each session and each moment is complete.

TALMON: Therapists will not feel like "failures" when they realize that it is not their job to "complete the work in one session," as you suggested, but rather, to join patients in one (or more) points in time in order to facilitate helpful solutions—most of which will be worked out long before and long after the particular session (or therapy).

Q: It seems that doing SST would be an ideal model for training new clinicians. In other words, it is clearly confined to a particular time; it has a beginning, a middle, and an end; it requires the therapist to concentrate his or her thinking. Have you used it as a training model with new clinicians? How has this worked out?

HOYT: Training clinicians, whether beginners or experienced pros, to think about promoting change and empowering patients within a brief framework would be attractive, although SST can demand an eclectic innovativeness and flexibility that may require clinical experience and seasoning. We have produced a professional training videotape (Talmon, Rosenbaum, Hoyt, & Short, 1991) and have begun to offer workshops in SST methods. So far, the response has been enthusiastic and mostly positive, although some clinicians either find the SST approach too much of a stretch from their own theoretical predilections and/or mistakenly think we are claiming SST to be a panacea or cure-all or replacement for other forms of psychotherapy that may be required. We hope to teach clinicians ways of working efficiently and appropriately to help patients get unstuck, to make a shift or pivot. For most cases, the model of "cure" is of dubious value and may interfere with the search for enhanced coping, new learnings, and growth (White & Epston, 1990). SST is not a "cure."

ROSENBAUM: Training clinicians in SST is more a question of inculcating a certain attitude than it is of passing on a set of techniques. This applies to both beginning and experienced clinicians. If any clinician goes into a session saying, "I will make this an SST," he or she is likely to fail, from trying too hard. Instead, we encourage beginners and experienced professionals alike to realize that when a client doesn't return, it may not indicate failure but rather success. Thus, we try to help clinicians approach each session with a certain openness to change in both themselves and the client, with curiosity and a willingness to let go and appreciate the experience that comes to them.

TALMON: New clinicians might be more open minded and flexible and therefore require less "unlearning" than we required ourselves as "products" of many years of therapy for ourselves with deeply ingrained psychodynamic "frames of mind." On the other hand, without the appropriate training in mental status examinations, psychodiagnostic testing, and ruling out critical signs for issues like psychosis, abuse, and intoxication, new clinicians may be too anxious and too insecure in their knowledge to effectively and *selectively* employ SST.

Q: At my HMO, often a somewhat knowledgeable patient will come in and state that he or she "knows" that you rarely get what you need or want from an HMO. Have you had any patient complaints regarding the SST program?

TALMON: If by "knowledgeable patient" you mean a patient who has been through a long-term therapy in a fee-for-service setting and now comes to your HMO clinic and asks for "more of the same" without having to pay for it, then it becomes a therapeutic issue to help the patient realize that every choice in life has a price and a time frame attached to it. I often refer this kind of patient to a highly reputable (and often expensive as well) fee-for-service private practitioner. At times the patient returns with a better targeted and more realistic expectation. It is my observation that often all long-term therapy produces is simply more therapy.

ROSENBAUM: Getting what you want is different from getting what you need. Both "needs" and "wants" are concepts. By meeting clients at their view of the world—acknowledging and accepting their needs, wants, and disappointments—we can help them realize that these are but mental constructions and help engage them in an immediate, deep search for their true self.

HOYT: SST is certainly not for everyone, and patients who truly want to engage in prolonged insight-oriented therapy will not be satisfied in SST. We try to educate patients regarding what is available as part of their health plan coverage. We do not have an "SST program" as such, but rather, we try to help each patient as efficiently and parsimoniously as we can. Someone who already "knows" they will be disappointed may be bringing an agenda (transference) that will undermine successful therapy unless recognized and appreciated (addressed and worked through and/or utilized therapeutically). Because patients are not forced into a single session, we have had very few complaints. Interestingly, one patient was offered more therapy but declined; on follow-up, she complained of treatment being too short. You can't please everyone, it would seem.

Q: What percentage of your patient population do you feel is appropriate for SST? What percentage of patients will accept one session as their treatment?

HOYT: Studies around the country suggest that 20–50% of patients are, *de facto*, seen for one session. In our preliminary prospective study of nonemergency outpatients in our predominantly working- and middle-class HMO suburban clinic, 34 of 58 (58.6%) chose to complete their therapy in one session. More studies with therapists oriented toward the possibility of successful SST will be needed before extrapolating these findings to the larger population.

TALMON: In specific settings such as community mental health services, SST may reach 80% of the served clients. The acceptance of one session as sufficient treatment does not have to be determined in advance. We advocate both presession screening as well as follow-up phone calls as integral parts of our SST approach. The condition and state of mind of the patient in the follow-up call are likely to be the determining factors in making an appropriate decision if SST was sufficient or if further therapy is required. The follow-up call is important to help patients consolidate their gains (when SST is sufficient) as well as helping the therapist to be better informed when patients need (or don't need) further therapy. This is especially important in large and busy clinics like ours.

ROSENBAUM: All therapies, even those several years in length, consist of a series of SSTs. Whether clients come in for a single session or many, by definition 100% of clients are appropriate for SSTs—it is the *only* form of therapy a clinician can ever deliver.

Q: What would you have done if the patient, rather than being pretty friendly and compliant, was resistant and unfriendly? Would you have recommended longer brief therapy (or, would you have shortened the session to 8 or 10 minutes)? Is lack of compliance a contraindication to SST?

HOYT and TALMON: Therapy can be more straightforward (and more pleasant) if the patient is compliant and cooperative, but resistance is often in the eye of the beholder. The capacity for independence in the face of authority can be a great strength, as paradoxical therapy methods appreciate. Our goal is to assist the patient in finding a solution that he or she finds useful and acceptable. Patients can always defeat us. The challenge sometimes is how the therapist can "fail" without having the patient fail, also. Are we willing to "fail" and be "wrong" if the patient comes out a "winner"?

ROSENBAUM: To talk about compliance is to impose a comparative value set on a fluid situation. I don't want clients to comply with me, but to be themselves. A client can never "defeat" me since I am not trying to "win." If I find a client "resistant" or "unfriendly," I try to ask myself what I am attached to in myself that makes such terms arise. Generally, the best approach at such times is to treat these feelings as a signal that there is a valuable opportunity for me to learn something, and to treat the client as my teacher. (I often fail at doing this, but it is important for me to recognize that it is my—not the client's—limitation.)

Q: SST seems to reflect a set of assumptions for approaching mental health problems from a positive, optimistic, and strength-oriented perspective. With that in mind, how do you incorporate these assumptions into your work with some of the "contraindicated" populations that you mention in your chapter?

HOYT: Our experience has been that so-called contraindicated populations have such difficulty accessing their resources and finding a useful solution through the course of one meeting that therapy is seldom successful after only a single session. The overall approach with such patients, however, is much the same—respect for their strength and capacities, facilitation of their abilities, and concern for their well-being. Patients in psychiatric dire straits usually require more attention in port before returning to the open seas.

TALMON: Yet, even among the contraindicated we found ourselves surprised. For example, a person with long-term abuse of cocaine was able to use the single session as a significant turning point toward sobriety. In short, when contraindicated populations are offered a second appointment and fail to keep it, we don't assume that they are "bad patients" who have failed us. We simply follow up with an open mind to find out if further therapy is indeed necessary.

ROSENBAUM: Patients who are acutely suicidal may not be appropriate for SST. Just because they are suicidal now, though, does not mean they will be suicidal next week, or even tomorrow. We are not "Pollyannas": doing SST requires acknowledging what is really happening *right now*.

Q: Why would you *want* to see someone for just one session? Now, I can understand that this may be necessary at some settings or under some circumstances, but is there any real reason(s) why it would be better to treat someone this way rather than perhaps seeing them over several sessions?

ROSENBAUM: My desire is not to see everyone for one session; my desire is to see everyone for one full moment, as long as that takes.

HOYT: Many (if not most) patients want the most parsimonious and least expensive treatment that will help. The "light touch" of a single visit may help renew the patient's self-respect for his or her own innate capacities. One visit may minimize fostering dependency. Sometimes "less would be more," as the architect Mies van der Rohe once said. Some therapists suffer with the suspense of "here today, gone tomorrow," while others enjoy the stimulation of new challenges. What is most important is that the patient's needs be served—the choice for therapy being a single session should ultimately rest with the patient, not the therapist or setting.

Q: How are we to make a living providing successful SST?

TALMON: When you recall that the majority of people with psychological problems never go to see a therapist, you may realize that there are many, many more people who can be helped by us. If being helped by a therapist is less expensive, more positive, and a safer experience than many of us were led to believe, then we are more likely to have our satisfied SST patients return for a checkup, another brief therapy, or even extended treatment sometime down the road—as well as referring many more patients to us.

Q: How did you become a brief therapist?

HOYT: I was born to be a brief therapist. My mother, a loving and wonderful woman bless her soul, was a major-league worrier. I often consoled her, and soon learned to do it quickly. When the story got old, I told her not to be such a worrier (my first second-order intervention) and began to find ways to enhance her self-understanding as well as to anticipate, outflank, and redirect her. This involved my whole family, including myself. My academic pedigree includes a Yale PhD, extended training with Whitaker, Horowitz, and the Gouldings, numerous long-term and short-term therapy courses and workshops, plus lots of side trips through various psychospiritual schools of enlightenment (est, Zen, the Sufis, Hasidic Masters, etc.), bodywork, and personal therapy. By temperament and attention span, I prefer the "action" and excitement of brief therapy. As staff psychologist and Director of Adult Services at a large HMO (Kaiser), my delight in new problems, stimulating contact and human experience is constantly aroused. Now, if I could only get my mother to stop worrying!

ROSENBAUM: Discovering the world of information theory and cybernetic epistemology, at first through Bateson's work, and attempting to find a career where I would not be actively causing harm to people or the environment, I decided to become a clinical psychologist. I attended Boston University's clinical psychology program because I wanted training in psychoanalytic psychotherapy. While very much influenced by the process orientation of psychodynamic work, I soon found, working in community mental health centers, that many clients had less fascination with examining process for process's sake and would leave therapy earlier than the books said was appropriate. Realizing my clients were interested in brief therapy, I thought it might be a good idea to accommodate them. I began by working within James Mann's model, and also began studying family systems therapy. I continued working in a combined brief dynamic/information theory/family systems model when studying with Mardi Horowitz at UCSF.

When I began working at Kaiser Permanente 10 years ago, it soon became clear that what seemed like brief therapy to me and most of my professors (e.g., a planned treatment of 12 to 30 visits) seemed interminably long to most of my clients. I began working more strategically and used more of Milton Erickson's methods. Over the last 10 years I have become more impressed that technique is more necessary to alleviate the anxiety of the therapist than the distress of the client; consistent with research findings, my clinical experience indicates that about the same percentage of clients improves regardless of what techniques from whichever theoretical school of psychotherapy are employed. So my major professional affiliation now is with the Society for the Exploration of Psychotherapy Integration.

But why brief therapy? My Zen practice teaches me that brief and long are illusions, mere concepts. To quote Zen Master Dogen: "The way the self arrays itself is the form of the entire world. See each thing in this entire world as a moment of time. . . . Thus the self setting itself out in array sees itself. This is the understanding that the self is time. . . . Each moment is all being, is the entire world. Reflect now whether any being or any world is left out of the present moment."

TALMON: One becomes a brief therapist if and when one treats people from all walks of life and does not limit his or her practice to treating other mental health professionals or highly sensitive, articulate, and psychologically minded people (preferably with sufficient financial resources). I don't see myself as a brief therapist per se. I try to provide appropriate and necessary treatments that meet patients within their worldview and available resources. We pretend in the last 10 years as if we have discovered brief therapy. As far as I am concerned, therapy was and is likely to continue to be (on the average) a very brief process (ranging from three to seven sessions with the mode being a single session). This was true long before we wrote books about it. Ancient healers treated many of their fellow men in a single healing ritual. Let therapy last the required length with more respect to our available resources and our patients' needs and choices. Our pocket, our egos, or our pet theories should be secondary.

ACKNOWLEDGMENT

Support for this project was partially provided by the Sidney Garfield Memorial Fund (Michael F. Hoyt, principal investigator), administered by the Kaiser Foundation Research Institute. The opinions reported here are those of the authors and do not necessarily reflect any policies of Kaiser-Permanente.

NOTES

1. A treatment may be one session in length by one of three ways: (1) patient stops but therapist wants to continue; (2) therapist stops but patient wants to continue; (3) mutual agreement of patient and therapist to stop. We designate our approach "planned SST" to emphasize that the treatment is brief by design. Our intention is that both parties, patient and therapist, be mutually satisfied and come away feeling that the one session has been useful and sufficient.

2. A related idea about readiness comes from Alexander's concept of the "corrective emotional experience" (Alexander & French, 1946, pp. 66–70; Marohn & Wolf, 1990). Alexander cited the classic example, from Victor Hugo's Les Misérables, of the convicted thief, Jean Valjean, who stole from the bishop who befriended him. As may be recalled, when the bishop forgave him, Valjean had a conversion experience, apparently transforming from sinner to saint. To understand this apparent "SST," we need to consider two items that Alexander does not mention. First, we should recognize why Valjean was in prison in the first place: for stealing bread to feed a hungry child. Second, later in the story Valjean himself offers unexpected forgiveness to the sadistic Javert, who has been his jailor and persecutor. Rather than triggering another happy conversion, Javert commits suicide by throwing himself from a bridge. Why does one kind act succeed while the other doesn't? The story is fictional and such motivations are usually multidetermined, but an important key might be the existence of underlying cognitive schemata. Brief therapy is more likely to produce dramatic shifts if favorable latent mental images are already in place, waiting (ready) to be reevoked. The bishop's kindness toward Valjean (a "good thief" who had stolen to feed a child) reminded him of his own goodness, whereas kindness toward Javert only met a hard heart and evoked more shame and rage. The experience might only be "corrective" if the recipient is open (ready) for healing. (A somewhat different analysis of Valjean's dramatic change has been offered by Andrews, 1991, pp. 222–229. He emphasizes the importance of the bishop's disconfirming Valjean's expectations, as we do, but Andrews sees Valjean's transformation as the "evocation of new responses" rather than a "reevocation" of an earlier and more positive latent or repressed self.)

3. This conveys the essence of getting started in an SST, not necessarily the exact wording. The key is to convey the belief that change can occur immediately (indeed, is inevitable), and that the patient has the power to seize the moment and make a difference. Technical nuances abound. With one

patient the therapist might say, "Let's get right to work so that we can figure out a helpful solution"; with another patient it was helpful to remark, "So, it's finally gotten bad enough that you're going to do something to get rid of this. You're ready to deal with it" (Hoyt & Talmon, 1990, p. 81). Other patients might like to think about what they want to "learn" or "create," avoiding the word "change" with its implication that something is wrong or bad.

4. A follow-up phone call seems to have a further therapeutic effect with many patients, as well as providing useful information for the therapist. Some patients remark that they feel remembered and cared about, and many are pleased to review and recount their strengths and successes. Knowing that a follow-up call will be coming may also promote internalization of the therapist and the SST work.

5. The patient and case material have been disguised to protect confidentiality. Aspects of this case and a family therapy case are dramatized in the professional training videotape, *Single-Session Therapy*, by Talmon, Rosenbaum, Hoyt, and Short (1990). Numerous additional clinical examples can be found in the book *Single-Session Therapy: Maximizing the Effect of the First (and Often Only) Therapeutic Encounter* (Talmon, 1990) and in chapters by Hoyt (1990, in press), Rosenbaum (1990, in press), and Rosenbaum, Hoyt, and Talmon (1990).

6. Because this was a research project, the follow-up interview was conducted by a clinicin (Hoyt) other than the treating therapist, to avoid biasing the patient's report. However, in normal clinical practice, it is often useful for the therapist to make the follow-up call.

REFERENCES

Alexander, F., & French, T. M. (1946). *Psychoanalytic therapy*. New York: Ronald Press.

Andrews, J. D. W. (1991). *The active self in psychotherapy: An integration of therapeutic styles*. Boston: Allyn and Bacon.

Austad, C. S., & Berman, W. (1991). (Eds.). *Psychotherapy in managed health care: The optimal use of time and resources*. Washington, DC: American Psychological Association.

Austad, C. S., & Hoyt, M. F. (1992). The managed care movement and the future of psychotherapy. *Psychotherapy, 29*, 109–118.

Baekeland, F., & Lundwall, L. (1975). Dropping out of treatment: A critical review. *Psychological Bulletin, 82*, 738–783.

Barber, J. (1990). Miracle cures? Therapeutic consequences of clinical demonstrations. In J. K. Zeig & S. G. Gilligan (Eds.), *Brief therapy: Myths, methods, and metaphors* (pp. 437–442). New York: Brunner/Mazel.

Bloom, B. L. (1981). Focused single-session therapy: Initial development and evaluation. In S. H. Budman (Ed.), *Forms of brief therapy* (pp. 167–216). New York: Guilford Press.

Brehm, J. W. (1966). *A theory of psychological reactance*. New York: Appleton-Century-Crofts.

Breuer, J., & Freud, S. (1955). Studies in hysteria. In *The Standard Edition of the Complete Psychological Works of Sigmund Freud* (Vol. 2). London: Hogarth Press.

Budman, S. H., & Gurman, A. S. (1988). *Theory and practice of brief therapy.* New York: Guilford Press.

Cummings, N. A. (1990). Brief intermittent psychotherapy throughout the life cycle. In J. K. Zeig & S. G. Gilligan (Eds.), *Brief therapy: Myths, methods, and metaphors* (pp. 169–184). New York: Brunner/Mazel.

Cummings, N. A., & Follette, W. T. (1976). Brief therapy and medical utilization. In H. Dorken (Ed.), *The professional psychologist today.* San Francisco: Jossey-Bass.

de Shazer, S. (1985). *Keys to solution in brief therapy.* New York: W. W. Norton.

Follette, W. T., & Cummings, N. A. (1967). Psychiatric services and medical utilization in a prepaid health care setting. *Medical Care, 5,* 25–35.

Frances, A., & Clarkin, J. F. (1981). No treatment as the prescription of choice. *Archives of General Psychiatry, 38,* 542–545.

Goulding, M. M., & Goulding, R. L. (1979). *Changing lives through redecision therapy.* New York: Brunner/Mazel.

Gustafson, J. P. (1986). *The complex secret of brief psychotherapy.* New York: W. W. Norton.

Haley, J. (1973). *Uncommon therapy: The psychiatric techniques of Milton Erickson, M.D.* New York: Ballantine Books.

Haley, J. (1977). *Problem-solving therapy.* San Francisco: Jossey-Bass.

Hoyt, M. F. (1985). Therapist resistances to short-term dynamic psychotherapy. *Journal of the American Academy of Psychoanalysis, 13,* 93–112.

Hoyt, M. F. (1990). On time in brief therapy. In R. A. Wells & V. J. Giannetti (Eds.), *Handbook of the brief psychotherapies* (pp. 115–143). New York: Plenum Press.

Hoyt, M. F. (in press). Two cases of brief therapy in an HMO. In R. A. Wells & V. J. Giannetti (Eds.), *Casebook of the brief psychotherapies.* New York: Plenum Press.

Hoyt, M. F., & Austad, C. S. (1992). Psychotherapy in a staff-model HMO: Providing and assuring quality care in the future. *Psychotherapy, 29,* 119–129.

Hoyt, M. F., & Talmon, M. (1990). Single-session therapy in action: A case example. In M. Talmon, (Ed.), *Single-session therapy* (pp. 78–96). San Francisco: Jossey-Bass.

Lazarus, A. A. (1971). *Behavior therapy and beyond.* New York: McGraw-Hill.

Malan, D., Heath, E., Bacal, H., & Balfour, F. (1975). Psychodynamic changes in untreated neurotic patients. II: Apparently genuine improvements. *Archives of General Psychiatry, 32,* 110–126.

Margulies, A., & Havens, L. L. (1981). The initial encounter: What to do first? *American Journal of Psychiatry, 138,* 421–428.

Marohn, R. C., & Wolf, E. S. (Eds.). (1990). The "corrective emotional experience" revisited [entire issue]. *Psychoanalytic Inquiry, 10*(3).

O'Hanlon, W. H., & Weiner-Davis, M. (1988). *In search of solutions: A new direction in psychotherapy.* New York: W. W. Norton.

Rockwell, W. J. K., & Pinkerton, R. S. (1982). Single-session psychotherapy. *American Journal of Psychotherapy, 36,* 32–40.

Rosenbaum, R. (April, 1989). *Music and mind: Forms of stability, change, and integration.* Paper presented at the symposium, "The Lively Arts and Psychotherapy Integration," Fifth Annual Conference of the Society for the Exploration of Psychotherapy Integration, Berkeley, CA.

Rosenbaum, R. (1990). Strategic psychotherapy. In R. A. Wells & V. J. Giannetti (Eds.), *Handbook of the brief psychotherapies* (pp. 351–403). New York: Plenum Press.

Rosenbaum, R. (in press). Strategic single-session hypnotherapy. In R. A. Wells & V. J. Giannetti (Eds.), *Casebook of the brief psychotherapies.* New York: Plenum Press.

Rosenbaum, R., Hoyt, M. F., & Talmon, M. (1990). The challenge of single-session therapies: Creating pivotal moments. In R. A. Wells & V. J. Giannetti (Eds.), *Handbook of the brief psychotherapies* (pp. 165–189). New York: Plenum Press.

Sifneos, P. E. (1987). *Short-term dynamic psychotherapy: Evaluation and technique.* (2nd ed.) New York: Plenum Press.

Spoerl. O. H. (1975). Single-session psychotherapy. *Diseases of the Nervous System, 36,* 283–285.

Talmon, M. (1990). *Single-session therapy: Maximizing the effect of the first (and often only) therapeutic encounter.* San Francisco: Jossey-Bass.

Talmon, M., Hoyt, M. F., & Rosenbaum, R. (1990). Effective single-session therapy: Step-by-step guidelines. In M. Talmon (Ed.), *Single-session therapy* (pp. 34–56). San Francisco: Jossey-Bass.

Talmon, M., Rosenbaum, R., Hoyt, M. F., & Short, L. (1990). *Single-session therapy* [videotape]. Kansas City, MO: Golden Triad Films, Inc.

Whitaker. C. A. (December, 1990). *Symbolic experiential family therapy: Model and methodology.* Paper presented at The Evolution of Psychotherapy: A Conference. Anaheim, CA.

White, M., & Epston, D. (1990). *Narrative means to therapeutic ends.* New York: W. W. Norton.

Wile, D. B. (1984). Kohut, Kernberg, and accusatory interpretations. *Psychotherapy, 21,* 353–364.

Winnicott, D. W. (1958). *Through paediatrics to psychoanalysis.* New York: Basic Books.

Wolberg, L. R. (1965). The technic of short-term psychotherapy. In L. R. Wolberg (Ed.), *Short-term psychotherapy* (pp. 127–200). New York: Grune & Stratton.

CHAPTER 5

Time-Limited Dynamic Psychotherapy

STEPHEN F. BUTLER
HANS H. STRUPP
JEFFREY L. BINDER

Time-Limited Dynamic Psychotherapy (TLDP) was developed by Strupp and Binder (1984) as an approach to individual psychotherapy that emphasizes analysis of the patient–therapist relationship (transference) as the central task for the psychotherapist. TLDP is rooted in contemporary psychoanalytic conceptions (e.g., Gill, 1982; Sandler & Sandler, 1978: Schlesinger, 1982) and reformulations by interpersonal theorists (e.g., Harry Stack Sullivan, 1953; Anchin & Kiesler, 1982: Levenson, 1972). Empirical research (e.g., Strupp, 1980a, 1980b, 1980c, 1980d) suggests that major deterrents to the formation of a good working alliance are not only the patient's characterological distortions and maladaptive defenses but, equally important, the therapist's personal reactions to these difficulties. Thus, TLDP attempts to specify principles and strategies geared to the assessment and management of potential problems in the therapeutic relationship.

The interpersonal problems that emerge in treatment with the therapist are assumed to be similar in form to the chronic, maladaptive interpersonal patterns that underlie the patient's difficulties in living, sometimes expressed through symptoms such as anxiety and depression. In this view, the patient's resistances to the therapeutic work are seen as manifestations of his or her difficulties in establishing a meaningful, collaborative, and successful relationship with the therapist and are not fundamentally different from problems establishing satisfying relationships outside therapy. Transference, in our view, refers to the patient's tendency to reenact problematic interpersonal scenarios within the therapy. The therapist's task, then, consists of identifying the problematic interpersonal patterns that increasingly influence the therapeutic relationship and helping the patient to understand rather than repetitively act them out. Accordingly, therapeutic change is hypothesized to occur as a result of (1) the patient's developing *awareness* of his or her self-defeating patterns, and (2) his or her *experience* of a different outcome within the therapeutic relationship itself. In order to achieve this goal, the therapist uses the role of participant observer, both to participate, in an unavoidable yet limited extent, in the patient's problematic patterns and to reflect on and interpret the maladaptive scenario. Repeated efforts along these lines help the patient identify and correct the assumptions that underlie maladaptive interpersonal patterns. If the therapist remains unaware of his or her recruitment into reenacting the patient's "typical" scenario, the latter's interpersonal expectations are confirmed, and the maladaptive patterns become more deeply entrenched.

TECHNICAL INTERVENTIONS OF TLDP

TLDP emphasizes various technical considerations for examining the therapeutic relationship, understanding the role of countertransference, making interpretive links to current and past relationships, understanding the meaning of interpersonal behavior, and identifying and dealing with resistances. TLDP also outlines a procedure for selecting and organizing clinical material into an identifiable therapeutic focus. This procedure serves as a heuristic for defining a central, cyclical maladaptive pattern (CMP) (Schacht, Binder, & Strupp, 1984; Butler & Binder, 1987). The CMP is collaboratively developed by the patient and therapist and, therefore, should reflect concerns that have tangible meaning in the patient's current life.

Specifically, the CMP is a working model of a central or salient pattern of interpersonal roles in which patients unconsciously cast themselves and others. The focus characterizes the patient's maladaptive interaction sequences, self-defeating expectations, and negative self-appraisals. This focus organizes maladaptive patterns into a cycle consisting of (1) *Acts of Self*, which refers to actions of the self toward other people; (2) *Expectations of Others' Reactions*, which refers to the imagined reactions of others to one's own actions; (3) *Acts of Others Toward Self*, which refers to observed acts of others that are viewed as occurring in specific relation to the acts of self; and finally, (4) *Acts of Self Toward Self* (*Introject*), which refers to how one reacts or behaves toward oneself (self-controlling, self-punishing, self-congratulating, self-devaluing, etc.). These four categories are used to create a narrative description that characterizes the rigidity, chronic repetitiveness, and self-perpetuating nature of neurotic and characterological problems. The CMP is a particularly useful guide, not only for understanding the patient's maladaptive scenarios but also for anticipating the therapist's reciprocal (countertransference) reactions (Butler, Flasher, & Strupp, in press).

THE ROLE OF TIME LIMITS IN TLDP

Use of the term "time limit" in TLDP may be somewhat different from the other treatment approaches described in this volume. Thus, some explication of how the therapeutic time frame is conceptualized may be useful at this point. The TLDP therapist's attitude toward time reflects an attitude of realism and rationality. The emphasis rests squarely on the patient's current life, the manner in which he or she relates to significant others in the here and now, including the therapist, and the extent to which unresolved problems from the past exert a disturbing influence on present-day adaptation. By this reasoning, insight that fails to modify the patient's contemporary functioning is valueless. At the same time, the TLDP therapist recognizes that some forms of psychopathology are deeply ingrained and may require prolonged and skillful effort to achieve results. We understand as yet too little to make accurate predictions about the amount and kind of therapeutic work required for a given case. Some workers in the short-term area unfortunately continue to hold out the hope—which is avidly seized on by a public wishing for magical solutions—that time-limited therapy can offer unique and inexpensive solutions to the perennial problems facing psychotherapy. Our clinical experience and cumulative research tell us that this is improbable. The achievements of psychotherapy are usually commensurate with the amount and quality of therapeutic work, modulated by the nature and extent of the problems to which it is addressed.

The potential contribution of TLDP, as we see it, is to be found in its emphasis on sharpening the therapist's thinking and therapeutic practice. The TLDP therapist should have a clear sense of direction, and the dynamic focus forces the therapist to keep in mind a destination and a broad outline of the territory to be traversed. This should be the case whether the therapist is practicing time-limited or more prolonged therapy. In either event, the TLDP therapist does not "push" the patient, yet he or she firmly guides the course of therapy. TLDP fosters an image of the therapist as *actively* working, from the first session, to identify chronic, maladaptive interpersonal themes and *actively* monitoring the state of the therapeutic alliance, especially as problems in the alliance reflect maladaptive interpersonal patterns. In addition, the patient's defensive responses to the time frame of the treatment are treated as any other enactment of the CMP that chronically interferes with the patient's functioning.

Time, per se, is recognized as always a factor in any psychotherapy, often characterized as relevant to issues of separation–individuation (Mann, 1973; Hoyt, 1990). Avoidance of intimacy because the relationship "will soon be over anyway" is a common resistance around treatment termination. It should be remembered, however, that issues related to autonomy are equally likely to be played out around time concerns. Managing these resistances is no less difficult for the therapist than other time-related resistances. Who controls the time frame and who submits are fundamental negotiations in any relationship. Monitoring allusions to the transference for reactions to a predetermined time limit, if one exists, or an impending termination is of interest to the TLDP therapist because of what this tells the therapist about the patient's focal concerns—not because it is the therapist's agenda to achieve a rapid cure. Movement ahead in therapy is always encouraged, with a sense of hope and optimism for the future. However, the TLDP therapist is also aware that the best of intentions, unchecked, can run headlong into a countertransference impasse. Time issues can be as easily overemphasized as underemphasized.

In the case described below, a time limit of 25 sessions has been stipulated by the research project. In another setting, such a time limit might be set by insurance coverage or limits imposed by the clinic. These limits are treated as real-life issues not fundamentally different from other "givens," such as the quality of parenting the patient received, whether the patient is rich or poor, attractive or plain, or whatever "limits" emerge as justifying and maintaining a maladaptive interpersonal stance. In the early sessions, the therapist might or might not make explicit reference to the time limit. This typically depends on the nature of the concerns expressed by the patient, usually as allusions to the transference. The therapist's main task is to develop the CMP, regardless of the manifest material with which it emerges.[1] As termination approaches, the issue of time limits typically emerges in the patient's allusions. His or her concerns are, thus, explored within the context of the salient maladaptive patterns that have been the focus of work throughout treatment.

CASE ILLUSTRATION

The remainder of this chapter is devoted to a case presentation illustrating some central principles and strategies of TLDP in the early stages of an outpatient therapy.

The patient, whom we will call Lynn, was a 37-year-old white married female who responded to an announcement for low-cost psychotherapy at the Vanderbilt Center for Psychotherapy Research Clinic. Lynn was seen by an interviewer who conducted the Structured Clinical Interview for DSM-III (SCID) (Spitzer, Williams, & Gibbon, 1987). She met criteria for Major Depression and Dysthymia. She also met criteria for Axis II diagnoses of Avoidant Personality, Dependent Personality, and Paranoid Personality. After pretesting, she was assigned for therapy to a senior clinician (SFB) who knew only her sex, age, and diagnoses. The following discussion is based on videotaped sessions with the therapist.

The First Session

In a "typical" first session in TLDP, the clinician begins by obtaining a history of presenting complaints, including symptoms and precipitating event(s) that led the patient to seek treatment at this time. The TLDP therapist listens carefully for and inquires directly about the interpersonal context in which the symptoms appear, thus beginning the process of developing a dynamic focus. While this is an important early task in TLDP, like all technical interventions, it is subordinate to the therapist's clinical judgment regarding the patient's emotional state and expectations at the moment. This point cannot be overemphasized and is substantiated by psychotherapy research, which consistently reveals the importance of the quality of the patient–therapist bond (e.g., Orlinsky & Howard, 1986). This therapeutic bond far outweighs specific interventions, length, or type of therapy. In practice, this quality of the relationship is often based on the patient's feeling of being listened to and understood. This, above all else, impresses us as the essence of therapy, and the effectiveness of any dynamic therapist, brief or otherwise, is ultimately limited by his or her ability to establish this connection with the patient.

Lynn's first session exemplified this fundamental rule. The therapist determined, in the first few minutes of interaction, that she needed to tell her story. What she needed at that moment was someone to listen to this story. She reported being depressed for most of her life, but especially so for the last 8 months. She related this exacerbation of her depression to an event that occurred just prior to her recent move to Nashville. She had discovered that her husband of 16 years was having an affair with a coworker. As the patient could no longer ignore the mounting evidence of the affair, she confronted him, and he acknowledged that he was in love with another married woman and no longer loved his wife. Eventually, he decided to give up the girl friend (or she decided to give him up—it was never clear), and the family moved to Nashville where he had secured employment.

The patient sought treatment at the Center because of the low fee. She described herself as very depressed, feeling blue, and preoccupied with the idea that her husband was a "time bomb," despite the fact that things seemed alright between them now. There had been previous times when he had told her that he no longer loved her. The patient had been in therapy several times, which she described vaguely as "helpful."

The Second Session

During the second session, the patient's presentation was more relaxed and the therapist and patient spent much time discussing old and recent history. The therapist listened for consistent themes in the patient material, using the categories of the CMP to actively explore and flesh out the patterns. Toward the end of this session, the therapist tentatively presented the emerging CMP by noting that the patient seemed to expect to be abused by important people, such as her father, previous boyfriends, and her husband. She seemed to feel resigned to abuse, because if she protested, she risked losing relationships that were experienced as essential to her well-being. In addition, an excessive lack of confidence in her own resources made loss of these relationships intolerable.

The therapist could have related these patterns to the therapeutic relationship. Indeed, it is not uncommon for an exploration of the patient's reaction to the therapist to occur within the first session (see, e.g., Butler & Binder, 1987). However, as with any intervention, the therapist must judge when the introduction of a certain line of inquiry will make sense to the patient. Premature or out-of-context references to the therapeutic relationship may do more harm than good (Butler & Strupp, 1989). In this therapy, it was during the third session that material emerged that illustrates most clearly how a TLDP therapist might work to develop the CMP and its connection with the therapeutic relationship early in treatment.

The Third Session

As the patient and therapist enter the room, the patient is making some small talk:

Lynn: I really wasn't real sure about today. I believe this is the right day. . . .

Therapist: You weren't sure?

L: I had one of those feelings that I might be wrong. I didn't write it down, and if I don't write something down, it's not much good to me. (*chuckle*)

In TLDP, detecting subtle reactions to the therapy and the therapist requires special attention to initial, supposedly off-the-record comments. The therapist suspects that such comments might reflect some ambivalence about coming to therapy.

T: How do you feel about coming today?

L: I need to come every day.

T: Every day?

L: Yeah. (*chuckle*)

T: What do you mean?

L: It gets me through the week.

T: How does it get you through the week? How do you mean that?

L: I don't know. Maybe I just come and unload, and go on.

T: You mean, talking about what's been going on?

L: Yeah, 'cause I don't have anybody, that I would be willing to talk to. So, it does help.

T: When you don't come here, then you just have to sit on all this yourself?

P: Yeah, I do. Nobody wants to hear it . . . I wouldn't swap places with you for anything. (*chuckle*)

Clearly, embedded in the small talk regarding her appointment are important messages about the evolving relationship with the therapist as well as underlying interpersonal assumptions about herself and others. Thus, a picture begins to emerge regarding a perception of her needs as too great to be fulfilled (i.e., wanting to come every day). To talk with someone is to "unload," suggesting that she somehow burdens those whom she feels she needs. At the same time, her comments reveal expectations of others (including the therapist) as unwilling or uninterested in meeting those needs.

T: Why? Why do you say that, Lynn?

L: I think it would be depressing to listen to people's problems and hear the worst side of everybody. I wouldn't like it, it would bother me.

This might be her way of saying, "I am afraid that you will see me as a burden." The therapist then provides an opening to discuss her hopes and fears about the therapist directly.

T: When you talk with me, do you have some sense of how I react?

L: Not really. I haven't seen any reaction (*chuckle*) at all. Sometimes I go out and think, "Why did I say that? He must think I'm a nut." Most of the time, it just doesn't seem to matter.

T: What doesn't matter?

L: How you feel about it.

T: How do you mean that?

L: Sometimes it bothers me when I'm talking to a friend and I don't get a response, but I don't really expect you to respond. I've had therapists before, and I know they don't respond much.

Prompted by the therapist's questioning, she goes on to describe how she restricts her expectations of the therapeutic relationship. That is, therapists will not tell her what they think, and they probably think that she does not handle "life's problems" well.

T: It sounds like you like to come in and talk, and there's something about coming here that is good. But you see me as kind of distant and sort of uninvolved.

L: Yeah.

The theme developing here is that she "sometimes" fears the therapist will believe something bad about her because of what she discloses about herself. Thus, intimacy is threatening, and her expectations of the other (in this case the therapist) are that he will be withholding and uninvolved. At this point, the therapist makes a decision to explore these patterns in other relationships in the patient's life. This can be useful in providing the patient with a rationale for examining the therapeutic relationship. However, the therapist misses here an opportunity to explore the patient's assumptions about his view of her as defective and about him as uncaring and uninvolved.

T: Is that true with your husband too?

L: Yeah. (*chuckle*)

T: It sounds like you are thinking of something.

L: Well, I'm afraid to say what I think with him. I try to keep peace. Like he says, he wants a real laid-back (*chuckle*) person, and I try to be what he wants me to be. For Christmas I gave him some cologne. He wouldn't wear it to work. I knew he liked it. But, then this thought came in my mind: He wore Giorgio when he was going with this girl in [city name]. And he just stopped as soon as she stopped [seeing him] and has not worn it since. And I thought, "Why don't you ask him why he didn't wear the Giorgio?" But I'm afraid to ask him.

T: The problem with those kind of questions or expressing your concerns about stuff is that it could upset the balance?

L: Yeah. He says he never thinks about this girl unless I bring her up. I would like for him never to think about her as long as he lives, so I don't ask questions that I would love to ask. There's a lot of things that have come up that I've wondered about that I'm not allowed to ask. . . . I always go along with the rules. Sometimes I get real upset, and I just have to be bad (*chuckle*) and ask questions. Then I feel guilty for asking him.

Here it becomes clear that it is her responsibility to keep the peace, to maintain the balance, despite the fact that she was the one who was wronged by the affair. The man sets the rules, she abides by them, or fails to and is responsible if he feels bored, angry, or burdened. At the same time, her passivity conceals a strong desire to control her husband, even his thoughts. Perhaps she can achieve this control if she can only follow the rules he sets down. She further elaborates on this theme in a discussion about her father, who beat her with a whip when she was a child.

L: I must be a lot like him if I don't like him, cause I don't like myself very well either. (*Chuckle*) I don't like myself not liking him. I would like to like him, but I don't. I don't like his jokes, I don't like him ignoring people, I don't like the way he treats my furniture (*chuckle*) when he's visiting. I don't like him. (7-second pause) He's kind of boring to me. (*chuckle*)

T: You keep wincing when you say these things.

Observations about the subtle aspects of a patient's behavior in the here and now are critically important.[2]

L: Whew, I'd hate for him to know that.

T: Yeah? What would happen if he knew it?

L: I think it would hurt his feelings.

T: You're afraid to hurt his feelings?

L: Well, I care about him. I don't want to hurt him. But I just really don't want to be around him, either. I don't want to offend him, although he's real offensive. He'll put his feet on my coffee table. I don't like that.

T: You don't say anything?

L: I'm scared of—him. He would say something real sarcastic, or he would make me wish that I had ignored the feet on my coffee table.

It's better just to let Daddy do what Daddy wants to do. Keep peace and—

T: Sounds like you've heard that somewhere: Let Daddy do what Daddy wants to do?

L: My mother always taught me to not say anything back to Daddy.

T: Somehow, if there are difficulties either with your parents or with your husband, the message is to ignore that. If you were to not go along with that rule, that's somehow dangerous. Things can get worse.

L: Yeah, that's it. You bring it on yourself unless you just go with the flow.

T: Anytime you express yourself, especially anything critical or demanding, you cause trouble.

L: Yeah. Sometimes when I'm really down on myself, I feel like it was a lot of my responsibility.

A pattern is emerging that repeats itself with the important men in her life: She is hurt in some way by those she cares about, but she cannot protest strongly or directly without risking further hurt or abandonment. The implications for the therapeutic relationship are clear: she has already acknowledged the importance of the relationship to her, yet the very fact of that importance puts her at risk for abuse. The conflict is that she wants the relationship but at the same time, fears it.

Later, she risks expressing further grievances against her husband. The therapist notes the hint of emotion and gently draws her attention to it.

T: How do you feel now, as you start talking about [these things your husband has done]?

L: Mad. (*chuckle*) Mixed up.

T: You said "mad" at first.

The therapist reinforces the use of the stronger, more emotional word. This conveys his comfort with strong emotional words and a message that such feelings are acceptable.

L: Yeah, mad.

T: What's it like for you to be mad?

L: It's, uh, kind of agitating [sic] like. It's dangerous.

T: What are your thoughts about that?

L: If I get mad enough, I might do something to embarrass him. Like something that I would regret later.

T: So you've got to keep pretty close reins on that—on feeling angry—with him.

L: Yeah.

T: Is there anybody that you get angry with, that you feel like you can let them know when you're angry or when you're disappointed with them or upset with them?

L: I don't think so.

T: Do you get angry with yourself a lot?

L: Mm-hm.

T: What do you do when you're angry with yourself?

This is a direct inquiry about the patient's introject. The effort here is to focus on what she does to herself when she is angry. By framing the introject in terms of something she does, the therapist subtly fosters the idea that her reactions are due to something she does to herself, rather than something that happens to her (over which she has no control).

L: I do self-destructive things like eat a lot of food, or (*chuckle*) I deny myself certain privileges. (*chuckle*)

T: Does this make you uncomfortable to talk about it like this?

L: A little bit. It's sort of embarrassing. (*chuckle*)

T: What's embarrassing about it?

L: It sounds selfish to be thinking about yourself and talking about (*chuckle*) yourself. People don't like to hear that anyway.

Although deflected away from the here and now, this is another reference to concerns about the therapist's reaction to her emotion. The therapist begins gently to explore the patient's assumption that he is bored or upset by her feelings by raising directly the issue with her. This also communicates that it is acceptable to discuss such feelings directly with the therapist.

T: [For three sessions] you've come in and told me things about yourself. Things that you've not told many other people. Then today, a couple of times, you've mentioned that people don't want to hear this stuff, or that you should not be talking about this. So, I wonder if it seems like I am bored, or if it seems like I don't really want to hear this stuff, or if I think that you should not be talking about this?

L: No, I think what makes the difference is that you are listening and you're trained to listen. To talk like this with other people, though, they're thinking, "Oh boy, this girl's got a real problem, she talks about herself all the time. She must feel real sorry for herself." But you're—trained to listen . . .

While the patient backs away from this "invitation" to acknowledge or work with negative feelings directed toward the therapist, she immediately goes on to provide some important evidence that he is on the right track.

L: . . . I had a therapist one time that went to sleep all the time. And I kept going back!

T: The therapist went to sleep—during your session?

L: She really went to sleep. Yeah. I never said anything to her, because I thought it was a thyroid problem. It bothered me when I was there, and I'd think, "I'm not going to come back. This woman's (*chuckle*) asleep." I don't know why I kept going back. I didn't want to tell her that I thought she was too (*chuckle*) sleepy to hear me.

T: You didn't want to hurt her feelings—or upset her.

L: Yeah.

T: You know, we talked last time about, I think you put it this way: that repeatedly, in different relationships, you get abused. That it is something you sort of allow to happen.

L: Yeah.

T: Partly, it seems like you allow that by sort of ignoring what's going on—I mean its kind of abusive, if you're being charged for a session and then the therapist goes to sleep on you.

L: Oh, yeah.

The therapist is aware that, despite his efforts, this statement carries negative or blaming connotations (that she allows the abuse) that could confirm her expectation that the therapist believes she is unworthy and to blame for her ills. As the TLDP model emphasizes, this kind of bind is commonplace in therapy and cannot be avoided. As previously stated, the therapist's task is not to avoid such entanglements but rather to remain as vigilant as possible to detect and explore such binds in terms of the CMP. While the therapist could have raised this issue, his response is to reinforce the collaborative nature of their exploration by asking:

T: Is that going too far?

L: No, I don't think so. 'Cause sometimes I would get angry about it. Just like I get angry about what I've let other people (*chuckle*) do. I think you're right.

Although it may be unlikely that this patient would actually reject the therapist's statements, her response suggests she is beginning to identify maladaptive behaviors across different relationships.

T: But a relationship is based on your not being too much of a burden.

L: I've always thought the ideal relationship would be to allow that person to do anything they wanted to and not let it bother you.

T: So ideally, you don't make any demands on anybody.

L: That's right.

T: You don't say, "I want you home, I want you to listen to me, I want you to get your feet off my coffee table."

L: Right. I want people to be real comfortable and real happy.

T: The problem is that it ends up bothering you, in spite of yourself.

L: Yeah, mm-hm, yeah.

T: And it does matter—

L: Yeah, it does.

Here, the therapist has helped her to see her style of trying to accommodate to difficult interpersonal situations by "trying not to care" and making no demands on the other, as she did earlier in the session with the therapist. Thus, by the third session, the therapist has (1) begun to develop an interpersonal or dynamic focus, (2) enlisted the patient as a collaborator in this endeavor, and (3) begun to present the focus in terms she can understand and acknowledge. Finally, (4) by moving back and forth between past, current, and therapeutic relationships, the therapist helps her build plausible connections between her relationship patterns.

THE CYCLICAL MALADAPTIVE PATTERN

In the course of therapy, the CMP developed with this patient revolved around her view of herself as an unworthy and guilty person who is totally responsible for the bad things that others have done to her in her life. Briefly, her Acts of Self were efforts to minimize the chances for abuse and abandonment by not being a burden, following the rules, and making no demands on the other. As she says, she tries to be what the other wants her to be. Her Expectations of Others were that others would be uninterested in her and see her as a burden and unworthy of their love and attention; they would be ready to abuse, neglect, or abandon her and would attribute the blame to her. Several Acts of Others were described in this session: her husband's affair and withdrawal of love, her father's indifference to her furniture, the indifference expressed by the therapist who fell asleep, and even the subtly blaming comment by the TLDP therapist (that she allows herself to be abused). These actions could all be construed as consistent with her expectations and as confirming her Introject: She must keep her needs and emotions (like getting angry) in check, suppress urges to make demands, tell herself that unmet needs do not matter, and punish herself with guilt and depression as the penalty for having unacceptable needs. Thus, the Introject completes the cycle, leaving her to try harder to not be a burden, follow the rules, and make no demands.

ASSESSMENT OF OUTCOME

While not all technical aspects of TLDP can be exemplified in this chapter, it is useful to present an illustration of what therapeutic changes look like in this form of time-limited treatment. The following excerpt is taken from session 10.

L: I'm trying to change . . .

T: Okay. What are you doing that suggests to you that you are trying to change?

L: I'm doing things differently, trying to be a little bit more independent, making decisions, taking a little bit more control of what happens. Making things happen that I want to happen.

T: Can you give me an example of that?

L: Okay. Let's see. Well, I had a birthday last week, and I decided that my birthday was going to be remembered (*laugh*) this year. I've always tried to pretend like it didn't happen, because I always thought we didn't have the money to celebrate. So this time, I decided that I was making my child [her 8-year-old son] feel that I was not important by letting everybody ignore my birthday. So, I told him that it was going to be my birthday and that I wanted him to make me something. And then my husband . . . I usually say, "Don't give me anything." Well, I decided I would say, "Give me what you want me to have, and I don't care about how much it costs." (*laugh*).

On my birthday, he didn't have anything, because he worked the day before, so I said, "We'll spend the whole day celebrating. We'll go to the mall, and we'll eat out." So we went to the mall, and he started going into his record store, and I turned around and walked out. I said, "This is my birthday, this is going to be my day."

And he goes, "oh, Okay." He looked a little shocked. So we shopped, and he bought me a dress, and he said, "I'm taking you out to lunch." I decided I was making them think I was unimportant by always saying, "Don't get me anything."

At Valentine's day, I really took control. I got paid [for playing organ at church], and I said, "We're going out to eat." I decided I was going to take my entire check and blow it. I always wait [for someone else to decide where to eat], and then I'm usually disappointed. So I said, "I'm picking [the restaurant] this time." For me, that was major, because I never make a decision. I always wait for things to happen, and they usually don't. I felt more important and less like I was forgotten. I realized people were going to forget as long as you let them forget your birthday, Valentine's day, and things like that. They will usually forget it if you make it seem unimportant. You teach other people that it is unimportant.

T: So, part of what you're saying is that if you think of yourself as unimportant other people will too.

L: They usually do. My mother was the most humble person in the world. She would go out of her way to make sure nobody remembered her birthday. I'm trying to be different.

A few moments later she added:

L: My husband bought four books. One was, *Dating Your Mate*, one was *Romance Rekindled*, one was *Bedroom Language*, and one was *Falling in Love Again*. That really shocked me.

T: What do you make of that?

L: I think he is really making an effort to prove to me that he means it to be different now.

T: Why, why now?

L: Being able to tell you and to get mad, and being able to talk about it. I found that through getting mad and letting him know that I can get mad, and that I could also tell him, "Okay, I'm mad about this, but this is what I want now." That was the hardest part, getting mad and letting him know that I was mad. When I was able to do that, then it was easier to tell him the good things I wanted too.

T: Were you afraid that if you got mad, he would just say, "Forget it?"

L: Yeah.

T: So far, has he said that?

L: No.

T: It sounds like maybe, he's saying something else, that he is *more* interested.

L: Mm-hm. Yeah.

Such reports are expected as patients begin to make headway on both understanding their CMP and experiencing a different outcome of those maladaptive patterns in the therapeutic relationship (corrective emotional experience).

During the 25 sessions, the patient showed significant improvement in her depression and in her relationship with her husband and family members. However, as the termination approached, she increasingly expressed the feeling that the decision to end the therapeutic relationship was completely out of her control. This mirrored many other losses in her life, where she perceived the other person as in control. What also emerged was her plan to not bother the therapist with these fears, but instead to put up a front. In effect, the termination was viewed by the patient as meeting the therapist's needs rather than her own: The therapist was in control of the termination, and her only available response was to hide her feelings. At the same time, she was evidencing greater efforts at risk taking, along with an increased ability to assert herself. Thus, it was viewed as a good sign when she stated her desire to continue beyond the 25 sessions (i.e., she risked making a demand on the therapist). After consultation with a colleague (JLB), the therapist agreed to extend the treatment for 10 more sessions.[3] This compromise reflected the recognition in TLDP of time as a universal issue in psychotherapy, and at the same time permitted the patient to experience a greater sense of control over the ending of the relationship. These last 10 sessions focused specifically on impediments to termination, and the patient was encouraged to examine her tendency to see endings as terrible and as her fault.

At termination, the patient evidenced a 33-point increase on the Global Assessment Scale (GAS) (Endicott, Spitzer, Fleiss, & Cohen, 1976) as rated by an independent clinician, from 47 (serious symptoms, impairment in social, occupational, or school functioning) to 80 (if symptoms are present, they are only transient and expectable reactions to psychosocial stressors; no more than slight impairment in functioning). Two self-report instruments also showed improvement: the Beck Depression Inventory (Beck, Ward, Mendelson, Mock, & Erbaugh, 1961) dropped from 28 to 4, and the Global Severity Index of the Symptom Checklist 90-Revised (Derogatis, 1977) evidenced a 15-point drop from a T-score of 55 to 40.

SUMMARY

In this chapter we have attempted to achieve several objectives. First, we wanted to present a relatively clear demonstration of how a TLDP therapist might begin to develop an interpersonal focus and to work with that focus early in therapy, both within the therapeutic relationship and outside relationships. Second, the vignette illustrates that the therapist cannot avoid reenacting the patient's maladaptive interpersonal scenarios. The object is not to avoid completely being drawn into these scenarios but to maintain a vigilant stance with respect to the state of the relationship so as to minimize inevitable reenactments and use them to therapeutic effect. The final objective was to depict how TLDP combines dynamic and interpersonal principles, the concept of focused therapy, and a time-limited format to achieve circumscribed but clinically important goals with a significantly disturbed patient.

In any TLDP therapy, the therapist adopts a time-limited attitude which fosters active exploration of the patient's experience of herself and her interactions with significant others, including the therapist. In this way, the therapist helps the patient understand her maladaptive interpersonal patterns. The essence of psychotherapeutic change, however, is not merely the patient's comprehension of abstract "patterns." Rather, the therapeutic process must promote an *experience* of more adaptive relating within the therapeutic relationship itself. It is this experience, sometimes called "corrective emotional experience" (Alexander & French, 1946; Strupp & Binder, 1984), that creates the conditions for interpersonal learning and therapeutic change.

EDITORS' QUESTIONS

Q: How would you briefly distinguish your TLDP approach from other forms of short-term psychodynamic psychotherapy?

A: TLDP incorporates relevant concepts and principles of contemporary psychoanalytic psychotherapy, ego psychology, object relations theory, interpersonal theory, and systems theory. In developing TLDP, a concerted effort was made to stay close to clinical and observational data, avoiding higher-level inferences and complex theoretical constructs. The overarching aim was to develop an approach that is practical, effective, and teachable.

TLDP attempts to treat chronic interpersonal difficulties by defining them as the focus of the therapeutic work (cf. Anchin & Kiesler,

1982). The basic principles and procedures defining TLDP as a distinctive form of time-limited treatment may be summarized as follows:

1. TLDP formulates problems and conflicts in terms of specific patterns of recurrent transactional behavior. Therapists pay systematic attention to salient maladaptive relationship predispositions defined in interpersonal terms (CMPs).
2. There is an emphasis on early and rapid identification and examination of the enactment of these predispositions in the therapeutic relationship.
3. Therapists are taught to examine and confront the patient's attitudes and behaviors ("resistances") that interfere with the formation of a collaborative therapeutic relationship and open communication. Similarly, therapists are instructed to use their own reactions ("countertransference") as potential sources of interpersonal diagnostic information.
4. The time-limited nature of the therapy calls for examination of the patient's reactions to termination, particularly as these reactions reflect how the patient construes termination in terms of the CMP. However, a concrete limit to treatment duration is not required. Rather in TLDP, time limitations refer primarily to an attitude on the therapist's part that involves a disciplined, active, and focused effort directed toward maximizing the efficient use of available time and immediately addressing obstacles to therapeutic progress that arise within the patient–therapist relationship.

Q: Does the patient's style of functioning or "personality" change? Is this a typical goal for TLDP?

A: By emphasizing the patient's patterns of relating to others, TLDP, virtually by definition, addresses the personality of the patient. As a CMP is worked through, one expects the patient to behave more adaptively and to avoid repetition of the CMP both in therapy and in the patient's external life. In this sense, personality change is expected to occur. It is our belief that for some patients extensive personality change can occur in a relatively brief period of time, but certainly not for all patients.

Q: What do you usually tell patients about the course and prognosis of treatment? Do you give patients any instructions about their role or how to "do" therapy?

A: It is important to socialize patients to the tasks of psychotherapy by explaining in simple language its *modus operandi*, the roles to be played by patient and therapist, and the kinds of changes that may be expected from TLDP. Such explanations should be realistic and down-to-earth. The therapist should maintain a cautiously optimistic attitude, but the future cannot be predicted.

Q: What if a patient seems to be doing well quickly—will you still proceed for 25 visits? Why that number, what is the rationale for length of TLDP treatment?

A: Ideally, patient and therapist should mutually agree on the best time of termination. The patient is, of course, free to terminate at any time, and there is nothing "magical" about a contract of 25 weekly sessions. At the end of 25 sessions patient and therapist may agree on another 25-hour block or a smaller number of sessions. We recognize that many patients do not desire long-term or intensive psychotherapy. If a time limit is set, it can be a calendar date rather than a specific number of sessions. As previously discussed, our position regarding time limits is that the therapist's attitude toward the use of time is crucial.

Q: For many community and HMO settings, 25 to 35 sessions would require a great deal of limited resources. How might the TLDP process be condensed to make it more useful for more patients and settings?

A: As stated, the 25-hour time limit represents merely a convenient rule of thumb. Many patients can benefit from a shorter course of therapy; however, whatever number is agreed on, patient and therapist should have realistic expectations. Being viewed as a growth process, the process of TLDP can usually not be expedited, but goals can be adjusted.

Q: In TLDP, do you ever assign homework; for example, in a case similar to the one presented, might you instruct the patient to ask people to do something for her? Do you ever use active strategies (such as directives outside the session)? Did you consider bringing the patient's husband in for conjoint work? Is such a strategy permissible in TLDP?

A: The TLDP therapist does not assign "homework" but rather works toward a better understanding of CMPs as they emerge in the patient–therapist interaction and other relationships. An important goal of TLDP is to help the patient achieve greater autonomy. We believe it best to avoid most forms of directiveness by the therapist. There are no rules against conjoint work; however, TLDP techniques and principles appear to be best suited to individual psychotherapy. In the present case example, the husband's reluctance to be involved in treatment (per the patient's report) limited the option of conjoint treatment. Since the husband routinely responded positively to the patient's efforts at greater self-assertion, the therapist chose not to push for a change in the therapeutic strategy.

Q: In the case presented, if the patient had not responded well, what are some of the issues you might have considered? How might you change your approach? Given her fitting the diagnosis of Major Depression, when might medication be involved?

A: TLDP has no prohibitions against pharmacotherapy. The TLDP therapist recognizes that the treatment of patients suffering, for example, from major depression may be significantly aided by antidepressant medication. If the TLDP therapist is a non-MD, collaboration with a knowledgeable psychiatrist is clearly indicated. Such collaboration may be suggested relatively early in treatment. When this course of action is indicated, no major changes seem to be called for in the psychotherapist's approach. The current case illustrates, however, that depressive symptomatology, not accompanied by serious suicidal concerns or debilitating neurovegetative signs, can be treated quite adequately with psychosocial interventions (i.e., without the potential side effects and other problems associated with taking powerful pharmacological agents).

Q: Are all or most patients suitable for TLDP? If not, what are the parameters?

A: Psychodynamic therapy of all kinds seems to work best with patients who are well motivated and have reasonable ego resources including prominently psychological-mindedness, that is, an ability to reflect on one's difficulties in psychological terms. In our experience, TLDP is most promising with patients who in the initial few sessions demonstrate the potential to view their unhappiness (in whatever symptomatic and/or behavioral form it takes) as the consequence of interpersonal conflict.

Q: How did you become a brief therapist?

BUTLER: My answer to this question must be that I do not identify myself as a "brief therapist" per se. My connection with time-limited psychotherapy began when I accepted an NIMH postdoctoral fellowship at the Vanderbilt Center for Psychotherapy Research under the direction of Hans H. Strupp. This group of researchers has for years emphasized scientific investigations of psychotherapy in order to achieve greater specificity of what the therapist should be doing or not doing in a session. Consistent with this approach, my professional goal has been to understand, empirically, what constitutes the skillful conduct of psychotherapy and to strive to achieve this ideal in clinical practice. The research with which I have been associated, as well as my clinical experience, invariably points to the importance of being consistently mindful of expected goals of treatment and how these goals relate to what is going on at the moment. It stands to reason, therefore, that the skillful therapist makes maximal use of the time available and minimizes time spent in directionless and tangential activity.

Despite a recognition of time as a crucial element in any psychotherapy, I do not particularly emphasize brevity. As with any potential countertransference issue, a therapist's overinvestment in brevity can result in therapeutic interventions that appeal to the needs of the therapist rather than address the needs of the patient. A healthy emphasis on maximizing use of therapeutic time can work to the benefit of our patients. Yet, as I view recent changes in the mental health care delivery system, I see the expectation growing that *all* therapy, regardless of context, should be exceedingly brief. While recognizing the potential influence of our own economic interests, those of us associated with brief therapy should work to ensure that scientific and clinical work on brief therapy are not misused by cynical economic interests to erode access to adequate treatment for our patients.

BINDER: My discovery of brief therapy was an act of necessity. In the early 1970s I was on the faculty of the University of Michigan Department of Psychiatry, and one of my responsibilities was to help institute a mental health service for medical school students and trainees. We had to respond rapidly and efficiently to service needs. My deepening involvement with brief therapy was an act of faith. I became acquainted with the works of the brief dynamic therapy pioneers (Balint, Ornstein, & Balint, 1972; Malan, 1976; Sifneos, 1972; Davanloo, 1980) and attended the first international symposium on brief dynamic therapy, held in Montreal in 1975. I was duly impressed with descriptions of their approaches and subsequently broadened my activities by developing a brief therapy outpatient clinic in Virginia and teaching brief dynamic therapy at the University of Virginia Department of Psychiatry. The evolution of my own approach to brief dynamic therapy resulted in part from witnessing successes and failures with brief therapy, my own as well as those of therapists whom I supervised. It also evolved from intensive empirical study of therapeutic processes and outcomes associated with this form of treatment. This most recent phase in my growth as a brief therapist has been the most rewarding because it has involved a long collaboration with Hans H. Strupp at the Vanderbilt Center for Psychotherapy Research. He taught me the importance of empirically scrutinizing the theoretical and clinical assumptions that influence our performance as therapists.

STRUPP: For almost 40 years I have been keenly interested in the problem of what constitutes psychotherapeutic change and how it is achieved. Indeed, this has been the *leitmotiv* of my career as a researcher, therapist, teacher, and consumer of psychotherapy. I became attracted to time-limited psychotherapy as a researcher who believes that significant change processes are amenable to intensive study and analysis in the shorter as well as the longer forms of therapy, and that they can be studied with considerably greater parsimony in time-limited forms. Although I remain convinced that significant therapeutic change, which I conceive of as a process of personality growth, usually requires substantial periods of time, I am also open to the idea that lasting therapeutic change can and does occur over shorter periods. With Harry Stack Sullivan I agree that we should avoid wasting time in therapy, which means that we should pursue relatively specific goals and remain focused on these goals. In the final analysis, my interest is riveted on *good* therapy, which in practice can occupy shorter or longer periods of time. In any event, I do not believe that, under ordinary circumstances, we can expect to accomplish as much in time-limited therapy as in the more extensive forms. Furthermore, the outcome of therapy is typically commensurate with the nature of the patient's problems and the participants' commitment to sustained work. Above all, we should not deceive ourselves—and our sponsors—that we can obtain stupendous results with minimal efforts. In the field of psychotherapy, no one should expect miracles.

ACKNOWLEDGMENTS

The authors would like to thank Dr. Herbert Demmin for his helpful comments on an earlier draft of this chapter. The work reflected in this chapter was supported, in part, by National Institute of Mental Health Research Grant MH-20369, Hans H. Strupp, principal investigator.

NOTES

1. To indicate the therapist's expectation of success in a brief amount of time as some authors endorse (e.g., Hoyt, 1990) is not a component of TLDP. The focus here is to determine the nature of the *patient's* expectations and his or her fantasies of what the therapist wants. For instance, it is more important to the TLDP therapist that the patient imagines that no one would want to spend much time listening to him or her. Thus, the therapist's enthusiasm for a rapid success might be secretly interpreted by the patient as confirmation that the therapist is bored and wishes this therapy were over.

2. Attending to the patient's subtle reactions in the here and now is intended to increase the patient's awareness of unstated and, perhaps, only dimly recognized feelings and thoughts. Although not explored in this vignette, such reactions often indicate the presence of thoughts and feelings the patient fears to share with another person. That is, one may be disgusted or shamed by particular thoughts or feelings, but to share these makes one vulnerable to the anticipated judgment of others (i.e., the therapist). Such judgments usually reflect an expected conclusion—for instance, that the patient is a disgusting, shameful person.

3. It should be pointed out that the complexity of such decisions renders no answer completely correct or without consequences. By acquiescing to her request, the therapist runs the risk of conveying the message that she truly is dependent on the therapist or therapy and thereby entrenching her dependency. Clearly, deciding whether or not to extend treatment is significant and deserves serious consideration. However, the therapist cannot avoid such dilemmas by making the "correct" decision or by blindly adhering to an arbitrary time frame. Rather, by seeking supervision, the therapist acknowledges the complexity of sorting out the transference–countertransference enactment. Regardless of the decision, the patient's interpretation of events must be explored and will certainly reflect the current state of her CMP.

REFERENCES

Alexander, F., & French, T. M. (1946). *Psychoanalytic therapy: Principles and applications.* New York: Ronald Press.

Anchin, J. C., & Kiesler, D. J. (1982). *Handbook of interpersonal psychotherapy.* New York: Pergamon Press.

Beck, A. T., Ward, C. H., Mendelson, M., Mock, J., & Erbaugh, J. (1961). An inventory for measuring depression. *Archives of General Psychiatry,* 4, 561–571.

Balint, M., Ornstein, P., & Balint, E. (1972). *Focal psychotherapy.* London: Tavistock.

Butler, S. F., & Binder, J. L. (1987). Cyclical psychodynamics and the triangle of insight: An integration. *Psychiatry,* 50, 218–231.

Butler, S. F., Flasher, L. V., & Strupp, H. H. (in press). Countertransference and qualities of the psychotherapist. In N.E. Miller, L. Luborsky, J. P. Barber, & J. Docherty, (Eds.), *Handbook of dynamic psychotherapy research and practice.* New York: Basic Books.

Butler, S. F., & Strupp, H. H. (1989, June). *Issues in training therapists to competency: The Vanderbilt experience.* Paper presented to the Society for Psychotherapy Research (SPR), Toronto, Ontario.

Davanloo, H. (Ed.). (1980). *Short-term dynamic psychotherapy.* New York: Jason Aronson.

Derogatis, L. R. (1977). *SCL-90: Administration, scoring, and procedures manual-I for the R(evised) version.* (Available from the author, Adolf Meyer Building,

Room 200, The Johns Hopkins Hospital, 600 N. Wolfe St., Baltimore, MD 21205).

Endicott, J., Spitzer, R. L., Fleiss, J. L., & Cohen, J. (1976). The Global Assessment Scale: A procedure for measuring overall severity of psychiatric disturbance. *Archives of General Psychiatry, 33,* 766–771.

Gill, M. M. (1982). *Analysis of the transference 1: Theory and technique.* New York: International Universities Press.

Hoyt, M. F. (1990). On time in brief therapy. In R. A. Wells & V. J. Giannetti (Eds.), *Handbook of the brief psychotherapies* (pp. 115–143). New York: Plenum Press.

Levenson, E. A. (1972). *The fallacy of understanding: An inquiry into the changing structure of psychoanalysis.* New York: Basic Books.

Malan, D. H. (1976). *The frontier of brief psychotherapy.* New York: Plenum Press.

Mann, J. (1973). *Time-limited psychotherapy.* New York: McGraw-Hill.

Orlinsky, D. E., & Howard, K. I. (1986). Process and outcome in psychotherapy. In S. L. Garfield & A. E. Bergin (Eds.), *Handbook of psychotherapy and behavior change* (3rd ed.) (pp. 311–381). New York: Wiley.

Sandler, J. & Sandler, A.M. (1978). On the development of object relationships and affects. *International Journal of Psychoanalysis, 59,* 285–296.

Schacht, T. E., Binder, J. L., & Strupp, H. H. (1984). The dynamic focus. In H. H. Strupp & J. L. Binder *Psychotherapy in a new key.* New York: Basic Books.

Schlesinger, H. (1982). Resistance as a process. In P. Wachtel (Ed.), *Resistance in psychodynamic and behavioral therapies.* New York: Plenum Press.

Sifneos, P. (1972). *Short-term psychotherapy and emotional crisis.* Cambridge, MA: Harvard University Press.

Spitzer, R. L., Williams, J. B. W., & Gibbon, M. (1987). *Structured Clinical Interview for DSM-III-R (SCID).* New York, New York State Psychiatric Institute, Biometrics Research.

Strupp, H. H. (1980a). Success and failure in time-limited psychotherapy: A systematic comparison of two cases—comparison 1. *Archives of General Psychiatry, 37,* 595–603.

Strupp, H. H. (1980b). Success and failure in time-limited psychotherapy: A systematic comparison of two cases—comparison 2. *Archives of General Psychiatry, 37,* 708–716.

Strupp, H. H. (1980c). Success and failure in time-limited psychotherapy: A systematic comparison of two cases—comparison 3. *Archives of General Psychiatry, 37,* 831–841.

Strupp, H. H. (1980d). Success and failure in time-limited psychotherapy: A systematic comparison of two cases—comparison 4. *Archives of General Psychiatry, 37,* 947–954.

Strupp, H. H., & Binder, J. (1984). *Psychotherapy in a new key: A guide to Time-Limited Dynamic Psychotherapy.* New York: Basic Books.

Sullivan, H. S. (1953). *The interpersonal theory of psychiatry.* New York: W. W. Norton.

A Time-Sensitive Model of Brief Therapy: The I-D-E Approach

SIMON H. BUDMAN
ALAN S. GURMAN

The interpersonal–developmental–existential (I-D-E) model of brief, "time-sensitive" psychotherapy was designed by us to be a broadly useful, practical approach that would take into account the great variety of patients seen in general outpatient therapy practices (Budman & Gurman, 1988). We consider our model time sensitive rather than brief per se because rather than taking place over a specific and circumscribed number of visits (e.g., less than 25), we emphasize the efficient and effective use of time.

Our definition of brief treatment differs considerably from the more common meaning given to the term. We have written elsewhere, "*What is, in fact, being examined in any discussion of brief treatment is therapy in which the time allotted to treatment is rationed*. The therapist hopes to help the patient achieve maximum benefit with the lowest investment of therapist time and patient cost, both financial and psychological" (Budman & Gurman, 1988, p. 5).

It is our belief that for some people time-sensitive/time-effective treatment may require a number of episodes of care spaced over an extended period of time. There are also cases of time-effective I-D-E therapy that may be interminable in that the patient may seek care at different periods for the rest of his or her life as the need arises (Budman, 1990; Cummings, 1986, 1990; Hoyt, 1990). [In this regard, Bennett (1983), describing a similar model of care, titled his paper

"Focal psychotherapy—terminable and interminable."] This form of intermittent, focused treatment over the life cycle may resemble the practice of family medicine as much as or more than it resembles traditional models of psychotherapeutic service delivery.

There are three essential elements of the I-D-E model. First, because it is oriented toward improvement rather than cure (while cure is rarely possible in psychotherapy, improvement is almost always possible), intermittent, focal courses of therapy are the preferred style of service delivery. Second, rather than emphasizing a specific set of techniques or fixed principles which are immutable, the I-D-E therapist maintains a set of *attitudes about change processes* in psychotherapy—these values then help to determine the ways in which the therapist will intervene. Table 6.1 presents a summary of the values we perceive to be pivotal in time-effective brief treatment and contrasts them with the values we view as being more associated with long-term, open-ended care. Relevant here, a recent study by Bolter, Levenson, and Alvarez (1990) surveyed over 200 psychologists using a measure that operationalized the contrasting values we propose. Their study, in general, confirmed that those who endorse brief treatment differ in their attitudes and values in many of the ways that we had hypothesized.

Finally, the model includes a variety of possible focal areas for treatment. Every model of brief therapy requires an area or areas of focus (Burlingame & Fuhriman, 1987; Hall, Arnold, & Crosby, 1990). Most limit the treatment focus to one discrete domain. The I-D-E model offers a variety of possibilities for selecting a focus and associated algorithms (recommendations) for treatment. The I-D-E foci subsume many of the possible areas of disruption for patients seeking care. The model, therefore, offers a flexible and broad array of possibilities for therapy. These treatment possibilities are unified by the nature of the model itself. That is:

> "The I-D-E approach in brief treatment is an attempt to capture and understand the core interpersonal life issues that are leading the patient to seek psychotherapy at a given moment in time, and to relate these issues to the patient's stage of life development and to his or her existential concerns. . . . The I-D-E approach is neither exclusively symptom-oriented nor exclusively intrapsychic or interpersonal." (Budman & Gurman, 1988, p. 27)

Figure 6.1 illustrates the five major areas of focus possible in an I-D-E brief treatment model. These foci are predicated on the central question, "Why now?" That is, why has the patient chosen to seek therapy at this point in life and at this particular time? Note that

TABLE 6.1 Comparative Dominant Values of the Long-Term and Short-Term Therapist

Long-term therapist	Short-term therapist
1. Seeks change in basic character	Prefers pragmatism, parsimony, and least radical intervention; does not believe in the notion of "cure"
2. Believes that significant change is unlikely in everyday life	Maintains an adult developmental perspective from which significant psychological change is viewed as inevitable
3. Sees presenting problems as reflecting more basic pathology	Emphasizes patient's strengths and resources
4. Wants to "be there" as patient makes significant changes	Accepts that many changes will occur "after therapy"
5. Sees therapy as having a "timeless" quality	Does not accept the timelessness of some models of therapy
6. Unconsciously recognizes the fiscal convenience of long-term patients	Fiscal issues often muted, either by the nature of the practice or the organizational structure
7. Views therapy as almost always benign and useful	Views therapy as sometimes useful and sometimes harmful
8. Sees therapy as being the most important part of the patient's life	Sees being in the world as more important than being in therapy
9. Views therapist as responsible only for treating a given patient	Views therapist as having responsibility for treatment of a population

we take very seriously the warning notice at the bottom of Figure 6.1. When the patient is actively alcohol or substance abusing, these issues *must* be considered simultaneously with or prior to any other focus being addressed.

Since the publication of *Theory and Practice of Brief Therapy* (Budman & Gurman, 1988), we have tried to amplify our model further and have incorporated a number of new elements. For example, we have further explored the issue of readiness for psychotherapy and have begun to employ a model of therapeutic readiness and change in treatment described by Prochaska and his colleagues (McConnaughy, Prochaska, & Velicer, 1983; McConnaughy, DiClemente, Prochaska, & Velicer, 1989; Prochaska & DiClemente, 1982, 1986). We have also been interested in the work of White and Epston (1990) on "reauthoring" and the personal narrative and have found elements of their thinking, as well as many of their techniques, to be quite useful and compatible with our model. A central aspect of our expanded model has been a growing interest on our part in Control Mastery Theory (Weiss & Sampson, 1986;

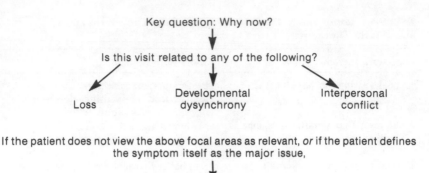

If the patient does not view the above focal areas as relevant, *or* if the patient defines the symptom itself as the major issue,

Symptomatic focus

If the patient has had repeated presentations around any or all of the foci above, without clear benefit, *or* if character issues preclude these foci because of constant interference with the therapeutic process,

Character focus

Warning: Under circumstances of active alcohol or drug abuse, this problem *must* be addressed before or simultaneously with the development of any other focal area.

FIGURE 6.1 Major foci in brief therapy. From *Theory and Practice of Brief Therapy* (p. 66) by S. H. Budman and A. S. Gurman 1988, New York: Guilford Press. Copyright 1988 by The Guilford Press. Reprinted by permission.

Engel & Ferguson, 1990). For purposes of this chapter, we briefly address only the issue of how we have incorporated Control Mastery into the I-D-E approach.

A NEW ELEMENT OF THE APPROACH: THE THERAPEUTIC RELATIONSHIP

All therapy takes place within the context of a therapeutic relationship. There are a variety of ways to understand and conceptualize this relationship. We have found Control Mastery Theory (Weiss & Sampson, 1986; Engel & Ferguson, 1990) to be an excellent way of thinking about the therapeutic relationship and to frame certain aspects of therapist–patient interactions:

> According to this model, patients come to therapy with the desire to master their conflicts and with a plan, which is often unconscious, for achieving mastery. The patient's plan may be thought of as a strategy for disconfirming pathogenic beliefs. . . . In testing a pathogenic belief, the patient carries out a trial action that is intended to provide information about that belief. (Silberschatz, Curtis, & Nathans, 1989, p. 41)

For example, a patient who came from a disorganized and chaotic family, in which there was little clarity regarding expected behaviors, might enter treatment and "test" (Weiss & Sampson, 1986) the therapist to see if the therapist will clearly elucidate and adhere to certain limits in the therapy. These tests might take the form of the patient's failing to come to sessions on time, "forgetting" to come to some meetings at all, or arriving intoxicated to a meeting. The therapist "passes" the test by being clear, firm, and direct about expectations and responsibilities in the treatment. On the other hand, if the therapist is circumspect about what is required of the patient and assumes that the patient is simply frightened or ambivalent about treatment and that pushing him or her "too hard" at this point in the therapy would not be useful, the therapist might then "fail" the test. There are also patients who manifest the same types of provocative behaviors but for whom it would not be useful to be very direct and firm. Such patients usually come from families in which one or both parents were often setting strict and arbitrary limits. Thus, identical behavior on the therapist's part might pass a test with one patient and fail a test with another. Control Mastery researchers have found that patients tend to make more progress in therapy when the clinician creates an atmosphere in which the patient feels safe because his or her pathogenic beliefs are being disconfirmed (Silberschatz, Curtis, & Nathans, 1989; Weiss & Sampson, 1986).

There are many aspects of the Control Mastery model that we have found to be useful in our work. However, for the reader to understand what was done in the case we are about to present, the brief overview provided should be sufficient. Control Mastery conceptualization is completely compatible with the I-D-E model and provides a frame for understanding the therapist's interactions with the patient. Within this interactional field, all aspects of the I-D-E approach may be applied. Control Mastery thinking offers an especially good fit with our I-D-E approach in its emphasis on the relational dimensions of therapy and on the therapist's need to be technically flexible and contextually relevant. The I-D-E approach is sensitive to a broad range of systemic cues and the patient's conscious and unconscious plans for achieving mastery of his or her symptoms and for testing the safety of the therapeutic encounter.

CASE ILLUSTRATION

(The therapist was Budman; commentary is by Gurman.)

Deirdre, a single 29-year-old woman, was referred to the mental health department of a large health maintenance organization because she had recently been plagued by severe panic attacks. These attacks were so severe that she had been unable to return to her job for the previous 3 weeks. The material presented below comes from her first therapy session. She had had a full physical exam a short time before her referral and there was no medical basis found for her complaint.

The First Session

Therapist: We spoke a little bit over the phone.

Deirdre: Yeah.

T: But maybe you could fill me in about what is going on for you.

D: Well, basically, what prompted me to call and seek some type of help was because starting probably the end of October, actually the beginning of November, one day I just went to work and I got this severe, really severe panic attack. You know, which sort of scared me. I mean at the time it was scary. So that was fine . . . I think I left work early or something.

T: Mm.

D: And, when I went back to work the next day the same thing happened and then I took some more time off and you know every time I went to work it just seemed to happen to me or I would get these panic attacks just walking down the street. So that's just basically it. (*Patient smiles.*) You know that's all I can tell you is that.

T: And it just came out of the blue?

D: Yeah, yeah. The severity of it came out of the blue . . . I mean I would have to admit that I probably am not the most confident person in the world. You know I've had varying degrees of this same thing happen to me before. You know? More severe, you know, at other times. I mean it's something I think that's probably been with me for 15 years.

An important question for the therapist to consider at this point is, "Why now?" If Deirdre has had similar symptoms in the past, some of which have been "more severe," why did she finally decide to seek treatment at this time? We have often heard, and ourselves engaged in, conversations about why people come to therapy. Different theoretical orientations emphasize different ideas about this fundamentally important question. We think that all, or nearly all, these ideas can be subsumed under three general categories of response: (1) "because the patient wants to change," (2) "because the patient doesn't want to change," (3) "because the patient has changed." Moreover, more than one of the above is usually true.

T: It was more severe in the past?

D: No, well, I did have one severe attack or bout of it, you know, a few, quite a few years back when I was in a totally different type of job. I was actually a caretaker in a house and I, it required that I spent a lot of time alone. I sort of built up this fear of going out at that time, you know, really just going out into the world.

T: So you wouldn't go out or you stopped going out?

D: Uh, I would go out when it was necessary, to cash a check or go to the bank or, a supermarket, but it would be, you know, feeling dread the entire time.

T: And how'd you get over that?

D: Time. You know, not actually, not really, not seeking any help. Which I don't think was the right thing.

T: It just got better?

D: Yeah. But after a long time. It got better but it was never explained (*sighs*). I mean I think it worried me but I just (*trails off*). I don't know maybe I just believed that it would get better.

T: How old are you now?

D: I'm, I'll be 30 in January.

Since this interview occurred in mid-December, the therapist is beginning to think about the possibility of a developmental focus for the treatment. The patient has had a similar problem in the past, but now, just prior to her thirtieth birthday, the problem is exacerbated and she chooses to seek treatment. The patient is then asked about her family and how they might relate to the current difficulty she is having.

D: Well, when I came here I was only 16 years old and basically I came out on a 6-week vacation with my mother because my brother was getting married and, uh, she brought me out here because she felt that I was going to elope with this guy that I was seeing at the time and he lived in Calgary. It's a long story (*smiles*).

T: So she was preventing you from being with him?

D: Yeah. Well, I, yeah (*laughs*). She more or less plucked me out of it, out of that situation and just you know, decided to bring me out here. Maybe it was her uh, design all along to you know, leave me here. But before the 6-week vacation was up she said, "Well, you know, what do you want to do? Do you want to go back? Back to a fairly miserable life." It was sort of miserable at the time.

T: And why was it miserable?

D: Because I was having a hard time at school and it had just become that way because I was seeing this guy and I guess my mother didn't like it and she had been in contact with the principal at my school. And, I had gotten kicked out of school for a week and there was just a lot of stuff . . .

T: So when you came to the United States [from Canada] with your mother at 16 she left you here?

D: Well, uh, I have a lot of family here. I suppose you were thinking, you were "zeroing in on" that word, "left me here." Basically, yeah, I was left.

T: Who did she leave you with?

D: Older brothers and sisters of which I have about you know, three to four elder brothers here and, you know, a couple of four or five older sisters at the time. I come from a large family.

T: How many people in your family?

D: Eleven kids.

T: Wow! That's a big family!

D: Yeah, outrageous. Too big!

T: And where are you in this, Deirdre?

D: Mm. I'm, let's see, there are four younger than me I think and that would make me, let me see, yeah, I'm number six from the from the oldest. Yeah that adds up doesn't it?

T: Can you tell me a little about your parents?

D: My father died . . . he died 5 years ago. Well he had a stroke about 9 or 10 years ago where he just progressively got worse. He never really recovered.

T: What kind of work did he do?

D: Not much (*laugh*). Well, he was a house painter most of his life but he didn't really do too much work anyway.

T: Why?

D: I don't know I . . .

T: Was he unable to work?

D: No.

T: Didn't want to work?

D: No. No, no he probably didn't want to work.

T: Was that a problem for your mother?

D: Yeah sure. Oh yeah, they had lots of problems (*laugh*).

T: She was angry with him?

D: I have everything.

T: You have everything?

D: No. I mean not everything. I don't mean I have everything. I have all of those things that you know, make a person seek out help.

T: Like what?

D: Well, my father was a drinker for one thing. You know, their relationship wasn't exactly right. There was no communications or anything.

The issue of substance abuse in the family has been raised and it is important that the therapist follow this up either now or at a later point in this session.

T: Do you drink or use drugs at all?

D: Mm (*clears throat*), yes I drink and I have been known to use drugs, also.

T: Uh, how much of each?

D: Mm, mm, not every day, but you know, if I start drinking I can drink more than moderately (*laughs*).

T: Do you get drunk fairly frequently?

D: Mm. No, no I wouldn't say that really. I would say if I if I start drinking at home or if I go out, yes, I mean I will drink more than two or three drinks, you know. I will get pretty sloshed.

T: How about Sam? [Boyfriend with whom she lives.]

D: He drinks, yes. Not, I wouldn't call him, he's not a heavy, heavy drinker or you know, mm, I mean neither of us drink excessively every day. You know, I'm not trying to make it sound like I like you know like we have a drinking problem. I don't think that's the way at all. I think we enjoy drinking.

T: Sounds like it could be by what you're saying.

D: Yeah, okay . . . Maybe you're right, actually. Maybe it is. I actually, lately, I've found that it hasn't been agreeing with me you know . . .

T: Mm.

D: If I uh, if I get drunk, I drink too much and I wake up the next morning with a hangover. You know, I feel terrible. You know I feel, just pretty, pretty goddamned awful . . . physically, I think, and emotionally . . .

T: Mm what kind of drugs do you use? Have you recently used?

D: Mm, coke.

T: Are you using coke now?

D: No.

T: When was the last time you used coke?

D: Mm, 3 or 4 days ago.

T: Three or 4 days?

D: Yeah.

T: And how much coke have you been using? Will you have?

D: Mm. Not a whole lot. Mm, I don't know. At the most we might split half a gram, you know, in one night.

T: Between you and Sam?

D: Or, or even less. I mean that's at the most even and at the height of our use it was probably about three times a week.

T: And how frequently have you been using it now?

D: Mm. Not too frequently. I've been making a conscious effort not to do it. I, you know, I've made a decision that I don't really . . . that it doesn't really agree with me. That I don't really care for its after-effects. So I will do maybe a smaller amount you know, uh, maybe once a week or something. This really is a realization which just started to happen to me over the last couple of weeks.

There now follows some discussion about other family members with drinking problems. It becomes clear that a number of Deirdre's sibs have had serious problems with substance abuse. Some are involved with Alcoholics Anonymous (AA) and some have been to detoxification facilities. It is clear to the therapist that regardless of what I-D-E focus is chosen, addressing substance abuse must also be part of the treatment.

The therapist then attempts to clarify how Deirdre is feeling about the session. Since the interaction is so important, it is often of value for the therapist to get some sense from the patient of how he or she is feeling in the interview. Deirdre describes herself as comfortable and surprised that she has been able to speak as much and as comfortably as she has. She also indicates that she has had no prior experience with therapy herself.

D: Yeah. I mean I've talked to therapists. I've known people in the profession. But Sam went through some therapy while he was going through a hard time some years ago. So he may have told me something about it. I mean he said that he went, he went to it as far as it was beneficial. But after the therapist started to tell him to do things that he really didn't feel was necessary that's when he decided well, you know, "Maybe I've had enough."

T: (*Smiling*) What if I tell you to do things that you don't think are necessary?

D: I'd have to wait and see (*laughs*).

T: All right, well I'll tell you the first thing that you won't think is necessary.

D: Which is?

T: Which is that I think that I'm probably not going to be able to do much for you while you're drinking and using drugs. It presents an absolute confusion of the situation. I can't tell how much has to do with the drugs and alcohol and how much has to do with other situations in your life. And I can do nothing about teasing those apart while you are using drugs and alcohol.

D: Mm.

T: And it may be a difficult thing for you to do . . .

D: Mm.

T: Not to.

D: Mm. Well, I mean are you saying that I should not drink anything period? (*Laughter*)

T: Yeah, that's what I'm saying.

D: Nothing at all? Not even a glass of wine with dinner?

T: That's what I'm saying.

The therapist has chosen to take a hard-line position regarding the substance abuse because he believes that one therapeutic test (à la Control Mastery Theory) in this case has to do with structure and clarity. Deirdre's prior description of her family sounds as though the boundaries and structure were extremely loose and confusing. Thus, one of her tests would be to see if the therapist were likewise unwilling to be definitive and clear about things. Substance abuse may be dealt with in a variety of ways in treatment. One possibility for a less hard-and-fast approach with a patient for whom the test was different might be to have her "play around" with her drug and alcohol use for a week or two, while she attempted to reduce it for several days at a time. This seemed not to be the desirable approach in this case since it would only delay the necessary and encourage viewing the therapist as erratic and unreliable.

D: Oh really? That sounds to me like it's an ultimatum. You know, you either do this or.

T: Well I'm not setting up an ultimatum for you. What I'm saying to you is that it's very difficult for me and I think any other psychologist or psychiatrist or social worker to really know what's going on with you while you're drinking and using drugs because at least part of what you're describing may very well have to do with alcohol and drug consumption.

D: Yeah.

T: Plus, I think that an important issue is, and again you may not want to hear this, it does sound to me by what little you've said that drinking was a problem for many of your family members as well and I'm sure that's had some major effects on your life.

D: I agree with, you know, as far as the drugs are concerned. I don't know if . . .

T: What about the alcohol?

D: I don't know if I've given you the impression that it's . . . and the alcohol too, okay.

T: Have there been periods of time during which you've not drank, or that you've not used drugs for extended periods?

D: Yeah.

T: When?

D: Gee, it's been a long time ago. Probably, I've been doing both on and off really in the past 7 years. You know. But mm, mm, I'm sure, I'm sure there was there was a point where I was first introduced to cocaine you know maybe in the, you know in '78, and there was probably . . .

T: '78? [This interview was being conducted in 1989.]

D: Yeah.

T: A long time.

D: Yeah. But I'm sure that there was a period in there where I didn't do it. You know I might, I think I had, you know, a sort of a fascination with it just for maybe a few months. Was it? Maybe, I think it was '79 actually.

T: Mm.

D: It wasn't '78, it was '79. But I think I probably didn't do it up until, I might have quit and then I you know I really didn't do any until like maybe '82. And ever since then it's probably been you know, just on and off, you know.

T: And the drinking has been since when?

D: Uh, probably always, you know, since I was 16. Actually, you know, I probably can remember taking a drink you know, at 15 or even earlier.

T: That's a long time.

D: Yeah. Yeah it is. It's horrible!

An important aspect of many I-D-E therapy sessions, but in particular the first one, is the session summary. In the summary, the therapist attempts to clarify cooperatively with the patient what has transpired over the course of the session examining the focus of the patient's presentation and perhaps the focus of the therapy. There is also planning for future sessions (if needed). We consider it to be unacceptable to end a session, especially an initial session, by merely saying, "Time to stop" or "See you next week." The session summary helps give form and structure to a meeting and helps the patient have some ideas (and hope) about the future course and direction of treatment. In the excerpts below the therapist presents the patient with his summary of the work that day and attempts to elicit her input and reactions to this summary.

T: Let me let me summarize a little bit with you and talk about how we might proceed from here. I do think that it's a very good idea that you came in to see a therapist.

D: Mm.

T: I think that there probably are a variety of issues and problems for you. It sounds to me like things in your background, things in growing up have not been easy and that you've not had an easy life in a variety of ways. But I think that, and this is just a shot in the dark, I think that part of the reason that you're here right now, has to do with the fact that you're going to be 30 next month . . .

"Why now?" "Because the patient has changed."

D: Mm.

T: and I think that part of what is going on for you, and correct me if I'm wrong, I think that you feel stuck in your life. I think you feel like you're going nowhere.

D: Mm (*looking very sad*).

T: I don't think you're very happy right now. And I think that there is a lot of fear and a lot of anxiety about where you are and where you're going.

D: Mm. Yeah. That could be right on. (*Begins to cry*)

T: Can you say something about that?

D: Mm, Mm, I th- it sounds like it could, you know, very well be, the case with me. But I'm stuck with it, you know, it's . . .

T: You're stuck with?

D: This is my life. This is, you know, that's it.

T: But people change things. People take control of things and change things for themselves. That I would assume is one of the reasons that you're here.

D: Mm.

T: That you want to change things.

D: Mm.

T: And the only way that change can happen is by you making some of the changes. It's not me. All I can do is to give you some input about . . .

D: Yeah, I know.

T: What I think or see.

D: Yeah, well, I think you're probably right, you know, I think I probably am, maybe I'm not very happy. Maybe I've never really been very happy you know, with myself or where I've been or, you know . . .

T: What are you feeling right now?

D: Uh, I don't know, just, I guess I'm just feeling (*pause*)

T: You look sad.

D: Mm?

T: You look sad.

D: Yeah, I guess I am sad a little bit.

T: I think that you find yourself in a very rough and painful position and as you're saying, it may be that there's been some of that throughout your life, but I think that . . .

D: I don't feel, I don't feel like I should complain about it either, you know.

T: There are people starving in China.

D: Yeah, or you know, it's just expected of you to pretty much handle this you know, type of stuff . . .

T: Without complaining.

D: Yeah (*crying*).

T: Let me suggest a couple of things for you and then we can schedule another appointment. I think that the fact that you're hurting at this point says to me that you want to do something about this problem.

"Why now?" "Because the patient wants to change."

D: Yeah.

T: I think you have some motivation to do something about the problem. As I said to you earlier on I don't think things are going to change . . .

D: Until I change them.

T: Until you change them. And one of the first things . . .

D: I don't know what to change.

T: Well, then . . .

D: I have to change myself, I guess.

T: Right. That can be done and people can do that. But one of the first things I think you're going to have to address is this issue of alcohol and drugs.

D: Okay, so (*laugh*) alright, fair enough. I can do that.

The therapist and patient then set up a plan for a six-session renewable contract. That is, there would be a reevaluation at the end of the six sessions whether, and if so how, the therapy should proceed. It was further planned that the first four sessions would be held several days apart (i.e., on a twice-a-week basis). The therapist felt that the period during the first 2 weeks that Deirdre was trying to remain "clean and sober" would be critical and that it would be very useful to meet more frequently than once a week. It was also planned that during one of the first four sessions, it would be helpful to meet with Sam as well as Deirdre in a conjoint session. The I-D-E therapist usually meets with the patient and a significant other(s) at some point early in the treatment.

Research has demonstrated that significant others who have no contact with the therapist over the course of treatment often feel resentful and excluded (Brody & Farber, 1989; Hatcher & Hatcher, 1983). Further, bringing in the significant others is frequently a very helpful and salutary process (Budman & Gurman, 1988).

When thinking about the patient's current motivation for therapy in terms of wanting to change/wanting not to change/having already changed, it is useful to consider further what is different now in the patient's experience and life. From an individual perspective, the therapist should consider that the symptom or complaint may now be different in terms of its frequency and/or intensity. Another possibility is that the patient's perception of the symptom or complaint may now be different than in the past (i.e., attributions about the meaning or significance of the symptom or complaint have changed).

At the interpersonal level, the therapist needs to consider the consequences of the symptom or complaint in two ways: the interpersonal consequences of the problem for the help-seeking patient, and the interpersonal consequences of the problem for others—in both cases, especially for people with whom the patient is intimately connected (e.g., family, lovers, close friends).

At the systemic level, it is also important to keep open the possibility that the help-seeking patient is in the therapist's office because of, in reaction to, or as an expression of changes in other people or even in other relationships (e.g., the relationship between his or her parents.) In all cases the matter of what has changed, what one wants to change, and what one wants not to change (or is reluctant to change) is relevant.

THE COURSE OF TREATMENT

After the second session the patient was feeling sufficiently better and returned to work. Her anxiety level was much lower and she felt able to do her job.

The patient began the third session by saying that she wished to talk about "the 'I' word." In this session she described to the therapist a long history of sexual abuse. It appeared that the initial therapy sessions had allowed her to feel quite trusting of the therapist and she was therefore able to begin talking about the abuse. Deirdre reported that she and several of her younger sisters had been sexually abused by some of her elder brothers. This abuse began at an early age and had continued until she was about 13, at which point she had been able to put a stop to it. She had "vaguely known" for some period of time about the abuse of

her younger sisters, although she could not recall any extended conversations with them about the abuse. Her father and mother appear to have
been too preoccupied with their own difficulties to have had any
knowledge of the abuse.

Once the sexual abuse became known to the therapist, the focus of
the treatment shifted to dealing with this issue. (In our model, we would
view sexual abuse as fitting in the category of "loss-focused" treatment.)
Throughout the course of the therapy, alcohol and drug use also continued
to be examined and discussed. As well as having Sam come in to a session,
at a somewhat later point, the therapist asked Deirdre if she would ask one
of her other sisters (who had also been abused) who was living in the area
to come in for a session with her. This proved to be a valuable session, in
that the sisters had never really discussed their thoughts and feelings about
the sexual abuse with one another at length. Therefore, each had been left
alone with her own feelings of pain, grief, anger, and fear.

FOLLOW-UP

During the first 3 months of her treatment, Deirdre was seen on a
weekly basis. After this period, the therapy moved to once every 3
weeks, then once a month and most recently to a five-times-per-year
basis. She has had some contact with the therapist for the past 2½ years,
during which she has had about 34 individual sessions.

Over this time she has been able to make enormous strides. She has
not had panic attacks. She is enrolled in college and hopes to eventually
get her BA degree. She has resumed running (something she was quite
good at as a teenager). In general, the outcome of treatment has been
most favorable. It is possible that the therapy sessions will continue on
an intermittent basis for quite some time or that we will gradually
reduce our meetings further and meet only if necessary. In any case,
Deirdre understands that the door is open and that she may return as she
needs in the future.

EDITORS' QUESTIONS

Q: In the case presented, what if the patient had not stopped
alcohol and drug abuse so readily? How might you have handled the
"ultimatum" issue?

A: This is certainly a key question for which no one answer will
suffice. There are a variety of creative possibilities that should be

considered. Were Deirdre to have indicated that she was fairly ambivalent about addressing her alcohol and/or drug use, we would try the following (most likely in the order indicated). [At the same time that the therapist is considering the options for intervention, it should be noted that it would be useful to try to "tailor" the particular interventions according to the ways in which the patient will be testing the therapist (à la Control Mastery Theory). As was indicated earlier, the particular patient's history and frame of reference would lead to differential effectiveness of the same general intervention.]

1. We would have her see a colleague who was a therapist with a subspecialty in substance abuse for a consultation. "Perhaps Dr. Smith, who specializes in such problems will have a distinct perspective on this issue. Dr. Smith is an expert in substance abuse and I have great faith in her recommendations." If our colleague also perceived the alcohol and drugs as a problem, she could follow the patient in regard to these matters. If the patient were willing to maintain intermittent contact with the substance abuse specialist this would be a constant reminder that the patient's substance use is not a trivial issue. Also, the problem cannot just be moved to the background. Each and every time the patient went to see the substance abuse specialist, her drug and alcohol use would again be brought to the forefront. In addition, if there were continued resistance (denial) in regard to the substance abuse issues, those could be dealt with parallel to the psychotherapy sessions, during the patient's sessions with the drug and alcohol specialist. During our sessions with the patient, we would ask her regularly how the alcohol and drug issues were going.
2. Along with the first option above, we would suggest to the patient that she attend an AA or a Rational Recovery meeting— "Could you try one of these meetings as an observer? Tell me what it's like for you. Did you learn anything about your substance use? Did anything relevant to your situation go on at the meeting?"
3. We would also recommend that the patient keep a drug and alcohol diary. In this diary she would examine when she was drinking or using drugs, how much she was using, whether there were any patterns to her use, and so on.

The three possibilities described so far are all ways to keep the patient thinking about her alcohol and drug use and to keep these problems from being ignored. They require that the patient have at least some willingness to comply and/or some nascent feeling that this may be a worthwhile area to address. These three possibilities are just a few of the varied options available if the patient has a willingness to reframe substance abuse as a legitimate concern.

Miller (1989) presents a variety of useful suggestions for increasing the motivation for change among substance abusing patients and indicates that it is most beneficial for the therapist to maintain a flexible, eclectic approach in treating alcohol and drug abuse.

4. Some severely addicted patients state quite clearly, "I have no substance abuse or alcohol problem! You are making a big thing out of nothing," or "I don't have any real interest in changing this part of my life. Let's talk about other things." Occasionally, under these circumstances, the therapist needs to move in the direction Cummings (1979) describes as "exclusion therapy." That is, the patient is told that he or she appears unready to address this aspect of his or her life at the present time. The patient should be free to recontact the therapist at any point at which he or she feels ready to begin to start to examine the substance abuse more closely. (There is no demand for immediate abstinence or request that the patient do exactly what the therapist says must be done. The request is for the patient to be willing to "open up" substance abuse as an important issue. A substance abuser so deeply committed to denying the problem that he or she needs to view it as a nonissue is unlikely to profit from therapy.) We have seen patients excluded from therapy for this reason, who later returned and indicated that the therapist's serious approach to drinking or drug use led them to reassess their position and to begin to address their drug or alcohol problems.

Clearly, there are a variety of ways for the therapist to address substance and alcohol abuse. What is critical, however, is that these problems not be forgotten or ignored. To do so is to risk an extended course of fruitless treatment.

Q: What is your reasoning in moving to get family background early in the interview? Why not simply deal with the problem at hand (i.e., the panic attacks)?

A: The therapist seeing a patient for the first time must make a decision about how much to stick with the here and now and how much to examine past history. Does one maintain an exclusive focus on the presenting problem and the current circumstances of the patient, or does one also clarify history and how the patient got to this point? Some models of brief treatment tend to deal very little with history (Friedman & Fanger, 1991; O'Hanlon & Weiner-Davis, 1989) and advise the therapist to deal exclusively with a search for solutions in the present.

Our interest in the past is mainly in regard to the ways in which a person's view of their history can inform us about the present. For example, what a patient tells us about his or her childhood may be quite helpful in clarifying the characteristics of the tests to which the therapist will be subject during the treatment (Weiss & Sampson, 1986).

Also, some sense of the patient's history also will help us to elucidate the nature of the personal narrative with which the patient enters therapy. Narrative psychology has recently been gaining prominence in the clinical area (Howard, 1991; White & Epston, 1990). There are a variety of ways in which the person's narrative may be important in the therapy. One of the most central is that the narrative tells us what in a person's history he or she sees as most consequential in helping make meaning out of their lives. That is, the therapist's request for history ("Tell me about how your family background might be related to your current problem.") is rarely met with a detailed chronological recounting of the patient's life from birth to the present. (If this type of ponderous, unselective response were elicited, the therapist would immediately have some ideas about the patient's characteristic cognitive and interactional style.) Rather, because organizing a narrative requires what White and Epston (1990) describe as "pruning," what most people respond with is an account of several notable events in their lives which they view as most central in leading to their current difficulty.

Our history taking tends not to be exhaustive (or exhausting); rather, it is oriented toward helping us to clarify the "why now?" question as rapidly as possible and to give us a clearer sense of the patient's expectations in regard to his or her relationships with significant individuals. It also can be quite useful in assisting us in identifying family members and friends who may be called into the treatment at a later point.

Q: Clinicians often consider the therapy of incest survivors to be long-term, ongoing treatment. What does an intermittent, time-sensitive approach like yours have to offer patients with such major difficulties?

A: First of all, it is important to understand that incest survivors should not be viewed in a unitary and undifferentiated way. Russell's (1986) excellent clinical research book, The Secret Trauma, makes it clear that there is great variation in the psychological sequelae of incest. This variation depends on the ages that the incest began and ended, who the perpetrator was, any supports the survivor had available at the time, and so on. It would be naive to assume that every incest survivor requires precisely the same type of therapy and can only be treated by weekly psychotherapy over an indefinite period.

In the I-D-E model, a patient like Deirdre can be treated over an extended period (chronologically) but with breaks during which she is able to work on various elements of the therapy outside of sessions. Bass and Davis (1988) indicate a number of important therapeutic events that take place in the "healing" of incest survivors. These events, such as "remembering," "breaking the silence," "grieving," and "confrontation" may be done during a continuous course of therapy or one or more may occur during an episode of intermittent treatment. As is often the case in psychotherapy, the patient may be able to do one or two pieces of work at a given time. Then she or he may need to consolidate gains in these areas before moving on to other areas. Recall that in the I-D-E brief therapy approach, the interpersonal experience of the patient is itself considered to have major healing and change-promoting power. Thus, with Deirdre, the therapist took advantage of the change-promoting leverage gained by the creation of a trusting relationship with her. He did this not by deepening the already present transference toward him but by bringing people important to Deirdre in her everyday life into the therapy. With regard to the incest, her sister's involvement in the therapy, albeit brief, was considered potentially to have greater direct therapeutic value than more removed discussions of those childhood experiences with the therapist alone. We believe that, in general, including in "individual therapy" those people with whom the patient has ongoing relationships and who are centrally involved in the patient's and therapist's ideas about "Why now?" leads to more lasting change than brought about via the substitutive relationship of the patient and therapist. It is also a strategy that is practical in helping to keep therapy as brief as possible, even in situations such as incest, that some therapists believe routinely require extensive (and intensive) treatment.

Q: Your response to the last question starts to get at some very fundamental ideas about the way change occurs in psychotherapy, or in different types of therapy. Of particular relevance to the work with Deirdre, aren't most of the assumptions and techniques of family therapists quite at odds with those of individual therapists?

A: It is interesting that our presentation and discussion of the work with Deirdre, including our response to that question, would help bring out such a question, since it is one that is often asked about the I-D-E approach.

Basically, we think that the question only really makes sense in the context of certain kinds of family therapy, or in terms of certain definitions of family therapy. One of us once said that what makes "family therapy" different from "individual therapy" is that in the former, one is at least as concerned about what happens between people as one is about what happens within people (Gurman & Kniskern, 1981). This would be true whether one is thinking about developing a treatment focus, selecting and using various clinical techniques, or evaluating the effectiveness of therapy. We recognize that in the more political domain of "family therapy," great efforts have been made to treat "family" and "individual" therapy as inherently antagonistic and incompatible. In fact, this is quite true when comparing the therapeutic aims and processes of treatment extremes, for example, Freudian psychoanalysis versus any of several influential "family" therapies that are almost exclusively interested in the overt transactional levels of people's lives.

On the other hand, we believe that the majority of practicing "family" therapists continue usefully to call on ideas from the psychology of the individual in their work, and so-called individual therapists find an ever-increasing coherence in using some of the therapeutic strategies of "family therapy" in working with one person. (A superb illustration of both of these patterns is found in Wachtel & Wachtel, 1985). The I-D-E approach is wholly consistent with the emerging integrative models of marital and family therapy, in which primacy is not given to any single level or domain of human experience. Rather, the fundamental "Why now?" question, when considered flexibly, will help lead the therapist and patient to the most treatment relevant areas for focused concern, be they intrapsychic, interpersonal, or both.

Q: How did you become a brief therapist?

A: As an undergraduate student, I switched majors five times in my first three semesters. Biology, chemistry, sociology, art, and english came and went as possible majors. I had a sense of confusion and apprehension (which is probably not uncommon for people in their late teens.) Finally, I decided to see a counselor at the university health service. I saw her for an initial visit during which she gathered history and busily took notes. At the end of that visit she said, "It sounds to me like the field that would really suit you is clinical psychology!" I had never heard of clinical psychology and was uncertain of what it entailed. The clinician (a vocational counselor) said that there was a young man on the staff of Student Health who had just graduated from a clinical psych program several months before and she was sure he would be glad to describe the area to me in detail. The next week I met with the new PhD and the rest is history. I can't remember the names of either of these fine single-session clinicians. However, these brief interactions changed the course of my life.

I trained as a clinical psychologist in the late '60s. Although the training I was receiving in graduate school was rather long term in orientation, the work I was doing at the Pittsburgh, Veterans Administration Hospital on my practicum with returning Vietnam veterans moved me in the direction of brief, time-effective treatment. Almost every clinical experience I had after completing graduate school indicated that many people coming in to treatment wanted to get as much as possible achieved at a low cost in terms of both time and expense.

My career as a clinical psychologist has been exciting and varied. What if I hadn't chosen to go to the student health service in 1965? I can personally attest to the power of a very brief intervention.

[Gurman's answer appears in his Chapter 9, this volume.]

REFERENCES

Bass, E., & Davis, L. (1988). *The courage to heal.* New York: Harper & Row.

Bennett, M. J. (1983). Focal psychotherapy—terminable and interminable. *American Journal of Psychotherapy, 37,* 365–375.

Bolter, K., Levinson, H., Alvarez, W. (1990). Differences in values between short-term and long-term therapists. *Professional Psychology: Research and Practice, 21,* 285–290.

Brody, F. M., & Farber, B. A., (1989). Effects of psychotherapy on significant others. *Professional Psychology: Research and Practice, 20,* 116–122.

Budman, S. H. (1990). The myth of termination in brief therapy: Or, it ain't over til it's over. In J. K. Zeig & S. G. Gilligan (Eds.), *Brief therapy: Myths, methods, and metaphors* (pp. 206–218). New York: Brunner/Mazel.

Budman, S. H., & Gurman, A. S. (1988). *Theory and practice of brief therapy.* New York: Guilford Press.

Burlingame, G. M., & Fuhriman, A. (1987). Conceptualizing short-term treatment: A comparative review. *The Counseling Psychologist, 15,* 557–595.

Cummings, N. A. (1979). Turning bread into stone: Our modern anti-miracle. *American Psychologist, 34,* 1119–1129.

Cummings, N. A. (1986). The dismantling of our health care system: Strategies for the survival of psychological practice. *American Psychologist, 41,* 426–431.

Cummings, N. A. (1990). Brief intermittent therapy throughout the lifecycle. In J. K. Zeig & S. G. Gilligan (Eds.), *Brief therapy: Myths, methods, and metaphors* (pp. 169–184). New York: Brunner/Mazel.

Engel, L., & Ferguson, T. (1990). *Imaginary crimes.* Boston: Houghton Mifflin.

Friedman, S., & Fanger, M. T. (1991). *Expanding therapeutic possibilities: Getting results in brief therapy.* New York: Lexington Books/Macmillan.

Gurman, A. S., & Kniskern, D. P. (1981). Research in marital and family therapy: Progress, prospect and perspective. In S. Garfield and A. Bergin (Eds.), *Handbook of psychotherapy and behavior change* (pp. 817–901). New York: Wiley.

Hall, M. J., Arnold, W. N., & Crosby, R. M. (1990). Back to basics: The importance of focus selection. *Psychotherapy, 27,* 578–584.

Hatcher, S. L., & Hatcher, R. L. (1983). Set a place for Elijah: Problems of the spouses and parents of psychotherapy patients. *Psychotherapy: Theory, Research and Practice, 20,* 75–80.

Howard, G. S. (1991). Cultural tales: A narrative approach to thinking, cross-cultural psychology, and psychotherapy. *American Psychologist, 46,* 187–197.

Hoyt, M. F. (1990). On time in brief therapy. In R. A. Wells & V. J. Giannetti (Eds.), *Handbook of the brief psychotherapies.* New York: Plenum Press.

McConnaughy, E. A., DiClemente, C. C., Prochaska, J. O., & Velicer, W. F. (1989). Stages of change in psychotherapy: A follow-up report. *Psychotherapy, 26,* 494–503.

McConnaughy, E. A., Prochaska, J. O., & Velicer, W. F. (1983). Stages of change in psychotherapy: Measurement and sample profile. *Psychotherapy: Theory, Research and Practice, 20,* 368–375.

Miller, W. R. (1989). Increasing motivation for change. In R. K. Hester & W. R. Miller (Eds.), *Handbook of alcoholism treatment approaches* (pp. 67–80). New York: Pergamon Press.

O'Hanlon, W. H., & Weiner-Davis, M. (1989). *In search of solutions: A new direction in psychotherapy.* New York: W. W. Norton.

Prochaska, J. O., & DiClemente, C. C. (1982). Transtheoretical therapy: Toward a more integrative model of change. *Psychotherapy: Theory, Research and Practice, 19,* 276–288.

Prochaska, J. O., & DiClemente, C. C. (1986). Toward a comprehensive model of change. In W. R. Miller & N. Heather (Eds.) *Treating addictive behaviors: Processes of change* (pp. 3–27). New York: Plenum Press.

Russell, D. E. H. (1986). *The secret trauma.* New York: Basic Books.

Silbershatz, G., Curtis, J. T., & Nathans, S. (1989). Using the patient's plan to assess progress in psychotherapy. *Psychotherapy, 27,* 40–46.

Wachtel, E. F., & Wachtel, P. L. (1985). *Family dynamics in individual psychotherapy: A guide to clinical strategies.* New York: Guilford Press.

Weiss, J., & Sampson, H. (1986). *The psychoanalytic process.* New York: Guilford Press.

White, M., & Epston, D. (1990). *Narrative means to therapeutic ends.* New York: W. W. Norton.

Launching Cognitive–Behavioral Therapy for Adolescent Depression and Drug Abuse

RALPH M. TURNER

During the past two decades cognitive–behavioral Therapy (CBT) has become an important short-term psychotherapy approach. Its origins are in cognitive psychotherapy (Beck, 1970; Ellis, 1962; Meichenbaum, 1977), social learning theory (Bandura, 1977a, 1977b, 1985), and behavior therapy (Lazarus, 1976). In addition, several of the founders of cognitive therapy were originally psychoanalytically oriented practitioners (i.e., Beck, Ellis, and Meichenbaum). Mahoney (1977) and Kendall and Bemis (1984) have described CBT as a hybrid, or integrative, form of psychotherapy. It is an amalgam of empirically established techniques and procedures drawn from both cognitive and behavioral research. Due to CBT's close ties to basic research, it is constantly expanding. So, in practice it is difficult to specify the exact procedures that are CBT. However, rather than being a flaw, this elasticity and permeability results in a model of treatment that is dynamic and robust.

THE BASIC ASSUMPTIONS OF COGNITIVE-BEHAVIORAL THERAPY

Despite this hybrid heritage, a consistent viewpoint about the nature of psychopathology and psychosocial treatment does characterize the cognitive–behavioral model. The basic premise of cognitive therapy is that our cognitive processes causally affect our behavior and emotions. This does not mean that the direction of causality is always from cognition to behavior and emotions. A recursive and reciprocal set of causal influences exists among the domains of cognition, behavior, and affect. However, what the pioneers in cognitive therapy did bring into focus for the first time is that our cognitive processes do impel our behavior and emotions in critically important ways.

A second assumption is that learning is a critical factor in psychopathology ontogenesis and the development of psychosocial treatments. Learning is more than Pavlovian and operant conditioning, however. The majority of human learning is cognitively mediated. Cognitive science, not classical animal learning theory, is the basis for the cognitive–behavioral approach.

A related assumption is that people's cognitive representations of themselves and the world, rather than the phenomenon of the actual environment, influence their reactions. These representations occur at both conscious and unconscious levels of awareness.

Cognition is an active process. People do not simply take in the world around them. They actively seek information and mentally construct it. Consequently, people often see what they want to see, hear what they are prepared to hear, and negate or circumvent information out of keeping with their expectations.

Understanding cognitive systems is essential for understanding psychopathology. Cognitive processes such as attitude formation, expectancies, causal attributions, conscious and unconscious self-statements, and expected scripts and roles for self and others are central to psychological functioning and emotional well-being or illness.

It is also assumed that reliable and valid findings in the cognitive, biological, and behavioral sciences are applicable for incorporation into the cognitive–behavioral perspective. So, cognitive–behavioral theory and practice need to accommodate advances in cognitive psychology research.

The task of the cognitive–behavioral clinician is to act as a diagnostician, educator, and technical consultant to the client. The therapist works with the client to design learning experiences aimed at lessening the symptoms of mental illness. CBT is a collaborative relationship between the therapist and the client. The goal is to teach clients enough knowledge and skills to be their own cognitive–behavioral therapist.

Taken together, these assumptions form the basis of cognitive–behavioral psychotherapy.

THE FRAMEWORK OF CLASSICAL
COGNITIVE-BEHAVIORAL THERAPY

There are several models of CBT. The model developed by Beck (1967, 1976) is the most studied and commonly used version.

Beck and his colleagues (Beck, Rush, Shaw, & Emery, 1979) focus on three interrelated concepts in explaining the cognitive theory of the genesis and maintenance of emotional disorders. These concepts are the cognitive triad, cognitive distortions, and the schema that undergird them.

The *cognitive triad* reflects the three domains of attributions individuals have to contend with to be emotionally stable. The first domain is the self. Persons can feel either positive or negative about their own self. The second domain is the individual's experience of the world. An individual can feel helpless or vigorous about his or her experience of the world. The third domain of the cognitive triad represents the individual's expectations for the future. An individual can feel pessimistic or optimistic. Clients are assessed regarding their status in each of these domains. Any given client might show negativistic thinking in one domain only, in two of the areas, or in all three. The function of the cognitive triad conceptualization is to permit the clinician to focus quickly on the domain or domains in which the client has problems with negativistic thinking.

Cognitive distortions are the common and habitual ways that persons pervert environmental information. The distortions are typically the central focus of therapy. Common cognitive distortions include dichotomous thinking, overgeneralization, biasing judgments, emotional reasoning, should statements, catastrophizing, disqualifying the positive, and personalization, to name several. Freeman (1990) provides a more detailed catalog of cognitive distortions. The cognitive distortions are pivotal in maintaining depressive and anxious states of mind. Educating clients about who they are and how they function is the principal task of therapy.

Beck has adopted Piaget's (1926) concept of the schema as a third pivotal element in his model. Schema are cognitive structures that propagate both the cognitive triad and distortions. Schema develop during our earliest experiences with the world. Schema store global generalizations about our self-worth and hope for the future. Cognitive therapy strives to illuminate the individual's schema, or core beliefs, and change them. Altering the deeply ingrained schema is essential and key for long-term therapeutic success.

THE DYNAMIC COGNITIVE-BEHAVIORAL THERAPY FRAMEWORK

Mahoney (1985, 1991) has championed the distinction between explicit (i.e., conscious) and tacit (i.e., unconscious) cognition. According to Mahoney, much cognitive processing occurs at the tacit level. It is automatic, overarching, and out of our day-to-day awareness. The tacit level consists of the rules and strategies that guide and direct information processing. It reflects basic assumptions, premises, and world hypotheses that act on the information available to us. Thus, cognitive–behavioral therapists now consider tacit, or unconscious, processes in their work with clients.

Integrally linked with the notion of tacit mental mechanisms is the concept of the feedforward mechanism. Working from recent findings in cognitive psychology, Mahoney stipulates that humans actively seek information and meaning structures by mentally creating a significant proportion of the environmental information they take in. This process is akin to a mixture of the mechanisms of projection and transference in psychoanalytic theory. Humans project and transfer meaning schema onto their experiences. This dramatically influences how and what they perceive of environmental events.

These phenomena have long been of interest to psychodynamically oriented researchers and clinicians (Turner, 1988, in press-a). Luborsky (1984) and Horowitz (1988) have developed measurement techniques designed to assess tacit interpersonal schema and their feedforward affects. The assessment procedure developed by Luborsky (1984) is called the Core Conflictual Relationship Theme analysis. Horowitz (1988) has produced a complementary approach called the Role Relationship Model analysis. Both models assume that distortions in the individual's tacit and feedforward cognitive strategies cause emotional disorders.

The approach to CBT described in this chapter integrates both psychodynamic assessment techniques to clarify clients' tacit and feedforward cognitive processes (Turner, 1983, 1988, 1989, in press-a, in press-b). Thus, in addition to the usual cognitive and behavioral assumptions, the current approach emphasizes the role of unconscious and active mental processing in human functioning. For these reasons I refer to this model as dynamic-cognitive–behavioral therapy (D-CBT).

The D-CBT approach stresses the significance of interpersonal relationships in human functioning. Change comes about through interpersonal interaction. The therapeutic relationship is the primary vehicle through which treatment works. Other factors such as performance of homework and education are critical for successful treatment, but the relationship provides the laboratory for changing cognitive distortions.

TECHNICAL INTERVENTION
IN COGNITIVE–BEHAVIORAL THERAPY

CBT is technique oriented. Freeman (1990) lists 18 cognitive techniques and 9 behavioral techniques typically practiced by cognitive–behavioral therapists. Understanding the role of technical intervention is important to an understanding of CBT.

The techniques are classified into two groups. One group of interventions makes clients aware of the explicit and tacit cognitions that affect their emotional and behavioral regulation. The second group of interventions is an aid to helping clients change their cognitive processes, behavior, and emotional experience.

The *triple-column strategy* (Beck et al., 1979) is an example of an awareness-enhancing technique. The therapist asks clients first to self-monitor their automatic thoughts and distortions in the context of emotionally upsetting situations. Next, they use the knowledge gained in sessions to challenge these thoughts. Clients try to define the type of cognitive distortion involved with their current situation and then to generate an alternative adaptive response to the distortion.

Externalization of voices is an example of a change intervention. People constantly engage in self-talk about their life experience. Clients' self-talk is analyzed by attributing a separate voice for the functional and dysfunctional elements involved in the thought. By having the therapist play the role of the dysfunctional voice, the client learns to identify negative self talk and respond adaptively to it. The therapist next models the adaptive response to the client's negative verbalizations. Then, clients practice stating their negative thoughts aloud using the adaptive voice. After rehearsal, the therapist arranges a series of increasingly difficult situations for clients to use the externalization-of-voices technique.

The practice of CBT requires a competent understanding of strategies for awareness and change. It also demands a skillful execution of the techniques. Freeman (1990) and Beck et al. (1979) provide a guide to the techniques commonly used in CBT.

THE INITIAL SESSION IN
COGNITIVE-BEHAVIORAL THERAPY

In the initial session in CBT, the clinician needs to get a clear description of the client's problems. The clinician should perform a formal diagnostic evaluation if the problems are symptomatic of a psychiatric disorder. Depending on the client's circumstances, a mental status examination might be necessary.

Typically, the cognitive–behavioral clinician will get some type of psychometric information on the client's symptom status. For instance, if the client is depressed, the Beck Depression Inventory (Beck, Ward, Mendelson, Mock, & Erbaugh, 1961) should be administered. In the case of obsessive–compulsive disorder or panic disorder, for instance, ask the client to self-record the frequency, severity, and environmental conditions surrounding the daily occurrence of symptoms. Virtually any reliable and valid psychometric assessment device can be used for assessment. In addition, the clinician needs to provide the client with an overview of the CBT approach. Many clinicians have clients read *Feeling Good: The New Mood Therapy* (Burns, 1980) to acquaint themselves with the cognitive–behavioral approach.

Although the cognitive–behavioral approach is short term, therapists do not always set a definite termination date. However, having a fixed end point provides a focus for the therapeutic work and helps to prevent regression.

An important task of the first session is for the clinician to check the capacity of the client to develop a sound working relationship with the clinician. The simplest means to accomplish this is to ask clients, at the close of the first session, if they feel comfortable working with you.

Assessment occurs over the first several sessions. The therapist's goal is to form a cohesive conceptualization of the case. The conceptualization includes specifications about the genesis of the problem, the types of schema and distortions involved, and a prescription for treatment.

The cognitive-behavioral treatment session typically lasts from 45 to 60 minutes. The therapist starts by asking the client to provide an overview of the previous week's events. The clinician helps the client to relate the recent experiences to the focus of treatment. Since homework is integral to this approach, the clinician next reviews the previous homework assignment with the client. The therapist ties these reports into the central focus of treatment and sets up a problem focus for the current session. The session problem focus serves as the basis for the next homework assignment. In closing the session the clinician briefly reviews the material discussed during the hour and links the session to the overall context of the therapeutic process.

CASE ILLUSTRATION

Cathy (a pseudonym) was first seen in the psychiatry emergency service. Rex, her boyfriend, brought her to the hospital because she had overdosed on Xanax and alcohol. Rex reported that she had threatened to commit suicide earlier in the evening. Cathy, however, stated that she accidentally took too much medication and that she had not intended to end her life. Cathy was kept overnight for observation. She was released from the hospital the next morning and referred to me for outpatient care.

The First Session

At the time of the first session, I had very little information about Cathy. The nurse from the psychiatric emergency service informed me that Cathy was 17, caucasian, and currently living with her boyfriend. The emergency room staff judged that Cathy had made a serious suicide attempt. They pumped her stomach and held her overnight for observation. The staff reported that Cathy and Rex were hostile toward one another. Cathy had consistently denied any suicidal ideation or intent, and she appeared stable after 8 hours of observation. The nurse reported that he felt Cathy was depressed and while not imminently suicidal, still at risk for another overdose.

I began the session by allowing Cathy to tell her story.

Therapist: Can you tell me what brings you to the clinic?

Cathy: I . . . I . . . I don't know if I should be here. I mean I've been feeling a little down, but I . . . I didn't try to commit suicide.

T: It sounds as if you do not want to be here. Is someone making you come in?

C: No. No, I wanted to come. I mean I have so many troubles. My parents. Rex, my boyfriend. The only thing that makes me feel better is my medicine. I don't ever think of suicide. I just took too much of my medicine and I had one little glass of wine with it, and Rex gets all worried that I'm trying to kill myself. I mean, I was just feeling good. . . .

T: Tell me please, what kind of medicine are you taking?

C: It's Xanax. I take one milligram three times a day. It's just last Friday night I was feeling bad, so I took six of them. That's what it takes to really work. Six or seven. Then I just had one glass of wine to help calm me down.

T: Are you sure that is all you had? After all, it was Friday night. A lot of people party on Friday night. No beer?

C: No, I don't like beer. Never have. I just had the one glass of wine, and Rex causes all these problems.

T: Have you and Rex been having problems?

C: Yeah! you could say we've been having problems. But, I love the guy, really I do. He can be so nice. I care for him. At least he cares for me, not like my family.

T: Problems with the family, too?

C: Yeah. There are always problems with my family. My parents, well . . . , they're not really my parents. I . . . I mean I . . . I'm . . . I'm adopted. They've always been good to me. It's . . . It's just that they are so conservative. They're real religious. I mean, well, my dad is anyway. My mom just goes along with it. She always goes to church when my dad is there. They tell my brother and me that we have to go when they're going. It's like . . . It's like she always just goes along with him, only she really plays it up. Like she's so pure and Christian. When dad isn't here she doesn't go; then she tells him she did. She just has to keep him off her back. They didn't use to fight, though. It was always real nice around home when I was little. But, ever since my dad got laid off from his job they've just seemed to be spending less and less time with each other. We have a house at the beach. Anymore, my dad spends all of his time there. He loves it, and my mom hates the beach. But he just stays there all of the time, anymore.

T: You said your dad had lost his job before all of this started to happen. Do you think he might be depressed?

C: He might be. I don't know. He really loved his job.

T: What kind of work did he do?

C: He's an engineer. He worked for an airplane company. He worked there all his life. Then, they just ran out of work and laid everybody off.

T: Has he tried to find another job?

C: No, I don't think so. He and my mom don't want to move. They moved a lot before, and they have the house at the beach. Besides, my dad says he's too old.

T: How old is he?

C: Fifty-nine.

T: Sounds like you are really worried about what is going to happen to them.

C: Well, yeah. But its more than that. They're just so religious and conservative. I mean, they just . . . they just don't care about me.

They treat my brother so much better than me. It seems like they love him more than me. They let him do what ever he wants. When I was his age I couldn't do anything. He can go wherever he wants. They're even buying him a car.

T: How old is your brother?

C: He's 16.

T: Is he adopted, also?

C: No, he's their real son.

T: Do you think they love him more because he is their biological child and you are adopted?

C: No . . . no. They've always treated me like their daughter. It's just that they're so conservative. They have different views about what boys can do and what girls can do.

T: So, you feel cheated and you are angry at them about that.

C: No, I'm not angry. I just feel hurt. I just wish they would love me like they used to. I would just like things to be like they used to be. They don't like anything that I do. They don't like Rex. They want me to live at home. They don't like where I want to go to school. Nothing I do can please them. And they're always bragging about Tom. How great he is at things. Meanwhile, he doesn't do anything. My mother does all of his homework for him. She is just supposed to help him, but she does it all. He doesn't do any of it. He'll never learn anything if she keeps doing it all for him. And they just expect me to do everything for myself; they don't help me at all. They just tell me what to do all the time. They just want to control me, not help me.

T: This is a lot of stuff to be having to think about. I think anyone would feel down and depressed if they felt deserted like you do.

C: (*Sighs and begins to cry*) And then there's Rex.

T: Yes, you said you two had been arguing. How is the relationship?

C: It used to be good. I mean when I first met him he was real good to me. Now, he just does his drugs and lays around all the time.

T: What kind of drugs?

C: Well, he's in a treatment program. He gets methadone there twice everyday. He's not supposed to do anything else, but he gets a lot of pills wherever he can. Then he just sleeps all the time.

T: How long have you and Rex been together?

C: A year. We moved in together this summer as soon as school was over.

T: How old is Rex?

C: Twenty-three

T: Do you love him?

C: I think I do. I . . . I . . . don't know. I used to. I mean he was so different when I first met him. He was getting straight and real full of life. We used to go everywhere. He was so nice to me. He was so good looking and it seemed like he knew everything. Now, he's just so mean to me. All we ever do is fight, or he's asleep.

T: Have you ever thought about leaving him?

C: I wanted to once, but I . . . I just couldn't. I don't want to hurt him. He couldn't handle it. His counselor says I should try to work it out. He says Rex needs me. He would have no place to go. I . . . I just would feel too guilty. I can't leave him alone. I don't know what would happen to him.

T: Sounds like you feel stuck.

C: I feel lost. Like I don't know where I'm going.

Following Cathy's initial presentation, which is rich in individual and family dynamics, I conducted a formal analysis of her depressive symptoms. She acknowledged sleep disturbance, depressed mood, loss of interest in sex, loss of interest in activities, and feelings of worthlessness. She did not experience crying spells often, but described herself as constantly on the verge of tears. I then had Cathy take the Beck Depression Inventory to assess her level of depression. She scored a 28 indicating a moderate to high level of depression.

I then turned the interview toward assessing her suicide potential. In particular, I needed to determine where she was obtaining the Xanax and if she was already in treatment. Cathy convinced me that the overdose had been accidental. She had wanted to get high, fall asleep, and avoid interacting with Rex that night. She did eventually tell me that she had told Rex that she would kill herself that night if he did not leave her alone. She said she was not serious in her threats and had wanted to frighten him.

When I questioned Cathy about her previous psychiatric care, she said that her mother had taken her to a therapist when she was 14 for nervousness and depression. Cathy had not wanted to go to therapy, but her mother insisted. After 6 months of talking and getting nowhere Cathy quit treatment. Her mother and father then arranged for Cathy to see their family physician. The family doctor prescribed the Xanax. Cathy had been taking the medication for approximately 2 years.

This set the stage for me to bring session one to a close. First, I needed to assess Cathy's status with regard to the elements of the cognitive triad. In addition, I needed to teach Cathy what cognitive–behavioral treatment would be like and to establish a contract for therapy. Also, I wanted to determine if she was comfortable working with me.

T: Cathy, I want to ask you a few more specific questions to help me get a handle on how to help you.

C: Okay.

T: When you think of yourself and your ability to deal with your problems which of these words best describes you, capable or helpless?

C: I like to think of myself as capable, but I just don't feel that way right now. I don't feel like I can do anything right, right now.

T: Sounds like you feel capable some of the time, but not currently.

C: I don't know. Sometimes I do, sometimes I don't. I guess, mostly I don't lately.

T: How about the future? What do you think of when you think of the future? Do you feel hopeful or hopeless?

C: It's . . . it's . . . hard to think about the future. I mean its like I can't see it. I can't seem to see beyond today . . . or right now. It just all seems black. Like . . . like I . . . I . . . don't know if there is a future.

T: Do you feel like the world is fair? Do you have a chance of dealing with it?

C: Yeah. I mean . . . I mean, everybody has got the same deal. I just wish it was like it used to be. Everything was so easy. It just seemed like everything was going my way. Now . . . I don't know. Everything is just so different.

T: How do you feel about being here today? Do you want to work on the issues you have brought up? I know you were not too interested in being here in the beginning.

C: I did want to be here. I just wasn't sure anybody could understand me, or would want to take the time to understand me. It feels good to just talk. I needed someone to talk to.

T: Do you feel okay working with me? The reason I ask is that our comfortableness in working together makes a big difference in whether we get anywhere or not. That is the most important thing: to get you to where you are feeling stronger and solving your problems.

C: Yeah, I like talking to you. Besides, coming to see you is out of my choice, not my mother's.

T: You need to understand, however, that we will not just be talking. We are going to be doing a lot of things to improve your skills at handling stress, solving problems, and changing the way you think about yourself and others. You are going to have homework assign-ments to do. I'll be asking you to try out new behaviors and ideas. Also, I am going to teach you how to observe your own thoughts and see how they affect you emotionally. I guess that is the first point I need to help you understand. It is our thoughts and beliefs that cause us to feel happy or sad. It is because we humans are such quick thinkers that we sometimes get into trouble. We are always thinking, even when we are not aware of it.

C: You mean like our unconscious.

T: Sort of. Except a lot that seems unconscious is actually just very quick conscious thinking. Because it is conscious that means we can learn to slow it down and evaluate whether our thoughts are correct or distorted. And we can do a lot of distorted thinking. Especially when we are depressed, it seems like we can put a negative filter on everything that happens to us. Then we miss even the good things. But it is all just a habitual way of thinking about ourselves, life, and the future.

C: It doesn't seem to me like I think about being depressed. I . . . I mean sometimes I'm not thinking about anything and I just feel bad. I think about my feelings after I feel them. If I just didn't feel this way then I wouldn't think about all this stuff. I could just go back to the way it used to be. I used to feel good all the time.

T: I understand. I understand what you mean that it seems like the feelings come first, but we know that is not the way it is. In a way, that is why there is psychology. We all, everyone of us, have our own personal theories about how we work and what makes us tick. Psychology's job is to figure out what and how we humans really operate. Almost all of us believe that we feel something first before we think about it. However, one of the things we know from psychological experiments is that it is just the opposite.

C: Are you telling me that my feelings aren't real; that I should just ignore them.

T: No your feelings are real, and I don't want you to ignore them. I want you to understand where they come from and how to have control over them.

C: But I can't control my feelings. They just come over me. All my life I've been trying to control my feelings and do what everybody else wants me to do. I've got to do what I feel.

T: But you sometimes feel ways that are unpleasant. Do you want to be trapped by those feelings?

C: No. I . . . I . . .

T: I think you are confusing being in control of your own life with having to let your emotions rule you. Letting your emotions rule you is just the same as losing your freedom to people. I think, also, that is what you like about the medication. It changes how you feel without you having to do anything. That is just a trap too, and you are not in control of it anymore. You do not have to behave just like you feel. Feelings and behaviors are different channels of being. You can behave and think differently than you feel. In point of fact, that is the key to good mental health. At first, it doesn't seem too real or easy to do, but with a lot of practice it becomes second nature. It is like playing a musical instrument. Have you ever played an instrument, or taken lessons?

C: Yes, piano.

T: Do you remember what it was like when you first started to take piano lessons? You felt awkward at first. But then after a while, the movements become smoother and eventually you do not even have to think about what you are doing. You are just on automatic pilot.

C: Yeah, you're right.

T: Managing our emotions, thinking, and behavior is just the same. You need to learn what thoughts lead you to feel certain ways and behave in certain ways. Then you can learn to analyze your thoughts so that the faulty ones can be removed. Then we will work on helping you to replace the distorted thoughts with rational thoughts. What makes all of this a little bit difficult is that our thoughts can occur so quickly we do not even realize they are happening. That is what gives us the feeling that we just feel things. In fact, some of our thoughts do exist at the unconscious level. In a sense we do not even have to think them. They are so deeply etched in our memories that we just take those ideas for granted. When we are growing up, particularly during our first 5 to 8 years, we learn attitudes about ourselves and others, particularly our parents, that are stored in our memories as undeniable beliefs. The problem is that a lot of times those beliefs are wrong. Usually those beliefs are tied to very important issues in life. For instance, I think that because you were adopted, and because your parents show more attention to your brother, you believe deep down inside of you that you are unlovable. That no matter what you do the people you want to love you will not give you the love you need. That basic belief colors everything you see in the world. There is a lot more to you than just this, but it does explain why you got involved in a relationship that sounds truly terrible. I think you just wanted to be loved by anybody, and it seemed someone like Rex was the only type of person who would care about you.

C: Why would anybody want to love me. Even he doesn't love me. He just wants to use me.

T: Once we have a clearer understanding of both your conscious and unconscious beliefs and thoughts about why you are in the relationship with Rex, I think you will be in a better position to decide what you want to do about the relationship. There is a lot of work to do, however. I would like to schedule for us to meet twice a week in order to really get you moving quickly. What do you think?

C: That sounds okay. I really feel like I need to talk and get things straightened out.

T: I do want you to discontinue taking the Xanax. As long as you have it around, you are in danger of overdosing again.

C: Okay.

T: After we are done here, I will have you talk to a psychiatrist colleague of mine to determine the best way to wean you off the medication. At the dosages you have been taking it is not wise for you to just discontinue. What we usually do is to move the client to valium, which is safer, in many ways, and then to take you off of it slowly.

C: I think I'm ready to stop it. I would like to get back to being me.

T: I do not tend to work for years with clients. I would like us to think about working for 3 months. At twice a week that would give us about 24 sessions. We can accomplish a lot in 3 months. However, you are not going to feel better right away or steadily get better. You will have some good days and some bad days for awhile. Our moods always seem to cycle. Just realize that because you have a bad time down the road does not mean you are getting worse again. There will be ups and downs.

C: I think I can handle it.

T: Okay, as your first homework assignment I want you to buy a copy of this book on the way home right after this session. It is called *Feeling Good*, by David Burns. I think you will be able to find it in just about any bookstore. It is like a manual for therapy. By reading it you will understand where we are going with therapy, and it will give you additional information on some of the homework assignments I will be giving you. I would like you to read the first three chapters before our next session.

Following our first session, I transcribed the session audiotape. I then reviewed the portions of the transcript in which Cathy discussed her parents, Rex, her brother, and any portion of the transcript that revealed transference phenomena. As I reviewed these interpersonal episodes, I scored them according to the procedure described by Luborsky (1984).

Cathy had a desire to be loved, taken care of, and directed. She also had an opposing desire to be independent and respected. This set of conflictual needs reflected her psychological developmental stage. Cathy was attempting to individuate from her family, but she was uncertain of her ability to function as an independent adult.

Cathy was blocked in the individuation process by tacit schema that predicted that if she acted autonomously, her parents and lover would castigate and abandon her. This schema was created by the pattern of behavior control exercised in her family. The rule was, to procure love be compliant, to be castigated and abandoned act self-reliant. Yet, she found herself aspiring to make her own life decisions. However, taking control of her life was frightening because she was not completely sure of the direction she wanted to take. She still retained a strong need for guidance. Consequently, she vacillated between obedience and depression and autonomy and anger.

The conflict produced severe anxiety. To cope with the anxiety, she often regressively wished for life to return to the period of tranquility she associated with her childhood. In order to realize this feeling, Cathy abused alcohol and drugs. Thus, Cathy had two types of reactions to these tacit schema: animosity and anger or resignation and depression. Since acting on her hostility and anger threatened her relationships, she often suppressed these reactions by abusing alcohol and drugs. However, she could also behave rebelliously. Two examples clearly delineated this coping strategy. First, she rebelled against her parents by living with Rex. Second, she acted out toward Rex by threatening suicide and becoming dangerously intoxicated.

The transcript of the first session was also evaluated according to Horowitz's (1988) Role Relationship Model analysis. This part of the assessment yielded a model of Cathy's tacit schema of self and others. In addition, this analysis revealed Cathy's expectations about significant others' actions toward her. These schema beget many of her cognitive distortions.

Cathy experienced herself as trapped in two omnibus roles in life. Some of the time she experienced herself as an "angry, incapable, and unlovable adult." When Cathy's significant others threatened to abandon her, Cathy's anxiety would increase. The elevated anxiety caused Cathy's self-perception to switch to the "downtrodden, but capable and lovable child." She was unable to consolidate her self-image because she interminably vacillated between these conflictual perceptions. Of course, these views were distortions of reality. Note that Cathy's cognitive distortion was not that everyone must love her. Cathy believed that she must allow others to domineer her to secure their love. This state of affairs was inextricably linked to depression. Entangled with this distorted cognition was another belief which declared that to act as an adult one had to be rebellious.

The therapeutic plan was targeted not only at Cathy's explicit cognitive distortions, such as "I must succeed at all tasks to be an adult, but also at tacit cognitions involving her experience of her self-identity.

FOLLOW-UP

The therapeutic work with Cathy went well. Treatment lasted for a total of 23 sessions. After 5 weeks, Cathy requested that we meet once a week. She successfully discontinued the medication, although she went through a period of resistance to giving up alcohol and sedatives. She energetically engaged in the homework assignments. Cathy became adept at recognizing her cognitive distortions, identifying their type, and refuting them. Assertiveness training plus five family sessions focusing on improved family communications enabled her to make her needs known to her parents. She broke off the relationship with Rex and moved back in with her parents for a month. Then she obtained an apartment of her own. Recently, she started her first year of college at a local university.

Cathy told me that she felt that changing her tacit distortions about her self-image was the greatest accomplishment she obtained in treatment. She described herself as no longer a slave to her emotions.

EDITORS' QUESTIONS

Q: In your introductory remarks you mention the importance of a "sound working relationship" between client and therapist, and you checked with "Cathy" regarding her comfort working with you. How might you have proceeded if, rather than being as comfortable and compliant as she was, Cathy had been difficult, resistant, or less motivated?

A: The pivotal criterion for me is whether or not the patient feels comfortable with me. If, for some reason, she had not liked or trusted me as a person, then I would have referred her to someone with whom she might get along better. On the other hand, resistance and difficulty would dictate a strategy of working through. I do not think any of us ever like to be rejected by clients, but it happens. This just has to be respected. Once, rather recently, I had a client who said she could not work with me because I have a stocky build. I really did not want to hear that! Such an issue could have been worked through, but her presenting problem was not related to this issue and she wanted brief therapy. I helped her with a referral.

Q: Applying some of the ideas of Luborsky (1984) and Horowitz (1988) to this first session and to the case, how might the therapist get entangled in Cathy's transference? Evoking related concepts, Butler, Strupp, and Binder (Chapter 5, this volume) suggest that the working through of such countertransference entanglements provides a context or crucible for the patient to have a corrective emotional experience. Was this part of the work done with Cathy? How so?

A: Yes, it is possible for the therapist to become entangled in Cathy's transference issues; I did. In the cognitive psychology literature, transference is referred to as the feedforward mechanism. We do not just take in the environment passively. We feedforward expectations for others' responses and our own responses onto ongoing interpersonal transactions. By and large, the phenomenon of the feedforward mechanism captures the phenomenon of transference and more. Indeed, Cathy alternatively reacted to me in the roles of "child" and "adult". Her behavior actually served as data to validate the assessment. I took these behavioral expressions as an opportunity to teach her about her tacit cognitive schema. I think the sessions ended up looking much like classic short-term psychodynamic therapy. The structure of the sessions, the assignment of homework, and the role-playing exercises give a different look. I find it of great interest that research in cognitive psychology and some aspects of object relations theorizing are converging. So, in answer to your question, working with the transference is a critical part of my work. Interpersonal behavior within sessions is a chance for behavior modification, par excellence.

Q: In the first session you recommended to the patient meeting twice a week for 3 months. Why that number? What is the rationale for the length and frequency of sessions? If a patient seems to be doing well quickly, will you still proceed with 24 sessions?

A: In general, I have found that 24 to 25 sessions is a good time frame for my patients and I to work in. I started Cathy with twice-weekly sessions because of the severity of her depression and the suicidal risk. I tend to schedule no more than two sessions per week in order to prevent too much regression; at least not in the short-term therapy mode. As soon as the patient and I feel he or she has reached the goal, we plan for termination. I have had clients reach their goal in four sessions. It depends on what the client needs.

Q: The elasticity and robust quality of your approach are evident in your multimodal use of assertiveness training and family sessions in addition to your individual work with the patient. What were some of the considerations with this patient that led you to directly involve her parents? What if her parents were not available?

A: In part, I wanted to assess the parents for what I call a "fascism" factor. If they had been unreasonable people I would have accepted that rebellion was the only solution to Cathy's individuation crisis. Luckily, they were not evil people determined to trap her in the family forever; overinvolved with Cathy and stuck in their own problems, but not bad parents.

Also, I felt that Cathy needed support and modeling in her attempts at adult conflict resolution. Bringing her parents into the sessions provided a marvelous behavioral laboratory to teach her skills as well as speed up the process.

If they had not been willing to come in, I would have role-played possible solutions for Cathy to try with them. However, I would have always felt that I was in the dark about her family reality.

Q: In the case presented, if the patient had not responded well, what are some of the issues you might consider? How might you change your approach? If she had resisted discontinuing her medication or had gotten more depressed without it, what might you have done?

A: Therapy just about always starts with enthusiasm. It is when the real day-to-day work starts that clients become lethargic. Therapy is like any other learning situation in life. We start out enthusiastic, but then the requirements of discipline and delay of gratification set in. I assume this will happen in every case. There is always a point when a discussion of the process of change is necessary. Following from M. Scott Peck, I call this part of therapy the presentation of the "Great Truths"—life is hard, it requires accepting responsibility for yourself and your wishes, it requires delaying gratification, and it requires discipline. These are the prerequisites for learning and living.

When I talk about changing cognitive structure, I mean really changing cognitive structure. The client's world view needs to be modified to a healthy adult perspective.

I expected Cathy to become more depressed; she did. In fact, she sporadically used alcohol and other drugs during the first several months of therapy. I used these events to illustrate for her the types of coping strategies (defense mechanism) she habitually used in certain stressful situations. Everything the client does is fodder for the therapeutic mill. My perspective is, I cannot lose. Every behavior, thought, and emotion fits into the pattern. The issue becomes how I can best help the client to see and understand the pattern and the tacit cognitive schema that dictate it. Next, I try to teach the client to become an expert self-monitor of his or her schema and patterns. If we get this far, then the goal becomes inhibiting the interpersonal responses to the schema and attempting new solutions.

The increased depression means we are on the right track. I do not change directions; I try to practice discipline and delay of gratification for myself. One of the reasons I am proud of the type of work I do is that it is difficult and requires so much discipline.

Q: How did you become a brief therapist?

A: My focus has always been short term. This is probably best explained by my theoretical orientation and my first job. Originally, I was trained in a traditional behavioral therapy framework. That approach has always emphasized a short-term focus. In addition, my first job was at the Pennsylvania State University Counseling Center. There, as in most university counseling centers, the accent was on brief therapy. Consequently, I have always taken the brief therapy view as the primary approach to treatment.

It is only after many years of working in a psychiatric outpatient department that I have seen the utility of long-term supportive psychotherapy. I think that brief treatment is the preferred approach to achieve substantial change for clients. It is only when the client is very fragile that I move to a long-term treatment plan.

ACKNOWLEDGMENT

Preparation of this chapter was facilitated by NIDA grant 1P50DA7697-01.

REFERENCES

Bandura, A. (1977a). Self-efficacy: Towards a unifying theory of behavior change. *Psychological Review, 84*, 191–215.
Bandura, A. (1977b). *Social learning theory.* Englewood Cliffs, NJ: Prentice-Hall.
Bandura, A. (1985). Model of causality in social learning theory. In M. Mahoney & A. Freeman (Eds.), *Cognition and psychotherapy* (pp. 81–100). New York: Plenum Press.

Beck, A. T. (1967). *Depression: Clinical, experimental, and theoretical aspects*. New York: Hoeber.

Beck, A. T. (1970). Cognitive therapy: Nature and relation to behavior therapy. *Behavior Therapy, 1*, 184–200.

Beck, A. T. (1976). *Cognitive therapy and the emotional disorders*. New York: International Universities Press.

Beck, A. T., Rush, A. J., Shaw, B. F., & Emery, G. (1979). *Cognitive therapy of depression*. New York: Guilford Press.

Beck, A. T., Ward, C. H., Mendelson, M., Mock, J. E., & Erbaugh, J. K. (1961). An inventory for measuring depression. *Archives of General Psychiatry, 4*, 561–571.

Burns, D. J. (1980). *Feeling good: The new mood therapy*. New York: William Morrow.

Ellis, A. (1962). *Reason and emotion in psychotherapy*. New York: Lyle Stuart.

Freeman, A. (1990). Cognitive therapy. In A. S. Bellack & M. Hersen (Eds.), *Handbook of comparative treatments for adult disorders* (pp. 64–87). New York: Wiley.

Horowitz, M. J. (1988). *Introduction to psychodynamics: A new synthesis*. New York: Basic Books.

Kendall, P. C., & Bemis, K. M. (1984). Cognitive–behavioral interventions: Principles and procedures. In N. S. Endler & J. M. Hunt (Eds.), *Personality and the behavioral disorders* (2nd Ed.) (pp. 1069–1109). New York: Wiley.

Lazarus, A. (1976). *Multimodal behavior therapy*. New York: Springer.

Luborsky, L. (1984). *Principles of psychoanalytic psychotherapy: A manual for supportive–expressive treatment*. New York: Basic Books.

Mahoney, M. J. (1977). Reflections on the cognitive–learning trend in psychotherapy. *American Psychologist, 32*, 5–13.

Mahoney, M. J. (1985). Psychotherapy and human change processes. In M. J. Mahoney & A. Freeman (Eds.), *Cognition and psychotherapy* (pp. 3–48). New York: Plenum Press.

Mahoney, M. J. (1991). *Human change processes: The scientific foundations of psychotherapy*. New York: Basic Books.

Meichenbaum, D. (1977). *Cognitive behavior modification*. New York: Plenum Press.

Piaget, J. (1926). *The language and thought of the child*. New York: Harcourt, Brace.

Turner, R. M. (1983). Cognitive-behavior therapy with borderline patients. *Carrier Foundation Letter, 88*, 1–4.

Turner, R. M. (1988). The cognitive–behavioral approach to the treatment of borderline personality disorders. *International Journal of Partial Hospitalization, 5*, 279–289.

Turner, R. M. (1989). Case study evaluation of a bio-cognitive–behavioral approach for the treatment of borderline personality disorder. *Behavior Therapy, 20*, 477–489.

Turner, R. M. (in press-a). Cognitive therapy for the borderline patient: Cogito ergo sum. In A. Freeman & F. Datillio (Eds.), *Cognitive therapy casebook*. New York: Plenum Press.

Turner, R. M. (in press-b). The utility of psychodynamic techniques in the practice of cognitive–behavior therapy. *Journal of Integrative and Eclectic Psychotherapy*.

Therapy with Direction

MICHAEL D. YAPKO

My approach is a direct consequence of having carefully considered these two questions: What, if anything, do all the various approaches to psychotherapy have in common? What must any approach to psychotherapy do if it is to be successful in alleviating client distress?

My response to these questions is this: Each approach must interrupt existing problematic patterns and build new ones that are more adaptive and life enhancing. Thus, my definition of psychotherapy is a simple one: pattern interruption and pattern building (Yapko, 1988). Where the various therapies differ dramatically is in the content of patterns on which they focus as the targets for intervention. For example, cognitive therapy focuses on interrupting limiting thought patterns ("cognitive distortions") and building new ones ("rational thinking") (Beck, 1967; Beck, Rush, Shaw, & Emery, 1979). Interpersonal psychotherapy focuses on relationship patterns, while behavioral therapy focuses on patterns of behavior (Klerman, Weissman, Rounsaville, & Chevron, 1984).

Although the content of therapies may differ dramatically, the underlying structure remains pattern interruption and pattern building. Likewise, the content of a client's problem is one dimension of consideration, while the structure of the problem is another dimension to consider. In my practice, the structure of the problem is the focal point of treatment; the associated content is used merely as a means for identifying the underlying structure. Thus, the emphasis is not on abstract issues but on the specific patterns underlying those issues, whether they be cognitive, affective, relational, behavioral, contextual, or physiological.

A MULTIDIMENSIONAL DISSOCIATIVE MODEL

A fundamental element of my model is the role of dissociation in the client. Dissociation is likely to be present to one degree or another in at least two ways. First, clients experience their symptoms as happening to them as a result of some unknown and consciously uncontrollable mechanism. The automatic nature of the symptomatic patterns represents a dissociative experience (Gilligan, 1987). Second, clients often already have skills and resources that they could, in theory, use to resolve their problems (Zeig, 1980). However, these resources are not available to the individual in the context(s) where he or she needs them—they are dissociated (Lankton & Lankton, 1983). The clinician's role, therefore, is to associate the desired resource to the appropriate context through the mechanisms of the therapy.

THE HYPNOTIC FRAMEWORK

The best framework for understanding client problems and therapeutic solutions is rooted in an in-depth knowledge of hypnosis (see Yapko, 1990). The hypnotic model identifies and characterizes virtually all of the essential components of both individual and interpersonal dynamics of therapeutic relationships. Any therapist skilled in communicating ideas can be observed to utilize aspects of hypnosis, even without recognizing it as such. Skilled communication requires using words and gestures to deliberately convey meaningful ideas. The hypnotic and strategic work of Milton H. Erickson is a powerful influence on my ideas and techniques, particularly his emphasis on the therapeutic use of what he called the "everyday trance" and the role of active, experiential learning (Erickson & Rossi, 1979, 1981; Rossi, 1980). Such methods require utilization of communication skills encompassing interpersonal dynamics (acquiring rapport, joining the client's frame of reference, utilizing client values and interests, defining the relationship as collaborative, communicating respectfulness and an intention to help, etc.) and an appreciation of individual subjective experience (the various individual patterns regulating the client's experience and his or her relevant utilizable resources).

The emphasis in a therpeutic intervention is on changing the client's experience in some way (Haley, 1973). Thus, in addition to the obvious exchange of ideas and outlooks between clinician and client (reframing), I view the role of the therapist as being the agent of therapeutic change who actively creates contexts for change. Creating a context for change means creating situations that interrupt existing client patterns and require the development of new ones that will prove more self-enhancing or self-valuing. Thus, two main methods of intervention are utilized: hypnosis (formal or informal, direct or indirect), with an intent to associate and/or reassociate dissociated resources, and directives, for the purpose of sending the client out in the "real" world to experiment (discover, challenge, confirm, disconfirm, etc.) with behaviors, relationships, perceptions, or whatever aspects of the individual are self-limiting. Simultaneously, of course, as the person has a pattern interrupted, the suggestion is present for an alternative way of responding that will be more useful (pattern building).

An emphasis of my approach is on results—an ability for the client to demonstrate new patterns in conjunction with a flexibility (selectivity) to know when and when not to employ the new pattern(s). Likewise, the client learns that his or her "old" patterns are not so much the problem as much as their rigid usage in inappropriate contexts simply for lack of a better, more effective response (Samko, 1986).

In sum, the key elements of my approach are the emphasis on the structure of client problems (how they do what they do rather than why) and the use of both hypnosis and directives to interrupt relevant dysfunctional patterns and build adaptive ones. While the majority of my interventions can be categorized as brief (ranging from 1 to 20 sessions), even in longer-term therapies I am using the brief therapy tactics associated with my outcome (skill-building) orientation.

GOALS FOR THE FIRST SESSION

Although virtually every session represents a potential turning point in the therapy, no session is as powerful in shaping the things to come as the first session. In this first meeting, I have a specific agenda of things to accomplish, none of which interferes with the spontaneity and normal flow of interaction one would want and hope for.

Specifically, I want to accomplish the following:

1. A comfortable rapport with the client, one that shows a mutual ability to be concerned, respectful, focused, intent on helping, serious, playful, and all the other components of a high-quality relationship.
2. A clarity about the client's frame of reference—interests, values, goals, and relevant resources I may want to access and mobilize, history of previous attempts at changing the presented problems, and interpretations and attributions about the problem.
3. A definition of our collaborative working relationship—my role as actively teaching and organizing resources for learning, the client's role as an experimenter with new or different patterns.
4. A building of expectancy—a future orientation that lets the

client know that the future will be different and better than the present or the past has been in some way.

5. A framing and reframing of the presented problem, having translated it (and negotiated it) into something treatable and changeable.
6. A clear impression of the level of distress of the client; hypnosis may be employed right away in the first session if it will help interrupt the experience of anxiety (or pain or rumination) and provide some immediate symptomatic relief.
7. A clear sense of priorities and sequence of the therapy process; which things to focus on first (because they are more urgent or are more likely to change and instill a sense of confidence or hopefulness) and which things can wait; which resources are immediately accessible and which need to be constructed; how direct or indirect I will need to be in my approach; how pervasive or compartmentalized the problematic patterns are; and how intra- or interpersonal the interventions need be.

My goals of treatment come from the client; how I help the person reach those goals is the product of how I conceptualize what he or she tells me, how I understand the structure of both the problem and the solution, and how skillfully I can identify the patterns to interrupt and the patterns to build (and do so).

Each of my therapy sessions is approximately 75 minutes in length. In the following edited transcript, I present portions of my first session with a client that illustrate many of the points that have been presented in this section.

CASE ILLUSTRATION

Lisa is a 29-year-old female who was referred for individual psychotherapy by the organizational psychologist at her worksite. I rarely consult with those who refer clients to me prior to my first meeting with a new client. The reason is a simple one: I do not want to be biased by the impressions of another when I conduct my interview. I want to arrive at my own impression of the individual without specific facts or diagnostic labels to (potentially) skew my perceptions. Thus, I had virtually no knowledge of Lisa or her circumstances prior to our meeting. Lisa arrived on time, and immediately began by asking for permission to tape our first session, having heard that I often tape my therapy sessions for the client's benefit. Naturally, permission was given, and the session began.

The First Session

Lisa: I was referred by [the organizational psychologist]; he's done some team building [with us]. He thought that a few sessions with you would put me on the right track. [He tells me that] I am the Queen of Dissociation. That's my forte. I just want to understand why and then I want to stop doing it. He also thinks that I'm blocking out a part of me—there's a part of me that's missing. Almost an intuitive side, he said. It could have something to do with a church that I went to long ago—it could be a hundred things. But, he knows that there's a part of me that was missing—that I was shutting off, and he thought it would be good if I got in touch with that. So, that's originally why I made the appointment. Since then, my life has fallen apart. Work is not bad for me; it's less stress than home. I'm in the midst of probably going through a divorce. (Briefly becomes teary-eyed) I'm not quite sure what to do about it. I've been to a marriage counselor three times with my husband—we're learning. I'm reading a book on codependency—it's interesting. I feel like I have a thousand issues in my head running around, and I can't focus in on them, I can't figure them out, which is unusual for me. I'm analytical. I can lay it all out, look at the facts, make a decision, and go with it. But now I can't—there's too much going on. So, you're going to help me sort out some of that!

Lisa informs me of the source of the referral and the reason for the referral. She presents his label for her behavior to me—the "Queen of Dissociation." What that means will need to be defined, but it is already noted that she has accepted that label enough to use it to describe herself. Labels are inherently self-limiting, so it will be necessary to delabel Lisa and instead focus on her experience.

Lisa could send me fishing for a cause like the church, but there is no need for me to do so since the goal is to focus on structure, not content.

Lisa indicates divorce is likely, but in a resistant manner. I do not yet know whether her hesitation is because she is ambivalent about divorce or truly wants one and just hasn't found the right reason yet.

This is a good description of the need to have a new structure for decision making besides what she currently does. Her current strategy results in confusion, not clarity.

Lisa describes herself as normally an analytical person. Whether that is true or not, it is clear that she has approached the resolution of her problems to this point in too global a manner to ever reach a clear decision.

Lisa defines my role as a collaborator, a realistic definition I accept.

The emphasis is on action from the start.

Therapist: And get through what needs to be gotten through.

L: Yes.

T: Where do you want to start? Marriage?

L: Yes.

T: You said that basically work is going okay?

L: Yes.

T: So, that's not an area that requires immediate attention?

L: No. I'm dealing with work. It's a hell of a lot less stressful than home. I've come to deal with the problems at work and kind of put them all on the right track, I think. So, that's going on alright. Boy, a brief overview of the marriage. . . . I've been married . . .

T: Well, before you go into that, I'm still trying to figure out areas [of concern], Marriage sounds like a first priority. But, there's one thing you said that I need to ask about: How does someone earn the title "Queen of Dissociation?" What does one do to deserve that title?

L: For a long time, I have been able to take myself out of a situation emotionally, stand back and look at it, and I always thought that that was a bonus. Being able to logically look at something rather than be an emotional wreck through it and not be able to do anything.

T: That's what you're calling dissociation?

Priorities must be established for where to begin our work. This models the skill of sequencing to Lisa from the very beginning of our relationship, a vital skill in effective problem solving, especially since she is confused and thinking globally about the "thousand issues in her head."

Clarifying priorities in terms of degrees of immediacy.

Resources Lisa used to resolve her problems at work will need to be identified and utilized (if they can help). Associating those resources to the context of her marriage may be a viable therapeutic strategy.

I purposely delayed Lisa from jumping into describing the marriage. Until I had some definition of her label "Queen of Dissociation," I would be unable to understand *how* she approaches the emotional issues of her marriage. Knowing *how* she would be likely to process information is important before I start to provide any.

Lisa defines dissociation as an ability "to take myself out of a situation emotionally, stand back and look at it." With that definition, she is describing an eminently useful capability. It leads to the obvious conclusion that she is simply misapplying that capability relative to the demands she faces in her marriage. Here is the "rigidity" that Erickson described as the typical basis for people's problems: rigidly applying a pattern in contexts where it is ineffective. The goal of facilitating Lisa's flexibility in dissociating from others selectively is now clear.

I want some definition of how she experiences herself, shifting away from a label that does not mean very much.

L: Well, that's what [the organizational psychologist] called it. Instead of participating and getting in there and feeling and being active in life, as a protection for myself I'm backing off, I'm dissociating. I'm not in there playing the game.

Lisa again lets me know the label was given to her by someone she assumed had the necessary expertise to make such a diagnosis. His label is a rigid one that does not serve her in any meaningful way. Her acceptance of the label is most probably an indication of her confusion about her problems.

T: You're doing that all the time, or you're doing that only in difficult situations?

How generalized or situation specific is this pattern she is calling "dissociation"? Is she doing this everywhere with everybody, or is she just emotionally pulled back in her marriage? Just how rigid a pattern is it?

L: I don't know. I do it a lot, I think. He thought it might have something to do with being hurt a lot—and that this is some sort of survival mechanism. I don't know. I had sort of a normal childhood; it had its ups and downs.

The organizational psychologist's labeling her and then suggesting reasons for the label is clearly not to her advantage, since it leads her to focus on her childhood, which is not relevant to interrupting and building patterns.

T: Some people just call it "being logical," not dissociated.

Here I test how attached she has become to the label in order to determine how much resistance I will encounter to removing it.

L: Yes.

T: Why isn't it?

L: I don't know. It might be.

T: How is it a problem?

She lets me know she is not very attached to the label.

L: [The organizational psychologist] told me it's a problem for me because I'm not participating, I'm not feeling.

T: Participating in what?

L: I guess maybe I'm just dissociating in the wrong situations and associating in the wrong situations and to the wrong people. There's one girl at work who I should be dissociating from and really closing her off. She's the one who can say things that really reach down and hurt me. She's the type of person who I shouldn't care what her opinion is and I should be dissociated from her and gap her off. I'm learning to do that. Maybe I need to associate more with people who are close to me and get in and feel what is going on. Rely on what I'm feeling, instead of putting up a wall.

Now Lisa has begun to recognize the label has more flexibility than previously realized—that it is more a situational reaction than a stable personality trait. She offers the example of being too attached to a coworker—disconfirming her title "Queen of Dissociation."

Lisa misinterprets her experience; she doesn't yet realize she is describing herself as too close to the situation rather than too detached from it.

T: Now you're telling me about a different problem. There the problem isn't one of dissociation. That's a question of context: When is the right time to dissociate, and when is the wrong time? The ability is okay, now we need to talk about where to use it and when to use it. That's a different kind of problem, isn't it?

I redefine for her what dissociation means while clarifying for her that dissociation is not inherently good or bad; it's a capability that can be applied well or poorly depending on context and the outcomes derived. This is a reframe.

L: Yes, it is. I'm trying to remember exactly what [the organizational psychologist] told me. Maybe it is the problem, and maybe it isn't. I always thought that was sort of an advantage in life.

Lisa grasps the notion that the value of dissociation is context determined.
Lisa is detaching from the label, paving the way for redefining her experience of herself.

T: Depending on the situation—it is. I think that you would like me in this situation to be detached and be a good observer and be objective about you and not get all emotional about you. Wouldn't you?

Reframing dissociation from negative to positive when used appropriately in a given context.

L: Right.

T: So, it's to my advantage to be distant—not nonsupportive and not cold, but far enough away to be able to see what's going on. So, am I dissociated right now if I do that?

Using our interaction as a concrete example of a context where detachment is not only desirable but necessary.
Facilitating the redefinition of dissociation.

L: I don't know—this is your job.

T: Am I dissociated in doing it?

L: No.

T: Am I cut off from my feelings?

L: No.

Encouraging Lisa to reframe her view of dissociation in light of our interaction. This paves the way for being able to later resolve feelings of detachment from her marriage more easily.

T: Am I unable to function well in the situation?

L: No. I think you function fine. That's interesting . . .

T: Well, obviously, I'm throwing a monkey wrench at what you're telling me for a specific reason: If you label yourself "Queen of Dissociation" and then you turn around and say that

A clear, conscious-level explanation of why I am poking at her rigid and negative view of dissociation. Lisa had previously stated she is analytical, indicating a preference there's something pathological about that, it will hurt you unnecessarily. It's a given that you have an ability to dissociate—and it's a good ability depending on where you use it. To be dissociated from your husband. . . . Well, how could you be unemotional to someone you've been attached with and invested in?

L: I don't know how I do it.

T: Is that why tears came to your eyes when you said you were going to get a divorce? Is that dissociation—unfeeling and uninvolved?

L: It's off and on.

T: Well, again, that's a different issue: You're not all of one or all of another.

L: Nobody really is.

T: Some people are. Healthy people aren't. What control is about and what health is about is knowing when to hold back and when to get involved.

L: Having the discretion to know what to do.

T: Selectivity. Being able to know that here's a situation where if I respond to my feelings, I'm going to machine gun 5,000 people; and here's a situation that if I don't respond to my feelings, I'm going to miss the fact that I'm really angry and not say anything to this person and then they're going to keep doing this to me.

L: So, I need to learn discretion?

for clarity and understanding, which I accept and utilize.

I reiterate that the value of dissociation is context determined, and then focus on the context of her marriage, where the dissociation is viewed as a problem.

A gentle challenge to her notion that she is dissociated from her feelings, when clearly she is not as emotionally detached as she seems to think. The rigid nature of her views needs to be made more flexible.

Lisa now acknowledges she is not fully detached from her circumstances, which is certainly different than where she began the session. It is now changeable, not fixed.

Confirming her now modified viewpoint of herself as a more accurate representation of her experience.

Educating Lisa to the fact that being fully dissociated *is* possible, but that she is not. The suggestion is implicit that she is more balanced and healthy than she has thought. A goal is established of learning to respond to each situation on its own merits rather than with a rigid pattern.

Lisa accepts the suggestion for that goal.

Offering "selectivity" as a goal and giving it definition through the example of sometimes responding to feelings and sometimes not, depending on the outcome it will likely lead to. This is the first suggestion of using an outcome (future) orientation in her decision-making process.

Lisa asks for clarification regarding the goal.

T: Well, at this point, I'm still trying to understand exactly what you mean by dissociation. But, I'm certainly raising the question of is it what you say it is?

L: I never knew what is was until I talked to [the organizational psychologist] and this is what he pointed out.

One last round of questioning to confirm that the "Queen of Dissociation" has reframed the label and associated experience.

This statement clearly reflects the potential dangers associated with dealing with labels rather than experience. It highlights how easily a pathological identity can be created and reinforced.

T: What he may be saying to you is that you're pulled back at times when it's to your disadvantage, and that you're too invested at times when it's to your disadvantage.

Reinforcing the redefinition of her dissociative experience as a question of how well it is applied in a given context.

L: Definitely too invested at times when it's to my disadvantage. I see that and I realize that. I probably do it in the reverse as well . . .

Lisa has clearly accepted the reframing and now is aware that she is not dissociated, but may be too much or not enough dissociated in response to specific life circumstances to her own detriment.

T: How long have you been married and what is the current situation?

Since her marriage is her first priority. I now proceed with obtaining information about this part of her life. It is predictable that she will now deal with the marital issue more realistically since "dissociation" has been redefined and associated to *any* context as a potentially useful resource.

L: I've been married 4 years. My husband's in the service, he's 26 and I'm 28. He's from the South, Alabama in particular, he moved out here and joined the service, we met after he was in the service for a year, we eloped to Lake Tahoe and got married. What basically started this whole mess was that he was transferred to sea duty—he went away for 3 months—came back and life was fine —no big deal, no changes. I missed him, he missed me. I was productive when he was gone. I lost weight. I exercised, I did my own thing. It was great! Five or 6 months later, he's going out for 6 more months. That 6 months was so utterly and drastically different from the first 3 months. We didn't do much in way of preparation, because he had already been gone earlier in the year and it was no big deal. So, we kind of assumed that him being gone for 6 months was no big deal. It was a disaster! (1) I changed, he changed. . . . I met someone while he

Lisa highlights in a general way that she has the resources necessary to manage her life independently. These are resources I may build on later in the event of a separation or divorce.

(1) Lisa's vision of the future is clearly a restricted one; she simply

was gone that started out as a friendship and slowly grew into something more. We never did sleep together, it was more of an emotional bonding. (2) It was someone I cared about, I don't know this person real well, I'm not tossing my marriage aside for this person. But I have a lot of confusion and a lot of dilemmas to solve as far as that goes. (3) . . . After meeting this other person, it opened up a lot of emotional needs that I had. I realized that I was very lonely and that I needed someone to talk to and this person was very interesting; he had a different outlook on life. (4) But most of all, this person was able to give me feedback which my husband doesn't do. (5) . . . It felt really good to have somebody who's almost on the same wavelength—I'm not saying my husband's stupid, he's not, he's a kind and wonderful human being, but he's different. He doesn't participate in that kind of conversation. He talks about the rodeo. He doesn't know anything about psychology. He's just different than I am. (6) I didn't realize that I really missed that until I talked and met this other person. . . . What I really want is to be happy and and if being happy to me means ending my marriage—that's what I should do. (7)

assumed an extension of the current situation, and did not anticipate any potential changes from an extended separation. This lack of a detailed future orientation amplifies any here-and-now problems and can lead to a trapped ("stuck") feeling, which Lisa experienced.

(2) The external factor of having met someone else undoubtedly was the catalyst for Lisa's surge in ambivalence about her marriage. Lisa further demonstrates a pattern of a high level of reactivity to external feedback (as suggested by her absorbing the label given by the organizational psychologist).

(3) Lisa's need for contact permitted her to establish a new relationship, which provided immediate gratification for many different needs. Her subjective feelings for this other man are her focal point, since she can acknowledge that objectively she really doesn't know him very well. Following her feelings in this context may be a poor strategy for deciding her future.

(4) The immediacy and power of the new relationship amplified Lisa's awareness that she could now get needs met that had previously been dissociated from her marital relationship.

(5) Lisa makes comparisons between her husband and the other man—a dysfunctional strategy for decision making since each currently has qualities she likes. Instead of making decisions about them by comparing them, she will need to orient to the future and the likelihood either one has for fulfilling her changing needs and desire of growth within a relationship.

(6) She claims he is just "different" but clearly devalues her husband's characteristics.

(7) Lisa suggests that she make the decision to divorce on the basis of whether it will make her happy,

yet she is so tied in to her ambivalent feelings in the *present* that she has not realistically assessed whether divorcing will, in fact, lead to happiness.

Lisa is oriented to the need to think beyond the feelings of the moment as the primary means for overcoming ambivalence. Guilt holds her back and fear keeps her from moving forward decisively. The solution is to go beyond the feelings of the moment in order to examine whether the consequences of a divorce will justify its undertaking.

T: The reason people end their marriage is because of what's going to happen afterwards. Now, that part you can control. When people get married, it's with the idea, "We're in love, we're always going to feel this way." Well, statistically, 70% of the marriages in California end up in divorce. So, that feeling doesn't stay with a lot of people, but no one says, "Gee, divorce is great!" Now, in this particular case, your husband hasn't knocked you around, he hasn't been a bad guy, he hasn't done anything wrong, he's just been him. . . .

It is suggested to Lisa that she approach divorce realistically, with an awareness that it is a difficult, usually painful, process.

Lisa has been looking for a dramatic enough, compelling enough reason to divorce. She must come to terms with having to make a decision to divorce according to criteria that are not extreme. Her thinking on this subject reflects a dichotomous, all-or-none style.

L: Then what makes it right for me to leave him?

Lisa wisely asks what an adequate justification for divorce is. She has not yet discovered one for herself, which has amplified her turmoil about what path to take.

T: There's only one justification: If you believe that you are better off without him than with him. . . .

She is told she must look to the future for an answer.

L: I don't know that.

She has been so oriented to the present turmoil, she has not considered the future in realistic detail.

T: Then, the question is: How would you know if you were better off? What could you achieve on your own or in other relationships that are not going to be possible in the context of this marriage? Now, the fact that he's a nice guy, clearly isn't enough for you, because if it was, you wouldn't have mixed feelings about it. You'd say, "He's a nice guy. I'm sold. I'm happy." It's clearly not

Lisa is provided with specific questions to ask herself to help her project into the future as a strategy for overcoming her uncertainty. In doing so, she must take more variables into account than just superficial compatibility.

enough. What you've said is that you basically really don't like a guy very much that you don't respect a lot. And that respect in someone really matters to you.

Feeding back to her statements she made about what is missing in her relationship with her husband.

L: Yes it does. Can I gain that respect back?

T: How do you gain respect back for someone that you've lost it for?

L: I don't know. . . .

She now has clarity that her lack of respect for her husband's limited way of going through life (according to *her* standards) is the pivot point in making the decision to divorce. She's asked to assess the possibility of regaining respect for him, and she sees no way to do that.

T: Now, I don't have an investment in whether you're with [your husband] or whether you're with this other guy. My job is to get the questions out, get your feelings out, and ask you to deal with them in a way that's realistic. Learn how to make decisions for yourself that you're going to have to live with later. This is a situation, I can tell you right now, where there is no correct path. You're going to end up having to make whatever happens—work. Your marriage is never going to be the same as it was. So, unless you have a new goal of figuring out a way to make the relationship livable and [future] growth oriented in some way, [then it doesn't stand a chance]. But, if you start to think backwards about, "Gee, what [in him] did I fall in love with?"—you won't get there. [Those feelings were] 3 years ago.

I make it clear that the path is hers to choose, defining my role as facilitating clarity in her thinking with an appreciation for consequences.

The direct suggestion is made that decisions need to be made according to desired consequences.

I want Lisa to be clear this is no longer a question of right or wrong, or of moral obligation. It is a question of realistically assessing potentials—personal and intrapersonal.

A direct suggestion is made to shift the focus from the past to the future since the past cannot be recovered.

L: I need to look at who the person is now. . . .

Lisa understands she must realistically assess her husband's potentials as they exist *now*, not how she viewed them when they married 3 years ago.

T: And what his potentials are and what ability and willingness he has to develop those things in himself.

A distinction is made for Lisa between a potential and a developed resource.

L: I fell in love with his potentials, and his potentials are his dreams and there's

Lisa indicates she understands that distinction, and that she is ac-a vast difference [between his potentials and what he actually does].

T: How well can a person take his potentials and make them into something? I mean, I can take any drug addict off the street and say, "This guy's got the potential to be President." So what? In the meanwhile, he's shooting up drugs and being useless.

cepting the suggestion to respond to him as he is rather than how she wishes he would be.

Reinforcing the notion that potential is only valuable to the extent that it is developed.

L: So, I need to look at my marriage.

Lisa is now clear she must resolve issues in her marriage as a first priority, and that the other relationship must receive secondary consideration.

T: What does [your husband] want? What does he understand about what you're looking for? How much does he understand about what you value that are things that don't apparently mean a lot to him?

L: Like . . . ?

T: Take the things that you were talking about having with this other guy; the psychological awareness, the higher consciousness, the ability to articulate ideas, your ability to banter back and forth, and his ability to challenge you and stimulate you intellectually.

I now turn my attention to how Lisa can more realistically assess her husband's potential to meet her needs by specifying her interests and values relative to his. I encourage shifting frames of reference to consider the relationship from his point of view.

Identifying the specific things she had stated were important to her. Notice how her focus on her confused feelings led her to forget what she has stated matters to her.

L: That's not who [my husband] is. He cannot be that person for me.

T: Because he doesn't have that ability?

L: No. I don't think he does. . . .

She is immediately clear that her husband does not possess the desired characteristics, and most likely never will.

T: If [your husband] said to you tomorrow, "I'm out of this relationship," how long would it take you to call this other guy and say, "Guess what? . . ."

L: Not long.

I question what would happen if the decision about the fate of her marriage were made for her by her husband's leaving her. It would then make it possible for her to be with the other man without having to actively bring that about. However, I want Lisa to make the decision proactively, rather than be a victim of circumstances.

T: As long as you keep the other relationship going, it remains an option for

By keeping both relationships going, if one fails (i.e., the man you. It's a guarantee you're not going to be alone.

L: It's a guarantee of another mistake.

T: Well, there's a price tag attached to everything, isn't there?

L: (Lisa laughs) Yes. So, I'm doing this to avoid being alone?

T: I wouldn't make it quite that simple. But, it certainly allows you to keep all your options open, doesn't it? It means that if you take calculated risks and play your cards right, you get to keep both things going.

L: Gee, I don't want to keep both things going. I know that.

T: Until something comes along and makes the decision for you. I think you have a guilt streak about 3 feet wide about the way you think you're supposed to be and what the integrity thing is to do. You keep talking about what's right and what's wrong.

L: Isn't that important?

T: I think if it wasn't for the guilt factor, you would have brushed [your husband] off about 3 months ago. He's a nice guy and you don't want to hurt him. He hasn't done anything wrong, he's just being himself. That's not a good enough reason to hurt him, in your view.

L: He's not.

T: That's what would make it wrong. That's what would make you feel really guilty. So, in order to not feel really guilty, you keep it going. You're not

leaves her), she will "automatically" have the other one to go to. This may prevent her from being alone, but it is no assurance that it is the right relationship for her in the long run.

Lisa understands that point.

The metaphorical statement suggests that taking control involves absorbing the consequences, a good reason to proceed intelligently.

Lisa starts to become aware that making no decision is, in essence, a decision to maintain status quo.

I am leading Lisa to appreciate the necessity of actively making a well-considered decision she can live with rather than letting circumstances run her. Empowerment is a dominant theme in my interventions.

A direct poke at passively letting the situation deteriorate out of control through inaction. The direct message is that she is trying to stay in an unsatisfying marriage out of guilt—a poor reason to stay married. I'm also detaching her from guilt feelings so her decision can be based on what's best in the long run.

Lisa is pushed to come to terms with her true lack of interest in her husband and to resolve her guilt over wanting a divorce. She is told going to be able to avoid making the decision. Even if the decision is made for you, then all you've done is decided not to decide.

L: I have to take control. . . .

T: If you want some eventual peace. Then, you can assume you're going to go through a period of days, weeks, months of pretty [uncomfortable] feelings.

L: Okay.

T: And, expect that and understand that that is going to be part of making very intense life decisions. So, it's not unexpected, it's not inappropriate, it's not unhealthy. Given the circumstances, that's the normal reaction.

L: I sort of feel the decision has been made. I need to stop thinking in terms of what's right and what's wrong, and start thinking in terms of what works, what feels good, what's positive. . . .

T: And not just right now, because what feels badly right now, might feel good later. That's what I was talking about when I said a divorce doesn't feel good. There are times when it's the best thing that can happen to two people. I happen to be a fan of relationships—I like it when it works out. I'm not one that's quick to say, "Hey, get a divorce."

L: Toss in the towel.

T: I'm not like that. I can only tell you what I see when I see couples that are in

she can let the situation deteriorate simply by doing nothing, and that is still a decision to let things eventually come to an end, but a passive one.

Lisa becomes clear she cannot assume a passive position when all passivity does is let the inevitable deterioration take place more slowly.

Lisa is again oriented to the reality that divorce is difficult, and that she will have difficult but normal hurtful feelings to deal with.

Reinforcing that some hurtful feelings are to be expected, and reframing them as a manageable, predictable part of the process. Given Lisa's pattern of all-or-none thinking and self-doubt, I want to anticipate and prevent her from experiencing unnecessary guilt and self-blame.

Lisa is much clearer about her feelings and the direction she must take. She has learned to judge according to feasibility, not some abstract moral principle unrelated to her feelings or circumstances.

Lisa has started to realize that right and wrong are relative, not absolute, terms.

Reinforcing a future orientation and suggesting a framework for dealing with her hurtful feelings: Keep your eyes on the goal. I also think it's important for her to know that divorce is not inherently good or bad but must be evaluated according to individual circumstances. This principle helps interrupt her pattern of all-or-none thinking.

here on the verge of divorce when the factor of one person not respecting the other is there—where one person is always telling the other person, "You're not enough." No matter what that person does, it's not enough. It's just not fair to do this to this other person. The stuff that you can't stand in this guy, someone else might think is fantastic.

Another reframing to help her make her decision is to have her evaluate the effect on her husband of continually being given negative feedback. It also utilizes her desire to protect him.

I'm now associating Lisa's dissociation from her husband to a well-intentioned protectiveness of his feelings. But, in doing so, she forces herself to try care about someone she doesn't really care for, a strategy doomed to fail.

L: I'm not even sure what I don't like.

T: It doesn't have to be anything specific. Although you have been . . .

L: Very specific.(*Lisa laughs*)

T: He's dull. He's not articulate. He's not quick. He's not psychologically sophisticated. He doesn't have the level of consciousness that you would want and the kinds of interest in things that you value. That's pretty specfic.

L: Holy shit!

T: Have you heard yourself say those things? Is it a shock when you hear them back? . . .

Lisa demonstrates her global thinking about her marriage by showing how quickly she can forget (develop amnesia for) the specifics of her own complaints. This is the pattern that keeps her from being decisive; it's almost as if every time she thinks about her husband's perceived flaws, she's considering them for the first time.

Lisa is surprised to hear how specific she has been in articulating her criticisms of her husband. Her surprise is genuine and offers insight into how she ruminates about the problems without getting anywhere in her thinking.

L: I don't feel comfortable delving into a relationship with someone else and still being married to [my husband].

T: The stuff that's going to happen with [your husband] is going to happen soon. You're going to go into marriage counseling and you're going to identify what the issues are and it's going to become very clear to you whether this relationship has growth potential or whether it's

Lisa has integrated the earlier suggestions that she must first address and resolve the issues in her marriage before shifting her focus to any other relationship.

Lisa is oriented to the expectation that when she actively addresses the issues, in contrast to her previous strategy of passivity, things will begin to resolve and a direction will become clear. Her role is defined, her "boyfriend's" dead in the water. You're not going to have to wait real long to find out about that. And, if this other guy is truly supportive, he is going to give you the room to do what you need to do. When you say to him, "I'm invested in giving this marriage every chance to work that I can, so I'm not going to be able to see you for a month or two or three until I know exactly where I'm at," [hopefully] he'll say, "Do what you need to do." Take care of the stuff with [your husband], and if that relationship goes on, the other guy is out. If the marriage doesn't go on, then you can [go from there]. You can't do both at once.

role is defined, and the expectation is that she will address and resolve her marital issues.

L: That's so funny, because I knew what I had to do, I knew what was best, and I know I'll feel better doing that. Why did it take you telling me to bring that out? It's something I already knew. Why?

It is made clear to Lisa that resolving the marital issues comes first. Her need for a concrete, linear plan of action is addressed, interrupting her previous patterns of global and abstract thinking about her problems.

T: Putting it into words. It's not just vague feelings anymore. It's clear and it's objective.

L: That's also going to reduce the stress. That's going to give me 50% less bullshit to deal with so I can focus in and shift aside the rest.

Lisa is in full agreement with all that has been said and verbalizes her sense of the viability of the plans established for addressing her problems realistically. Her comments reflect how global and abstract her thinking was to the point of creating her confusion and indecision.

T: You'll still be stressed. How do you feel about all that we've talked about and what you're approaching?

The session comes to a close with Lisa expressing relief at having a clear direction.

L: Utterly enlightened. I needed to know that question.

Lisa needs to know that while having a clear direction will help alleviate some stress, she will still have some stress present simply because of the complex and volatile nature of what she is dealing with.

T: Did you get what you came for?

L: Yes. I got more than what I came for.

Creating an opportunity for Lisa to give me feedback about our session.

T: Let's meet again in 2 weeks, okay?

FOLLOW-UP

Lisa filed for divorce 5 months after our initial session. We had four more sessions in the first 2 months following this first meeting. I did not see Lisa again until 3 months later, when she came in to say she had filed for divorce. The subsequent four sessions following our first meeting involved continuing with these goals in mind:

1. Establishing more realistic expectations of others on the basis of specific criteria. Interrupting the pattern Lisa had of assuming people are more capable than they really are (Yapko, 1992a).
2. Establishing more realistic expectations of herself. Interrupting the pattern of being self-critical and lacking in acceptance for her true feelings.
3.. Establishing a greater clarity of personal boundaries. Interrupting her pattern of putting others' needs ahead of her own and trying to avoid conflict.

I continue to see Lisa on an occasional basis, such as when work problems or issues about new relationships surface.

Lisa proceeded with her divorce in a straightforward and efficient manner. By the time she filed, she was absolutely clear that her marriage had no future. Her lack of guilt and her clarity that this was the right thing for her to do made it possible to move forward with her life in a manner she continues to feel good about to this day.

SUMMARY

The approach to therapy I advocate is one that places a great emphasis on problem solving and the building of necessary resources for responding effectively to life situations. Milton Erickson rarely, if ever, talked about pathology per se. Instead, Erickson talked about rigidity as the essence of the problems our clients present to us (Zeig, 1980). The case of Lisa illustrates this point well. Lisa's rigid belief that she *should* care about her husband and *should* be committed to the marriage flew in the face of the harsher reality that she didn't really love or respect him or feel committed to the marriage.

Lisa also demonstrated how vital a part of the therapy process the negotiation of the presenting complaint is (O'Hanlon & Weiner-Davis, 1989). Lisa's label, "Queen of Dissociation," was an inappropriate and self-limiting label that precluded the more flexible recognition that *any* pattern a person holds has equal potential to help or hurt, depending on the manner and the context in which it is applied. Thus, the need for the therapist to facilitate flexibility in the client and teach the client to move beyond current circumstances remains a constant of directive therapy.

Therapy with direction presupposes a willingness to strive for specific results measurable to the extent that our clients' lives are enhanced. It is my hope that this chapter has helped to elucidate some of the concepts and techniques associated with brief therapy.

EDITORS' QUESTIONS

Q: What was the role of hypnosis in this case? How would you distinguish your approach with this patient from cognitive therapy?

A: I make a distinction between formal hypnosis and informal hypnosis (Yapko, 1990). Only in about one out of three therapy sessions will I conduct a formal hypnosis session in which I separate the hypnotic interaction from the rest of the therapy session. In this first session with Lisa, informal hypnosis was used on a constant basis in my directing her attention to perspectives and ideas that would reassociate her inner experience and encourage greater clarity about the relevant issues in her life. In later sessions, formal hypnosis was used to facilitate the process of Lisa's acquiring and utilizing relevant ideas and skills for managing her problems. It is fundamentally true that whatever can be accomplished with the use of hypnosis can also be accomplished without the use of hypnosis. Why employ hypnosis at all? For its ability to efficiently consolidate and make use of client capabilities that are dissociated and, hence, unavailable to the individual for conscious and deliberate use. Hypnosis helps an individual access and utilize the relevant resources necessary for change.

In distinguishing my approach with Lisa from cognitive therapy, I acknowledge that there is a substantial overlap with a cognitive therapy approach. Clearly, I wanted to alter the way Lisa thinks about her experience and how she forms the conclusions she reaches. A cognitive therapist would likely have wanted to do the same. Cognitive therapy places a far greater emphasis on conscious understanding and rational thought than I do. Human beings are *not* rational creatures, and though learning to think rationally is often a valuable therapeutic goal, I believe it is also of great importance to be able to skillfully organize and utilize unconscious and nonrational aspects of the person's experience within the therapeutic context.

Hypnosis is compatible with virtually any therapeutic modality. Thus, hypnosis can be used to facilitate greater clarity of thinking and a higher degree of rationality if that is the therapeutic goal. Likewise, hypnosis can be used to amplify emotionally based experiences or, for that matter, *any* experience on *any* dimension. Hypnosis is a tool for amplifying and associating experiences.

Q: Does the patient's "structural" problem change? Is this a goal of your treatment? Is her style of functioning or "personality" different on follow-up? How well are the goals described on page 173 met?

A: The question whether a client's structural problem changes relates most closely to the notion of "strategy." Clearly, there are functional and effective strategies for doing things (such as forming relationships or making business decisions), and just as clearly there are dysfunctional strategies for doing things. In the case of Lisa, the strategy (i.e., the series of steps) that Lisa followed to make decisions about which feelings to acknowledge within herself and how to best respond to those feelings only produced confusion and agitation. Thus, it was a goal of treatment to establish a new sequence of steps for making life decisions.

Lisa has, in fact, effectively evolved a new structural approach to making important decisions in her life. She now places a considerable emphasis on the value of anticipation. She now thinks well ahead of current circumstances to anticipate not only how her decision will work in the short run but also how her decision will work in the long run. Previously, she did not do this. She is now able to more realistically assess the variables that influence her decision and whether these are variables to take into serious consideration, or whether they are irrelevant to the overall goal. Thus, Lisa has established a far more effective means for making decisions that she continues to rely on. Furthermore, she recognizes that her new strategy is *a* strategy, not *the* strategy for making all decisions. After all, some decisions can and should be made on the feelings of the moment. This idea reinforces the notion of "selectivity."

Lisa has done very well in meeting the goals established for our therapy. She is now much more realistic in her assessments of other individuals. She is more aware of the need to listen and observe more closely the degree of self-awareness and congruity in others. Furthermore, Lisa has come to terms with the recognition that she cannot always do as others wish. In line with that realization, Lisa was taught ways to avoid confrontations when possible, but to manage confrontations assertively when necessary. Lisa is much more accepting of her own needs and wants as legitimate and, consequently, is also far better at establishing and maintaining her sense of personal boundaries.

Q: What do you usually tell a patient about the course and prognosis of treatment? When and how do you determine and discuss length of treatment? How do you motivate the patient?

A: I want to establish that the therapeutic relationship is a collaborative one from the outset. Thus, after a client has described his or her problem(s) to me and I have some clarity about what specific pattern(s) I am going to want to interrupt and what specific skills I'm going to want to teach, I communicate to the client that the problems that he or she is experiencing are resolvable. In various writings (Yapko, 1988, 1992a), I have made a point of describing how vital a phase building positive expectations for successful treatment is. Thus, it is important in the course of the first session to make it clear to the client that the problem has clearly defined parameters and that there is a specific plan for accomplishing resolution. The client is informed that the majority of the clients that I see are treated within a brief therapy framework, ranging from 1 to 20 sessions, and I communicate my expectation that it's likely that the person's problem can be resolved within that range.

Motivation is directly tied to expectation. The need to build a positive expectancy in the client is vital to every aspect of treatment, including whether the person even decides to seek treatment; whether the person participates meaningfully in the treatment; whether the individual will have a partial or complete recovery and a fast or slow recovery; and even what the likelihood of relapse is. The techniques for building expectancy all revolve--to one extent or another—around the use of hypnotic age progression, a general strategy of orienting the client experientially to the positive possibilities that the future holds (Yapko, 1990).

Q: You indicate using about 75 minutes per session. What guides your decisions about length of sessions, frequency, and spacing? You mention continuing to see the patient on an "occasional" basis. How long have you seen the patient overall? How many sessions approximately? What are your views about interminability and intermittency? How and when might you more definitively terminate with a patient?

A: My therapy sessions are 75 minutes in length because I simply do not like to be hurried in my interaction with the client, nor do I like to give my client the sense that the speed at which my "meter runs" is more important than the client's problems. So, the length of my sessions is purely a product of wanting to take that little bit of extra time to reaffirm to my client that he or she has my attention in more ways than one. Frequency of sessions is dictated by the urgency of the individual's circumstances and the severity of his or her symptoms. The more urgent the situation or severe the symptoms, the more likely I am to see the individual more than one time per week. Normally, I space my sessions 1 to 2 weeks apart in order to give the person ample opportunity to review the tapes of our sessions (which I routinely provide) as well as ample time to carry out the structured task assignments I routinely give clients to conduct in between sessions.

I have continued to see Lisa on an occasional basis, approximately once every 2 to 3 months. I have seen her a total of 23 times in the more than 2 years since she first consulted me. Part of Lisa's therapy was to help her recognize that she could ask for what she wanted in her relationships with others. Lisa learned the value of "reality testing" with me, wisely recognizing that no one has a firm grasp of objective reality. Rather, we only have our own subjective interpretations of life experiences. Lisa sees a positive value in intermittently seeking an outside opinion about important life decisions that she makes. I view this intermittent contact as a manifestation of Lisa's recognition that one of the ways that she can take care of herself is to seek support or advice as needed with an eye on prevention. Most of the time, people seek therapy when disaster has already occurred. Lisa's life has been smoother and more satisfying because she has the wisdom to recognize preventative opportunities by reality testing with someone she trusts. She is highly independent, yet cognizant of the value of perspectives besides her own.

I am aware that there are some clinicians who have as an ultimate goal of therapy a final termination where contact with the therapist ends. This is most likely the therapist's agenda rather than the client's. My preference is to have the client make the choice about how to best use me and my skills. The termination as a point of finality in our relationship is not encouraged as a goal, nor is it discouraged. Rather, the value of occasional contact is simply one more choice for the client to make as he or she learns how to best manage his or her own life. A time that I would be most likely to definitively terminate with a client is when there is simply no positive contribution I can make to the overall quality of this individual's life. Otherwise, I leave it open as a possibility to continue contact to whatever extent the client feels it would be helpful, but only if I am clear that the individual is using me and my skills appropriately.

Q: In the case presented, if the patient had not responded well, what are some of the issues you might consider? How might you change your approach?

A: If Lisa had not responded well to my intervention, I would immediately examine what I had missed in Lisa's presentation of her problem that I failed to respond to appropriately and meaningfully. I am utterly convinced that it is my job as the therapist to use my communication skills to make meaningful contact with my client. The hypnotic principles for establishing rapport and conducting therapy can be reduced to a very simple formula, first described by Milton H. Erickson, MD: Accepting and utilizing the client's reality (Erickson & Rossi, 1979). Thus, when a connection is not made that facilitates the therapy, I first look at my approach for any oversights or errors I may have made.

I do not believe it is valuable to think about "resistant" patients who seek therapy but "really don't want to change." I believe that the individual wants change to occur but is limited by his or her beliefs and range of available resources. Thus, it would not occur to me to blame the client for the lack of rapport or the lack of therapeutic success. If I offer ideas or task assignments to a client and he or she does not respond to them in a way that I would have liked, I take that as a comment about there having been something inappropriate about what I have said or done. Although I may have the same therapeutic goal in mind for later suggestions or assignments, I never give the same assignments twice or offer the same idea in the exact same way. Flexibility is required in continually adapting myself and my approaches to the needs of the individual client.

Q: Are there any contraindications for using hypnosis?

A: Hypnosis is a therapeutic tool. Hypnosis is not good or bad; it is neutral in value. What gives hypnosis a positive or negative valence is how it is applied. Hypnosis as a model of influential communication teaches us to recognize that our words and gestures (as our only therapeutic tools) must be carefully considered and applied in the context of treatment. There are well-considered words that are purposeful and efficient, and there are haphazard and randomly utilized communications that yield unfortunate and undesired outcomes. Using communication skillfully and therapeutically represents the artistry of therapy.

There are no contraindications for the use of hypnosis that I am aware of. There are many ways to misapply it, however. Thus, hypnosis, like therapy, is something that must be well planned and sensitively applied if it is to benefit the client.

Q: How did you become a brief therapist?

A: I remember one pivotal day when I was sitting in my advanced psychoanalytic techniques class at the University of Michigan. This was in the early 1970s—still the "hippie" era. The professor, who saw symbolism and personal unconscious motivations in *everything* made the preposterous statement that "men who wear their hair long have an unconscious wish to be women and are usually latent homosexuals." He totally ignored social context. Something snapped in me, and all of a sudden I realized that almost everything I'd been learning was nothing short of delusional. I became interested in *change*—not unprovable theories that demonstrated their lack of utility with every patient who, years later, was still suffering. I became interested in interpersonal (systemic) aspects of people's problems, seeing them as far more relevant to therapy than hypothetical intrapsychic structures. This interest led me to the innovative work of

Milton Erickson and a deep appreciation for his many contributions to making therapy brief, practical, and results oriented.

REFERENCES

Beck, A. (1967). *Depression*. New York: Harper & Row.
Beck, A., Rush, J., Shaw, B., & Emery, G. (1979). *Cognitive therapy of depression*. New York: Guilford Press.
Erickson, M., & Rossi, E. (1979). *Hypnotherapy: An exploratory casebook*. New York: Irvington Publishers.
Erickson, M., & Rossi, E. (1981). *Experiencing hypnosis: Therapeutic approaches to altered states*. New York: Irvington Publishers.
Erickson, M., Rossi, E., & Rossi, S. (1976). *Hypnotic realities*. New York: Irvington Publishers.
Gilligan, S. (1987). *Therapeutic trances: The cooperation principle in Ericksonian hypnotherapy*. New York: Brunner/Mazel.
Haley, J. (1973). *Uncommon therapy: The psychiatric techniques of Milton H. Erickson, M.D.* New York: W. W. Norton.
Klerman, G., Weissman, M., Rounsaville, B., & Chevron, E. (1984). *Interpersonal psychotherapy of depression*. New York: Basic Books.
Lankton, S., & Lankton, C. (1983). *The answer within: A clinical framework of Ericksonian hypnotherapy*. New York: Brunner/Mazel.
O'Hanlon, W., & Weiner-Davis, M. (1989). *In search of solutions: A new direction in psychotherapy*. New York: W. W. Norton.
Rossi, E. (Ed.). (1980). *The collected papers of Milton H. Erickson* (Vols. 1–4). New York: Irvington Publishers.
Samko, M. (1986). Rigidity and pattern interruption: Central issues underlying Milton Erickson's approach to psychotherapy. In M. Yapko (Ed.), *Hypnotic and strategic interventions: Principles and practice* (pp. 47–55). New York: Irvington Publishers.
Yapko, M. (1988). *When living hurts: Directives for treating depression*. New York: Brunner/Mazel.
Yapko, M. (1990). *Trancework: An introduction to the practice of clinical hypnosis* (2nd ed.). New York: Brunner/Mazel.
Yapko, M. (1992a). *Free yourself from depression*. Emmaus, PA: Rodale.
Yapko, M. (1992b). *Hypnosis and the treatment of depressions: Strategies for change*. New York: Brunner/Mazel.
Zeig, J. (1980). *A teaching seminar with Milton H. Erickson, MD*. New York: Brunner/Mazel.

COUPLE AND
FAMILY APPROACHES

Introduction to Couple and Family Brief Therapy Approaches

STEVEN FRIEDMAN
SIMON H. BUDMAN
MICHAEL F. HOYT

In this section of the book, our focus shifts to models of time-effective therapy with couples and families. Doing effective brief treatment requires that the therapist "hit the ground running." To accomplish this the therapist must negotiate a focus with the client. This task is particularly challenging when there are two or more family members in the room at the same time—who may not always agree with one another on the reasons for being there. However, having multiple family members in the same place offers the therapist an in vivo opportunity to look at relationships in the context of the "here and now."

Each of the authors whose work is represented in this section has developed specific methods and strategies for working in a time-effective manner with couples and families. Each is an expert in juggling multiple realities and in developing a collaborative alliance that allows for construction of well-formed outcomes. Although coming from varied perspectives, all of these contributions reflect the therapist's sensitivity to the issue of time. One additional element that is very important centers on the therapist's ability to introduce something novel in the initial session that captures the attention of the client or client system and provides them with a revised view of their predicament. As we will see in the following chapters, novelty comes in many forms.

In the first chapter in this section (Gurman, Chapter 9), the author provides us with an example of his pragmatic treatment approach in working with couples. Combining both an intra- and interpersonal focus, Gurman tailors his methods to the particular couple seen. His integrative model draws on elements of psychodynamic, cognitive, behavioral, and systemic/strategic therapies. In the case presented, Gurman sensitively and persistently hones in on a specific area of the couple's relationship. He is able to effectively challenge the couple's distancing maneuvers and, by so doing, enables change to occur.

Susan Johnson and Leslie Greenberg (Chapter 10) describe how they create a therapeutic context that emphasizes the emotional dance of the couple. Combining a focus on both inner processes and relationship dynamics, the therapist helps each member of the couple to reclaim his or her internal affective experience and be more vulnerable with the other. By attending to the here-and-now experience of the couple, and taking a gentle yet persistent therapeutic stance in uncovering masked emotional expression, the therapist creates a positive climate for self-observation and for restructuring of the dynamics of the couple's relationship in a time-effective manner.

The chapter by Donald Baucom, Norman Epstein, and Robert Carels (Chapter 11) describes a treatment approach based on principles of social learning theory and social exchange theory. This model incorporates and integrates both historical information and current interactional data and tailors the interventions to the specific needs of the couple. One of the therapist's goals is to identify cognitive and behavioral factors that interfere with satisfaction in the relationship and to develop interventions that will alter these patterns. In the case described, the therapist generates a novel set of tasks for the couple that utilizes their playful tendencies in creating a context for change.

Judy Davidson and William D. Lax (Chapter 12) present a consultation with a couple that exemplifies use of the reflecting process, a paradigm developed by Andersen (1987) in Norway. Utilizing a cotherapy team, the authors share with the couple their ideas and thoughts as the therapy process unfolds. This conversation between the therapists, and between the therapists and members of the couple, has as its goal to perturb the meaning system that the couple has developed about their predicament. No attempt is made to impose the therapists' hypotheses on the couple. Instead, the therapists work to understand how the couple's issues are embedded in the meaning systems they have developed and then to generate conversations that stimulate the emergence of new perspectives. Obviously, this team approach provides an intrinsically engaging format for the couple who have the opportunity to "overhear" a discussion about themselves. This chapter is an excellent example of a collaborative model in which therapist and client work together in constructing new ideas leading to change.

Following in Davidson and Lax's footsteps, Steven Friedman (Chapter 13) also emphasizes the therapeutic conversation as a medium for creating change. The case described utilizes a solution-oriented model, the "possibility paradigm," and engages the family in a reauthoring process with the aim of liberating them from their plight. Although focused on the child in the family, the therapist's interventions (especially the use of letter writing) involve the other family members in the change process. Besides being time effective, this model serves to empower the client system by amplifying strengths and avoiding pathological assumptions.

Chapter 14 (Weakland & Fisch) demonstrates the usefulness of seeing one family member (the most motivated) as a way to create change in a family system. On the basis of work developed over the past 20 years at the Mental Research Institute, the authors demonstrate how to effectively disrupt behavioral cycles using strategic interventions. The therapist employs a "minimalist" approach in activating the "customer" to vary her usual mode of behavior with her son, resulting in a positive outcome.

In the final chapter in this section (Aponte, Chapter 15), the author draws on the principles of structural family therapy. He provides a consultation that creates an immediate shift in the typical family process. His interventions evolve out of the initial family enactments he observes. Aponte successfully joins with family members and then actively challenges them to change. He disrupts the family's old routine and creates a new experience for the family in the room. This approach requires that the therapist be personally and emotionally involved in the action and be comfortable taking charge immediately in directing the flow of the session. Aponte demonstrates how the therapist, as director and facilitator, can actively and sensitively intervene in a family system to create change.

REFERENCE

Andersen, T. (1987). The reflecting team: Dialogue and metadialogue in clinical work. *Family Process*, 26, 415–428.

Integrative Marital Therapy: A Time-Sensitive Model for Working with Couples

ALAN S. GURMAN

In this chapter, I discuss some of the major aspects of Integrative Marital Therapy (IMT) that characterize its typical brevity and, in fact, require that it be carried out in a time-sensitive manner. I state the task at hand in this way because IMT was not developed to be a method of brief work with couples per se. Yet, there are some characteristics of clinical work with couples and families that render perhaps all but the most depth-oriented object relational models (e.g., Scharff & Scharff, 1987) brief by the time standards of traditional individual therapy (Gurman, 1981; Gurman & Kniskern, 1981). First, therapy focused on interpersonal problems leads to a greater emphasis on the current determinants of behavior. Second, sources of resistance to change are more readily identified in the living laboratory of couples therapy than in the less ecologically valid context of individual therapy. Third, problematic behavior is more directly modifiable than in individual therapy. Fourth, since most couples enter therapy in a crisis situation, they often "want to back off from the enforced togetherness of the therapeutic session" (Brewster & Montie, 1987, p. 4) quickly, once the crisis has been resolved or at least its intensity has been reduced. Finally, terminating couples therapy rarely raises all the symbolic and affectively loaded issues seen in depth-oriented individual treatment, since the major interpersonal attachments of marital partners in therapy are each other rather than the therapist.

IMT itself is committed to three basic premises (Gurman 1978, 1981, 1985). First, it is held that the effective practice of marital therapy requires a broad explanatory basis of human behavior. Second, a singular focus on intrapersonal "versus" interpersonal aspects of human experience is believed to be arbitrary. Third, all levels and dimensions of human experience may potentially need to be attended to in clinical practice, from the cultural and social to the cognitive, affective, and behavioral to the biochemical and physiological. Given these premises, IMT asserts that different methods of therapy may be differentially helpful for different types of problems, and that, within a coherent integrative framework of marital dysfunction and the nature of therapeutic change (Gurman, 1985), techniques drawn from different models of therapy can be used in synergistic concert. Specifically, IMT draws heavily on the principles of social learning theory, object relations theory, and General Systems Theory.

It is assumed that marital conflict arises when the "rules" of an intimate relationship that are central to each partner's sense of self are in some way violated. These relational "rules" include both the conscious and unconscious expectations of, and anxieties about, intimate relating that are brought to the marriage by each partner. These rules may, of course, be shaped over time by the marital interaction itself and by other forces in people's lives. Furthermore, these rules refer to expectations of both oneself and one's partner. In this, it is assumed that people generally strive to maintain a relatively consistent sense of self and a relatively consistent perception of those to whom they are intimately connected.

In IMT, there are two essential principles that guide the therapist's decisions and actions: (1) since people shape each other's personalities, couples therapy can lead to individual change; and, (2) behavioral change can change the inner schemata of both one's self and one's partner that constitute the perceptual templates of central importance in marriage and other close, committed relationships. The general aims of IMT are: to identify and clarify the links between individual experience (conscious thoughts, preconscious "automatic thoughts," conditioned affective responses, etc.) and the marital interaction; to create therapeutic tasks that both challenge the couple's rule-governed problematic behavior and allow in new information about each partner, in order to restructure both self-perceptions and perceptions of the partner; and to teach interpersonal relationship skills (problem solving, conflict resolution, and communication skills) as needed. The most commonly used techniques in IMT, then, include interpretations, training in interpersonal skills, cognitive restructuring, enactment, and task assignment.

In the first session of IMT, there are three major aims. First, the beginnings of a therapeutic alliance with each partner must be established (Gurman, 1981). Since IMT is oriented toward action and problem solving and regularly calls on the interpretation of unconscious motivation rather early (by traditional standards) in treatment, a trusting patient–therapist relationship is essential to help foster a feeling of safety in the therapeutic context, within which challenges can be put forth and experiments can be conducted.

Second, a clear treatment focus must be aimed for, though it is not always possible to establish change goals that are both clear and phenomenologically meaningful in the first 60-minute encounter. The treatment focus is a guide for future action, not a box to limit the possibilities of change.

Third, the change process must be set (or continued) in motion early, usually by the therapist's assignment of out-of-session tasks. Early out-of-session tasks can vary from exploring the consequences of new marital behavior, to reflecting on particular themes identified in the first sessions as central to the couple's dilemma and discord, to each partner's pinpointing of concrete desires for change in his or her spouse's behavior. It may also include speculating about the ways in which each partner may be contributing to the continuation of the very aspects of the relationship he or she finds dissatisfying by unwittingly reinforcing the undesired behavior of the partner.

CASE ILLUSTRATION

Bob, a 36-year-old taxi driver/musician, initiated the first session for himself and Ruth, a 39-year-old dental hygienist. They were seen in the outpatient clinic of a university-based health maintenance organization (HMO) and were assigned to the therapist by a receptionist simply on the basis of his time availability. Before the first session, the therapist knew nothing about them as a couple or as individuals.

The First Session

Therapist: I really know nothing whatsoever about you, so just give me some idea of how you came to make this appointment, whose idea it was, and what's going on at this particular time that you called in.

Ruth: Well, I guess that we, our main problem is communication, we're having some trouble with that. I guess it was Bob's idea that we see someone.

T: Can you say some more about . . .

R: Well, you know, we've been seeing each other about 6 years and, you know, it seems like we've had a lot of turmoil in our relationship.

The first statement of the couple's problem is that it is one of "communication." This is a sort of all-purpose term couples use to refer to a wide variety of difficulties. A major clue as to the basic problem in the relationship is provided early on, when Ruth notes in passing that she and Bob have been "seeing each other about 6 years." To the therapist, the fact that a couple in their late 30s has not yet made a long-term commitment after so long ("Seeing each other") immediately suggests the possibility of both individual and relational developmental dysynchronies (Budman & Gurman, 1988) as major foci for concern. For these reasons, the therapist does not inquire further at this point about "communication" but hones in on the couple's tenuous mutual involvement. He still wants to know more about why the couple has sought help at this time.

The therapist finds out that Bob and Ruth have lived together for varying lengths of time, but now not for several months. Even then, Bob always "kept my own place," and would leave their apartment for different lengths of time when they fought. They now "see each other" two or three times a week. Their struggle, it turns out, is not whether they will marry, but whether to live together again, something Ruth has recently been pushing for ("Why now?"). All this is complicated, or made more understandable, by other developmental facts revealed in the first 20 minutes: Ruth is still married to a man from whom she has been separated for 9 years, and Bob is still married to a woman from whom he has been separated for 12 years. Ruth has an 11-year-old son who has Tourette's syndrome, and lives 5 days a week with his father ("because he is a better disciplinarian," Ruth explains). Bob's "marriage of convenience" has not been legally ended because "we just never got around to it," even though he feels "emotionally divorced." Ruth has not divorced her husband because neither were willing to pay the financial costs involved, she rationalizes.

Bob mentions that there had been physical abuse in his marriage, and the therapist immediately inquires about the place of violence in the relationship at hand (Budman & Gurman, 1988).

Bob: There's one thing I should throw in . . .

T: Sure.

B: My wife and I, when we did break up, what led to our breaking up was I had, I had an abuse problem with her most of the time we were married [sic]. There was a lot of physical abuse, a lot of fighting, a lot of physical fighting.

T: And how serious did that get?

B: Well, I mean, hospitalization was never required, but it could have gotten to that.

T: Emergency room visits, things of that sort?

B: No.

T: Visible bruises or cuts or . . .

B: No, I wouldn't say that bad, either.

As Budman and Gurman (1988) have noted, when substance abuse and/or spouse abuse is present, it/they must take precedence over all other treatment considerations. Bob acknowledges he had a drinking problem during his time with his wife, but that most of their violent episodes did not involve alcohol. He has been in an "alternatives to aggression" cognitive–behavioral "course" at a local social service agency. There has been no violence in his relationship with Ruth, Bob says, and Ruth confirms this ("No, he just yells real loud").

T: So, you know that sometimes when he leaves in the middle of a fight it's because he's afraid he might lose control?

R: Yeah, I know that, but it's really frustrating 'cause it seems like we never, once we approach the subject again it gets to that level of anger and I'm to the point where I'm almost afraid to express dissatisfaction a lot of time.

T: (*To Bob*) So, it's a short-term payoff, the benefit of leaving in case you're right, and in the long-term it's the opposite; it builds resentment and contributes to problems not being resolved.

Here, the therapist is aware that Bob is feeling embarrassed about his history of violence and decides not to challenge his way of describing his "protecting" Ruth from any danger he may present. Still, the therapist wishes to suggest that short-term gains may not justify the long-term losses, especially since he is privately hypothesizing that Bob's "protection" of Ruth is simply a (powerful and effective) rationalized maneuver to avoid the closeness that, in the therapist's view, is inherent in effective problem solving. The conversation now drifts, not surprisingly, back to various stories about how and why Bob and his wife have never legally divorced. One way to lengthen therapy is to not ask painful or anxiety-arousing questions of patients, and to set a pattern of not doing so in the first session. The therapist avoids this lengthening error.

T: Okay, now, so coming at this for the third or fourth time here, so why aren't you divorced?

B: Basically, the same reason that Ruth and Larry haven't. You just, you have, I think all of us have a tendency to just let things kind of roll on without, you know, doing much about them. I don't think either of us took the marriage very seriously, so it's kind of beside the point to get divorced. . . .

The therapist has clearly touched a very sensitive nerve in the quasi-committed relationship between Bob and Ruth that involves each of their elaborate sets of rationalizations for being separated from their respective spouses for so long. Sensing he has come upon a core dynamic of how the couple avoids adequately defining their relationship, the therapist returns to material that is phenomenologically closer to consciousness for the couple. Doing so will help to foster his alliance with each of them.

T: So, you notice I've studiously avoided asking you about what's actually going on day to day now because I had a sense that there was something complicating in the background here, but now that I've got sort of the frame around the picture, we can look at the picture a little bit more carefully. So, when you two are talking about the trouble you have "communicating," what does that mean?

B: Yeah, I mean she's told me, she doesn't, she's afraid to tell me how she's feeling about things. I know she wants to spend more time together and, you know, I take the relationship very seriously, I love her very much and, you know, I, but I have a lot of other things in my life that I'm interested in. I'm a musician and that takes time and I, you know, we're both working and, I mean, I think she gets frustrated because I don't always want, you know, to be together.

R: I guess two nights a week isn't enough and I feel like I need more, you know?

T: That's the typical week?

R: Mostly, yeah, it is.

B: No, no. *Two* nights a week?

R: That's the way I see it!

T: Well, we could probably start documenting or something . . .

R: Okay, Sunday night we spent together . . .

T: No, I was just kidding about documenting it! (*Couple laughs*)

In brief therapy, it is essential that extended nonproductive exchanges between patients not be allowed, and arguing about such facts as how often a couple spends time together is just such a topic. The therapist interrupts the exchange with tongue-in-cheek humor. Note that despite the therapist's direct and explicit request for a clearer description of the couple's "communication" problem, the conversation almost immediately returns to the closeness/distance issue.

T: Has this amount of time together been kind of difficult for you for the whole 6 years or was there a time when you were together a lot more?

R: Well, when we first started seeing each other, I guess it's always been an issue, because when we first started seeing each other, you know, he was at my house all the time. But I still wanted more, you know, I felt like I, I just felt like that wasn't enough. I wanted to live with him and . . .

B: At the time, you know, also when we first got together I was having, I was attempting to have a relationship with her son, Tommy, and it, you know, I, I mean from her point of view I guess I wasn't putting much into it. In my point of view, I was putting as much in as I could and I was, it was very difficult. Sometimes, he can be a pretty difficult kid and, you know, I don't think I have a whole lot of skills in that area, dealing with kids, so like right now I really don't have any kind of contact with him at all.

T: Do you work weekends particularly or . . .

B: No.

T: Oh, so how come you don't see her on weekends?

Again, the therapist challenges the couple's varied distancing rationalizations.

R: Well, I have Tommy on weekends, so . . .

B: I have a real rough time with him, you know, I mean I just . . .

T: Well, I'm more confused. You stay away on weekends?

B: Pretty much, yes.

T: So, you have time which you could see Ruth on weekends . . .

B: . . . if I chose to hang out with Ruth and Tommy but I seem to, you know, I don't, he gets real difficult when I'm around, I mean I don't know, he's, you know, the last time I spent a lot of time with him he was a lot younger.

T: But he in some sense is the reason you stay away on weekends? Is that, I mean, if he lived with his father, his biological father, in California would you go over there on weekends?

B: Yeah.

T: Oh, so there is something about what goes on when the *three* of you are together that's unpleasant?

B: Yeah. It's been quite a while since that's even happened, so maybe I better give it another chance.

B: (*To R*) What's the idea in your mind why we're staying away?

R: Well, I guess it is, yeah, well, you know, it's hard to get a babysitter and the time that I have Tommy on weekends I want to spend time with him, so . . .

T: So, it would be, so you might want Bob to be there, if he were there the whole weekend, say, that would create some tension for you to divide up your time and your attention and your . . .

R: Tommy has Tourette's syndrome, too, so he's, you know. . . . If I'm paying too much attention to him, then he does something to get our attention, that's negative, you know, so, it seems like we have to constantly be after him, you know.

B: Yeah, when we were spending a lot of time and I was, I'm sorry, go ahead.

R: Well, the time that Tommy and, well, us three were together it wasn't real quality time because we were . . .

T: So, everybody felt like they were kind of missing something in the situation.

B: Yeah, it seemed like it, you know, I found myself just, you know, not knowing how to deal with the role when we were seeing, when we were first seeing each other a long time ago. It was, it was difficult for me to know, you know, I think anybody who gets involved with somebody who's got a kid who's not their, you know, natural child is going to have that problem. I mean I knew, you know, I'd met Tommy and, you know, I didn't, you know, I felt like somehow I was supposed to be a surrogate parent and I just didn't know how to fulfill that role at all. I wasn't very good at it, anyway.

T: So, his Tourette's problem makes it difficult to be with him . . .

B: Basically, it seems like we're sort of, you know, like we get close, one gets closer, the other backs up, or vice versa.

T: Yes, yes, that's right.

B: I mean, well, I mean I can, I think basically a lot of the times I'm the one who's backing up and, you know, 'cause I do kind of covet the time that I spend by myself or with my friends and stuff. I mean I really enjoy our time together when, you know, when we're getting along well, but, you know, I do have other things I like to do and I guess sometimes I feel, I get to feel a little, you know, stifled or something if, and it's really got, I don't think it's got anything to do with her as a person, it's just, you know, I think I just maybe expect more freedom, you know, than, I don't know, than is natural . . .

T: So, if you were married right now, if you were unmarried from your spouses, of course, and then if you were married now, how would that change? Do you think that Ruth would be more insistent on your being together more?

B: If we were married?

T: Yeah.

B: Gee, I guess if we were married we probably would be living together so, I don't know if that, she'd probably want me to, she'd want me to like take off more then. Yeah, I suppose that she would feel like we should spend much more time together than two nights a week if we were married, that's pretty reasonable, I guess.

Some discussion follows of the new job Bob will soon be starting as a laboratory technician, and so on.

T: Okay. So, again, I'm not trying to get closure on something that's not appropriately closed off here at the moment, but is it fair to say that this issue of time together, of various ways of talking about time together, being involved with other people or things or activities, commitment to the relationship, and so on, that that's the biggest issue over which you have conflict?

R: I would say so. Yeah, I've thought about taking classes and things like that, too, to make, to fill in the time that I'm not with him and stuff, so, but then if I take a class and take time I set down to that, then it would be only like just a very few days a week that we can spend together, you know, so . . .

It is becoming very clear that there are a number of intertwined developmental issues at work here: neither Ruth nor Bob has completed his or her pseudodivorces; Bob wants to be close and now feels quite lonely but fears commitment, as well as his own anger; Ruth has not yet established clear generational lines with her 11-year-old son, such that she feels forced to act as though her adult relationship with Bob hardly exists; Ruth is somewhat conflicted about whether to pursue further education, given her concern that doing so would distance her from Bob still more; Bob has never really "made it" as a musician and, at age 36, is still switching among semiskilled and skilled jobs; he also feels quite inadequate in terms of (step-) parenting-type skills, and seems embarrassed that at his age, he is still so uncomfortable around children. So, now, when Ruth pushes for greater commitment, all these developmental matters are implicitly brought to the surface of the couple's relationship. The therapist is aware that the time for the first session is nearing an end, and so he attempts to pull together the various strands that have been mentioned, alluded to, explored, etc. In brief couples therapy, it is essential that an agreed-on, coherent statement of the central relational problem be arrived at before the meeting ends.

T: Let me back up here for a minute. I'm sure I'm glossing over something, but primarily what you describe as a problem of "communication" doesn't seem to me to be a problem of communication. That is, it seems to me that of most concern to you is how involved are you, are you going to be, and all the various questions that raises, like living together and marriage, you know, coming and going, and who's in control of what aspects of your being together. In general, it seems that you communicate and you've gotten across your ideas, your feelings, your preferences, your wishes to each other quite well. It's not that you don't understand where the other person is coming from, 'cause I think you do understand where each other's coming from . . .

R: I agree. It's not that we don't understand each other, it's that we don't know where we're going.

T: Yes. I also think you have a lot in common, there's a lot of mutual caring that comes through between you right here [in the session]. The basic issue, as I see it, is one of how involved you want to be, are comfortable being, at this point in your lives. It may be different somewhere down the road.

B: Yeah.

T: So, that's the main issue I think you need to deal with, and that's what I suggest we focus on if you want to come back.

The therapist and the couple agreed to meet every other week. Brief therapy with couples very often is held at less-than-weekly intervals. Just as students do not necessarily learn best in the artificially constructed 50-minute classroom unit of time, so, too, do couples not necessarily require, or even utilize well, sessions timed on the basis of therapists' work habits. Moreover, longer intervals between sessions seem often to allow a more selective and productive use of in-session time (vs. the familiar refrain, "What should we talk about today, Doctor?"). In addition, less-than-weekly sessions seem useful to couples (and others) in implicitly conveying that the real work of therapy takes place outside the therapy sessions themselves. In minimizing the couple's feelings of dependency on the therapist in this and other ways, another major therapy-lengthening trap may be avoided. The first session ends with the therapist's request that before the next session, Bob and Ruth independently reflect on what he or she, not the other, was perhaps doing that had kept the relationship on the fence for so long.

THE COURSE OF THERAPY

Unfortunately, but consistent with the couple's description and discussion of their relationship in the first session, Ruth appeared for the second session by herself. They had had an argument on her birthday. She was angry that he had arrived at her apartment late because he was practicing his music and, to make matters worse, brought her a birthday gift that, to her, showed little interest in what she valued and enjoyed and seemed to her just a perfunctory, last-minute gesture. The whole evening seemed to her to capture the essence of his limited involvement in their relationship. Ruth appeared to have reacted to her disappointment about that evening's events more forcefully than was typical of her. She told him that until she felt ready, she did not want to talk to Bob, and that she would be going to our next session alone. He did not object. My understanding of this was that we had, indeed, identified the core developmental issue in their relationship in our first session, and that, implicitly challenged to go one way or the other with his ambivalence, he had made his choice. Unfortunately (or fortunately, depending on one's perspective), he had done so in the context of a major and symbolically loaded life-cycle event, Ruth's 39th birthday.

Very often, when a relationship has been chronically characterized by an oscillating pursuer–distancer arrangement, forcing one side of the couple's shared ambivalence, either toward or away from the partner, is followed by a more defined, differentiated response by the partner. A style of therapy more content to slowly unravel relational dynamics might have allowed, or even required, a more gradual exploration of each partner's ambivalence about the relationship and each other, examined each partner's history of other relationships, and explored mutually reinforcing projections and collusive processes in a tentative fashion. Brief couples therapies, such as IMT, also require that the therapist be aware of such implicit processes and unconscious motivations, yet IMT requires that the therapist use his or her deep understanding of relational dynamics as a basis for action as well as reflection (Gurman, 1991).

The third session, Bob did appear, and the couple seemed quite toned down, compared to how intense they had been during the birthday fight. They both seemed to have been genuinely and profoundly scared by nearly calling their relationship to a halt as a result of the feelings that were generated that evening. Their fear seemed to motivate them to want to carefully reexamine what had happened that night, to better understand their own motivations for their ways of dealing with each other then, and to clarify their feelings, the assumptions each had made about the other person, etc. Their mutual exploration in the session was cautious, yet heartfelt, and by the end of it, they both felt both more at ease and in more emotional contact than they had been for some time.

My understanding of all this was that the implicit "rule" that intimacy and commitment were to be avoided by each of them, in his or her own turn, had been violated first by Bob's request that they enter therapy. This violation of their mutual distance dance was further intensified by my challenges to them in the first session, and that intensification was heightened still further by Ruth's refusal to back down from her anger at Bob in the context of the birthday row. The couple had now, between the second and third sessions, and in the third session, taken the frightening step of mutually exploring their fear of simultaneously opting for closeness and had found that they could, at least for that time, survive it.

While the therapist's interventions might have appeared to a naive observer to have been simple (and they were, at a behavioral level), they were based on a multileveled and multidimensional appreciation of the dynamics of the couple's relationship. In IMT, the therapist's capacity to understand complexity, yet intervene with simplicity, is at the core of keeping treatment brief. Certainly, with Bob and Ruth, the therapist's ability to feel comfortable challenging the couple's central dynamic contract was heightened by the personal comfort he felt with them in their sessions. His use of humor (and the couple's response to it) was also essential in forming the trusting alliances with each member of the couple that eased such direct, rule-violating challenges.

Several weeks passed until the therapist's next, and final, contact with the couple. Although they were scheduled to meet as a threesome, last-minute work responsibilities did not allow Bob to attend the session. Ruth was quite comfortable with this, and smilingly announced that they had decided to "take a chance" and try living together in the near future. While this course of therapy was briefer than most of the therapist's brief therapy, and while meaningful therapy with this couple could have continued for months, the therapist was comfortable exiting the scene when the couple wanted him to do so. In IMT, as in many types of brief therapy that are time sensitive rather than time limited (cf. Budman & Gurman, 1988), couples often return for further work, often on different issues than those about which they originally sought help.

EDITORS' QUESTIONS

Q: IMT is an eclectic model drawing on a variety of therapeutic approaches and ideas. Would you describe how your approach evolved as a method of brief therapy?

A: IMT evolved quite naturally as a method of brief therapy because of the fundamentally *integrative* (not eclectic) view it takes of both relationships and therapy. In this therapy, it is believed that change at one level of human experience often reverberates at other levels. Because wisely selected therapeutic interventions can effect change at mutliple levels of psychological, interpersonal, and systemic organization, a significant degree of clinical change will often occur in periods of time that are quite brief by traditional standards. Thus, therapy that considers problem-maintaining factors at all levels, and selects interventions with careful attention to the lifely effects at these different levels, inherently fosters brevity.

Q: Are there any contraindications for using the IMT model with couples? What kinds of couples are especially good candidates for IMT and which kinds are not?

A: The major contraindications are found in therapists, not in couples. Since IMT places an emphasis on the therapist's multileveled formulation (of problem maintenance and predicted patient responses to particular interventions), very few special patient characteristics preclude the use of MIT. Thus, for example, very concrete behavioral tasks may be the order of the day with highly educated, overly abstract, emotionally indirect couples, whereas exploring family history may be called for with a couple who approach life in rather practical and simple ways. Both kinds of interventions may be aimed at challenging an implicit underlying agreement the couples have not to reveal themselves in ways that feel unsafe. Unfortunately, many therapists limit their effectiveness, and the range of problems and people with whom they could work by not thinking at multiple levels. Some couples, of course, are not good candidates for any couples therapy, including IMT (e.g., those who are uncontrollably argumentative in sessions or physically assaultive at home and those whose Axis I psychopathology precludes focused, sustained, and coherent dialogue). Those best suited to IMT are couples who are open to examining life, problems, and solutions in varied ways (i.e., in both the behavioral and the cognitive–affective domains).

Q: Some marital therapy approaches engage the couple in a formal assessment process prior to beginning "treatment." Your interview— assuming it is representative of your method—seems to move directly and immediately toward intervention based on a minimum of background information. Would you talk about the importance of assessment in IMT?

A: Yes, this interview is quite representative. Of course, sizable sections of the transcript were omitted due to space limitations, and in those parts of the session more "background" information was addressed. Assessment in IMT is not "formal" in the sense of being artificially separated from a phase of the encounter called "treatment." The therapist constructs probes, prescribes tasks, offers interpretive reframings of meanings, poses challenges, and so on based on a fluidly evolving network of hypotheses about problem maintenance. In our brief therapy book (Budman & Gurman, 1988), we detail the areas of assessment that we find important to be aware of in most, if not all, couples therapy: presenting problems, attempted solutions, and the consequences of change; individual and couple assets and strengths; communication and problem-solving skills and styles; styles of influence; relational boundaries; life-cycle status and accomplishment; affection and attachment; marital (couple) relationship history; sexuality and sexual functioning; relationship commitment; spousal and substance abuse. I believe Bob and Ruth can be rather clearly described in most of these areas, even from the limited transcript. Also, keep in mind that "assessment" does not end at the end of the first session.

Q: Do you prefer, as in the case described, to have no information about the couple prior to the initial interview? In what ways is background information about the couple or the presenting problem useful? What information are you most interested in knowing prior to your first meeting with the couple?

A: In this case, I had no prior information about the couple, not because of my preference but because of the structure of the clinical operation in our department's HMO. Having some information about couples before the first interview can certainly be useful in forming some extremely tentative hypotheses about the family structure, the place of symptoms in the family, and so on. On the other hand, having a great deal of such prior information is not essential to me. Thus, when a couple calls me directly to request to see me, our phone conversation is almost always limited to a very brief conversation about what the person I am talking to sees as the presenting problem.

Q: What was telling you that you could continue to pursue, so early in the initial interview, the sensitive issue of why this couple has not formally severed their previous relationships, without endangering your therapeutic alliance?

A: As I alluded to earlier, my comfort in being humorous with this couple was *the* central signal that I could enter this sensitive territory. I am prone to punning, noticing, and commenting on absurdity and exaggeration, and so on. When I feel free to show this part of myself to a couple, it has almost never been a mistake to probe and push deeply, even in the first session. Conversely, when I feel very restrained and distant from a couple, early pushing on defenses seems never to be appropriate. I think that a lot of caring and warmth comes through in humor, and that perhaps serves as the anesthetic for the sometimes painful therapeutic operation. Humor is not a technique; it is a part of the therapist. When the self-aware therapist is intuitively stiff and cautious, I assume that to be a reliable index of the couple's anxiety about changing.

Q: In this interview, you immediately hone in on critical developmental issues for this couple: intimacy and commitment. Do you generally find that behind a couple's presenting problems there is some developmental issue that needs to be addressed?

A: Some therapists believe that virtually all marital and family problems reflect some kind of developmental issue. This is a vastly overstated position in that some problems create, or at least lead to, rather than reflect, such developmental issues (Gurman, 1983) (e.g., the primary wage earner is laid off from his or her job and gets depressed or the previous parental role structure changes) and the couple comes in because they are fighting too often. The life-cycle impasse idea should be a descriptive one but is too often used as though it were explanatory. On the other hand, contextualizing almost any type of presenting problem in developmental terms, as part of the clinical formulation and goal setting that are essential in brief therapy, lends a very important flavor of coherence to treatment planning in that it "makes sense" to most people. Developmental problems are not, in my view, "behind" presenting problems, in the sense of being either more "true" or more "basic." They are important parts of the landscape of marital and family life, but not necessarily the ground in which everything grows.

Q: Was there some reason you decided not to give this couple a task or homework assignment at the end of the initial meeting? Generally, how do you incorporate homework into your work with couples?

A: As I noted, "The first session ends with the therapist's request that before the next session, Bob and Ruth independently reflect on what they, not the other, were perhaps doing that has kept the relationship on the fence for so long" (p. 195). This request was not *en passant* but explicitly conveyed the therapist's expectation that the self-reflection activity identified above would occur. Out-of-session tasks need not be interactional to qualify as therapeutic tasks. Unfortunately, many family therapists have ignored individual psychology so much that tasks directed to individuals are underused. The purpose of this "individual" task with Bob and Ruth was to disrupt their collusive agreement to remain ambivalently connected, with each attributing his or her distance to the other person. In brief, this was an "individual" task designed to challenge the unconscious basis of the couple's everyday interaction. This assignment illustrates the use of a therapeutic task whose purpose is not self-evident and is not explained to the couple. IMT regularly also incorporates more straightforward tasks whose purpose is made totally explicit by the therapist (Gurman, 1981, 1985).

Q: How did you negotiate a treatment contract involving meetings on alternate weeks? Did you also suggest to the couple that these meetings last for some finite period of time (e.g., 3 months or 6 months)?

A: In general, brief therapy is facilitated by minimizing patients' dependency on the therapist, and spacing sessions at less than the traditional weekly (or more frequent) interval helps in this aim. Moreover, for couples who are not beginning therapy in a true crisis state, approximately biweekly sessions often seem to fit with the flow and rhythm of everyday life. When paired with out-of-session tasks (designed both to initiate change and to minimize dependency), biweekly sessions maximize patients' responsibility taking. In the case of Bob and Ruth, moreover, I judged that seeing them weekly would imply a sort of forced, too rapidly established closeness out of proportion to the closeness of the relationship. With this couple, I did not suggest how long we might continue to meet but rather simply informed them of the maximum number of sessions (seven) available to us through Ruth's HMO insurance policy.

Q: How do you generally decide when it is time to terminate treatment? What indices do you use to evaluate treatment success?

A: Treatment is terminated when the couple have reached their goals, in their view; when the couple do not find that they have fully achieved their aims, although there has been some real change, but have lost a significant degree of motivation for continuing work; or when the couple clearly do not think they are making any progress and/or when they find their "match" with me not to be a solid one. Largely, then, the decision to end therapy is the couple's, though I will also suggest "taking a break" from our work if I believe they are not committed to the therapeutic task. Finally, of course, with some couples we end (having planned to do so) simply as a function of their having very limited financial resources (e.g., a seven-session HMO limit paired with restricted personal funds). Quite often, in the sort of primary care style of my work (Budman & Gurman, 1988), I work with a couple for a rather brief period, say "adieu" rather than "good-bye," and pick up with them farther down the road, as new life circumstances arise for which they feel I may be helpful.

Q: Why do you say "unfortunately" in regard to the fact that Ruth appeared alone at session two? I have the impression that this couple was actively using you as a means to destabilize their dance of ambivalence. The therapy structure perhaps provided a way for them to safely push the limits of the relationship and test out the consequences. Do you ever get the feeling that couples are moving on their own evolutionary track and that the changes we see have less to do with our specific interventions and more with the couple's trajectory toward change?

A: No, I generally do not believe that the changes we see have less to do with our interventions than with the couple's "trajectories." If I believed that, I would probably stop practicing therapy! I certainly do acknowledge, however, that sometimes all we need to do to be helpful is a minor carburetor adjustment, rather than an engine overhaul, that gets a couple developmentally back on track.

I thought it unfortunate that Bob did not come to the second session for a very simple reason—it is almost always easier to do couples therapy with a couple than to attempt to bring about change in a couple through one individual. Your idea that they were using me to destabilize their ambivalent dance reflects an assumption that they came to therapy *in order to change*. While there is some evidence of this, two other possibilities also exist (see Budman & Gurman, Chapter 6, this volume). First, they also, I believe, came to therapy because they *had changed* (Ruth had recently been pushing for more of a commitment, so they were already "destabilized.") Bob's failure to appear can also be seen as an expression of his wish to be in therapy in order *not to change*. Elements of all three answers to the question, "Why now (have you come for therapy)?" (Budman & Gurman, 1988), are commonly present.

Q: How did you become a brief therapist?

A: Actually, I don't think I ever "became" a brief therapist. I think I was born that way. I am a very task-oriented and goal-directed person and often favor efficiency over elegance (actually, I find efficiency to *be* elegant!). I am by nature also very active as a therapist, in part because I enjoy working with people more when I am being that way than when I am primarily listening, empathizing, and interpreting. From my undergraduate psychology years at Boston University through my graduate years at Columbia, I thought that much of what went on in the highly esteemed long-term therapies of the day seemed quite unnecessary to achieve most of the goals for which most people sought out psychotherapists in the first place. I believe that people are extremely complex, but that our theories of therapy need to be only moderately complex, and that our actual interventions, while based on rather complex understanding, should themselves be relatively simple.

REFERENCES

Brewster, F., & Montie, K. (1987). A double life: What do family therapists really do in private practice? *The Family Therapy Networker*, *11*(1), 33–35, 37.

Budman, S. H., & Gurman, A. S. (1988). *Theory and practice of brief therapy*. New York: Guilford Press.

Gurman, A. S. (1978). Contemporary marital therapies: A critique and comparative analysis of psychodynamic, behavioral and systems theory approaches. In T. Paolino & B. McCrady (Eds.), *Marriage and marital therapy* (pp. 445–566). New York: Brunner/Mazel.

Gurman, A. S. (1981). Integrative marital therapy: Toward the development of an interpersonal approach. In S. H. Budman (Ed.), *Forms of brief therapy* (pp. 415–457). New York: Guilford Press.

Gurman, A. S. (1983). The virtues and changes of a life-cycle perspective in family therapy. *American Journal of Family Therapy*, *11*, 67–72.

Gurman, A. S. (1985). Tradition and transition: A rural marriage in crisis. In A. S. Gurman (Ed.), *Casebook of marital therapy* (pp. 303–336). New York: Guilford Press.

Gurman, A. S. (1991). Commentary on D. E. Scharff & J. S. Scharff, "Joining the family: Countertransference can be the therapist's compass." *The Family Therapy Networker*, *15*(5), 79–81.

Gurman, A. S., & Kniskern, D. P. (1981). Family therapy outcome research: Knowns and unknowns. In A. S. Gurman & D. P. Kniskern (Eds.), *Handbook of family therapy* (pp. 742–775). New York: Brunner/Mazel.

Scharff, D. E., & Scharff, J. S. (1987). *Object relations family therapy*. Northvale, NJ: Jason Aronson.

Emotionally Focused Therapy: Restructuring Attachment

SUSAN M. JOHNSON

LESLIE S. GREENBERG

In the last decade the nature of marital distress has been clarified and delineated (Gottman, 1979; Gottman & Levenson, 1986). The essential elements of this phenomenon are negative affect, negative attributions and perceptions of the other, negative content patterns such as criticism and blaming, and perhaps most significantly the organization of all of these elements into self-reinforcing rigid interaction patterns that take on a life of their own. The prototypical interaction is one of rapid escalating aversiveness resulting in hostility and/or withdrawal from the encounter. This pattern destroys trust and the capacity for closeness and fosters anger, fear, and alienation. Recent research suggests that the process of emotional engagement predicts marital satisfaction in the long term rather than the ability to resolve particular conflict issues (Gottman & Krokoff, 1989). The two elements that stand out here are the negative affective responses a distressed couple evoke in each other and the powerful interaction patterns that take over the relationship and define it in spite of the good intentions and insight of the partners. The approach to couples therapy described in this chapter, Emotionally Focused Couples Therapy (EFT) (Greenberg & Johnson, 1988; Johnson & Greenberg, 1987), focuses on two elements: compelling intrapsychic emotional responses and the organization of interactions into negative rigid patterns. EFT assumes that both these elements, which are seen as reciprocally determining and influencing each other, have to be reprocessed and reorganized to create a more positive relationship between partners. Both inner experience and relationship events have then to be expanded and redefined. The redefinition of the relationship in EFT is aimed at the creation of mutual responsiveness and accessibility. This goal, which implies a particular vision of what constitutes health in an intimate relationship, is based on bonding theory (Bowlby, 1969, 1988). A healthy partnership is viewed here as a secure bond rather than a rewarding quid pro quo contract or a relationship where partners are relatively free of past unconscious conflicts. Bonding theory views the emotional connection between partners and the management of proximity-seeking behaviors and separation anxiety as primary elements in a close, interdependent relationship (Johnson, 1986).

The EFT therapist, when seeing a couple for the first time, focuses on the emotional climate of the relationship, and the primary emotional responses he or she hypothesizes underlie the interactional positions of each partner. The emotional responses focused on most often are fear and vulnerability, sadness and pain, and anger and resentment. The focus on vulnerability is consistent with bonding theory, which suggests that security is the core motivational element in close relationships, and with the experiential theory of human functioning, which suggests that it is defensiveness, the desire to protect the self from vulnerability, and the subsequent disowning of experience that are essentially problematic. Empirical research also seems to suggest that defensiveness, the protection of personal vulnerability, is a key element in the organization of negative rigid interaction patterns (Gottman, 1991).

The EFT therapist also focuses on the process of interaction; the problem is not the issues that arise but how these issues are processed and how that process defines closeness/distance and control/dependence in the relationship. The EFT therapist watches the interaction to assess how the self of each partner and the nature of the relationship are defined by the process of interaction. The therapist is concerned with identifying the rigid positions each partner takes in the relationship dance, the most noted of which is the pursue/withdraw pattern (Greenberg & Johnson, 1988; Napier, 1978; Gottman & Levenson, 1986). The aim of the therapist is to use the experience and communication of reprocessed emotional responses to evoke new interaction patterns and, in a reciprocally determining fashion, to use new patterns to evoke new emotional responses in the session; for example, the expression of longing and loneliness underlying explicit hostility tends to evoke compassion and contact rather than withdrawal from the partner, and the expressed compassion allows for a more congruent request for contact from the previously hostile partner.

THEORETICAL PERSPECTIVES

The first fundamental assumption of EFT is that a distressed marital relationship is best viewed as a bond in which essentially healthy attachment needs are unable to be met because of rigid, negative interaction patterns. Second, emotion is viewed as adaptive and primary in the context of intimate relationships and as organizing attachment behaviors. The expression of emotion is seen as constituting a primary signaling system regulating social interaction and motivating interpersonal responses (Greenberg & Johnson, 1986; 1990).

EFT is a synthesis of experiential and systemic change strategies (Johnson & Greenberg, 1987). As in experiential therapies in general, the central focus of EFT is on the client's present experience and how the client processes that experience. The therapist is constantly involved in validating, heightening, and expanding whatever is poignant in each partner's experience (Perls, Hefferline, & Goodman, 1951; Rogers, 1951). Elements of ongoing experience that are not attended to are focused on, identified with, explored, and integrated into the client's sense of self. In experiential theory it is not feelings or needs that are problematic but the disowning or disallowing of these feelings and needs. EFT is systemic in that each partner's responses are constantly framed in terms of the pull of the interpersonal field; that is, in relation to the other's behavior and the reaction a particular response is likely to evoke. There is, then, a constant focus on the structure and process of interaction. The position each partner takes in this dance is made explicit, expanded on, and linked to underlying emotions.

At this point it seems appropriate to elaborate briefly on the implications of bonding theory for the practice of therapy. Adult love relationships are more and more being viewed in terms of attachment theory (Shaver, Hazen, & Bradshaw, 1988; Collins & Read, 1990). Attachment theory provides the EFT therapist with a map of the key features of intimate relationships and a language with which to understand and reframe responses and interactions. For example, it helps the therapist to legitimize the needs of the couple if these needs are viewed from an attachment perspective (i.e., as essentially innate and adaptive) (Johnson, 1986). Many of the problematic behaviors occurring between partners are viewed as symptoms of insecure attachment and the threat of loss and separation; this threat then evokes an intensification of attachment behaviors such as clinging and angry protest, followed by depression and detachment (Bowlby, 1969). Attachment theorists (Ainsworth & Bowlby, 1991) have specifically commented on the close relationship of anger to attachment-related anxiety and the intensification and distortion of attachment behaviors.

Bowlby (1969) suggests that the primary source of intense human emotion is the formation, maintenance, disruption, and renewal of affectional bonds. These bonds consist of an affectional tie and a set of proximity-seeking behaviors. Affect is viewed as organizing attachment behaviors, particularly when perceived inaccessibility or emotional unresponsiveness of the attachment figure threatens the security of the bond. In EFT the compelling emotional responses underlying the interactional positions of the partners are reprocessed so that the interactional patterns can be reorganized. Affect is then the target and agent of change.

The content of therapy, the focus of EFT, is closely tied to the attachment perspective. The language and the therapeutic reframes used by the EFT therapist heighten attachment-related experiences—such as isolation, abandonment, deprivation, and fear, which are evoked by interactions with the partner—and validate the need for safety, comfort, closeness, and protection. The metaphors that arise in therapy are typically those of contact, shutting out, letting in, vulnerability, wounds and weapons, helplessness and self-protection, or fears and longings of the childlike dependent aspect of each partner.

Attachment theory also suggests that it is in the process of emotional connectedness with intimate others that working models of self and other are operationalized and enacted. Relationship definition and self-definition are two sides of the same coin and are accessed in the process of interaction. The recognition and acceptance of intimate others are essential for the full expression and integration of different aspects of self, and the elaboration, integration, and revision of the models of self and other is a process which continues throughout life (Bowlby, 1988). In EFT, the accessing of new aspects of self enables these aspects to be integrated into the self schema and into the relationship. New emotional experience and new interactions challenge and modify the working models of each partner.

CHANGE STRATEGIES

EFT is usually implemented in 12 to 20 therapy sessions, two of which are usually individual sessions. These two individual sessions occur after the first conjoint session and are used to cement the therapeutic alliance, to explore sensitive issues, such as fidelity and commitment, and to expand hypotheses as to how each spouse views the other and experiences him- or herself in the relationship.

The sequence of steps in the process of treatment is presented below.

1. The delineating of conflict issues in the core struggle.
2. Identifying the negative interaction cycle.
3. Accessing the unacknowledged feelings underlying interactional positions.
4. Reframing the problem in terms of underlying feelings and attachment needs.
5. Promoting identification with disowned needs and aspects of self and integrating these into relationship interactions.
6. Promoting acceptance of the partner's experience and new interaction patterns.
7. Facilitating the expression of needs and wants and creating emotional engagement.
8. Facilitating the emergence of new solutions.
9. Consolidating new positions.

It is not possible in this chapter to elaborate on each step of therapy. The steps and the interventions associated with them are elaborated elsewhere (Johnson & Greenberg, 1987; Greenberg & Johnson, 1988). In all these steps the therapist is engaged in two main tasks: (1) accessing, validating, and reprocessing emotional responses, and (2) creating new relationship-defining interactions. The first task requires the use of techniques taken from gestalt and client-centered therapy. The moment-to-moment experience of the client is the key reference point in therapy. The therapist tracks how the partners construct their emotional experience and how this in turn creates their position relative to their partner. This is a process of discovery and creation; it is not simply more intimate self-disclosure.

The second task involves the reframing and restructuring of interactions toward accessibility and responsiveness. The reprocessed emotional experience of the partners is used to enact and expand negative patterns and to create new relationship events. Interactions are tracked and refocused, replayed, and restructured. As the nature of the dialogue between partners changes, previously unresolvable problems become less relevant and problematic because they are able to be addressed on a completely different level in the context of the newly defined relationship (Johnson & Greenberg, 1991). The treatment process described above has been evaluated in a series of outcome studies with generally positive results (Johnson & Greenberg, 1985; Johnson & Greenberg, 1985b; Goldman & Greenberg, in press; James, 1991; Dandeneau & Johnson, in press; Dessaulles, 1991). Change process research has also identified key processes and change events associated with positive outcome (Johnson & Greenberg, 1988).

The kinds of clinical issues that arise in the implementation of EFT are issues such as timing of interventions, the need for constant process diagnosis (Greenberg & Johnson, 1986b), the differentiation of levels of emotion (Greenberg & Safran, 1989), and the integration of intrapsychic and interpersonal interventions. The therapist has to nurture, and if necessary heal, any rifts in the therapeutic alliance and must be able to move from being directive to simply tracking and following the client's experience. A certain comfort with strong emotion is helpful in implementing EFT and aids the novice therapist in acquiring the skills of heightening emotion and using it to create new interaction patterns. A large part of the process of learning to implement EFT is understanding what emotion should be accessed, at what points in therapy, in what type of interactions, and what effects such expression will have.

CASE ILLUSTRATION

The first four sessions of EFT constitute assessment as to the nature of the relationship, and its suitability for marital therapy and for EFT in particular, as well as the setting of the stage for therapy, in terms of making an alliance with both partners and assessing each partner's openness to intervention. The mnemonic of three P's, present process, positions and patterns, and primary emotion, has been used in training therapists. The therapist focuses on present process, that is, on the moment-to-moment events that occur within each partner and between the partners, and the positions each partner takes in the interaction. The therapist also focuses on emotional responses and experience, paying particular attention to nonverbal cues such as the tone of voice and vivid images used by partners, asking questions such as "How do you feel as you say . . . ?" or "What is it like for you to hear your partner say . . . ?" The most important goal of the first session is to build a hypothesized map of the interaction and the way it is experienced by each partner; in the most reductionistic terms, to identify positions/ cycles and vulnerabilities/protective strategies. The rigidity and reactivity of positions and responses are particularly noted. At the end of the first session the couple is given a diagnostic picture and if appropriate, they are offered 15 to 20 sessions of therapy. At this time, provided it is clear, the therapist shares his or her view of the relationship, the problem, and the task of therapy in a manner that validates both partners' perceptions and sets the stage for the sessions ahead.

In the first portion of this interview the therapist obtained basic information such as the length of the relationship (6 years), health status, referral source, and scores on the Dyadic Adjustment Scale (DAS) (Spanier, 1976), which were 58 (male partner) and 69 (female partner). The norm for divorcing couples on this measure is 70, so this couple certainly scored in the severely distressed range. They were a well-educated professional couple with whom it was easy to form an alliance and who had been referred to the hospital clinic by their family doctor. Basic information as to factors that are contraindications for EFT, such as violence in the relationship or an intention to separate, had also been assessed. Positive indicators were that the couple seemed relatively nonreactive to each other for their level of distress and each seemed willing to take some responsibility for the problems in the relationship. They were motivated for therapy, stating that they were both very unhappy and something had to change, but they did not want to leave the relationship. The couple were in their late 30s and had one child who was 3 years old.

The problem was presented by the wife (Prue) in the following terms (this was related in a controlled but angry manner while her spouse remained quiet, reserved, and reasonable); they had both been mature independent people when they met; they married quickly because he had been asked to move to another city by his company. She did not want to leave the city (to which they had now returned) and had had to give up her job and her social life. When they moved he was very preoccupied with work and she felt lonely and depressed. They struggled through this and then she became pregnant and again, after the birth of their child, felt lonely, unsupported, and "depressed." They then returned to this city and when the husband (Mark) was asked again to move, Prue refused and the relationship went into crisis. Mark saw the problem as his wife's irritability, their fights, her lack of warmth, and her lack of commitment in that she had always given him the impression that she could leave anytime. He viewed the relationship as a "power struggle" with himself as the loser. He said this in a calm rational manner. Neither could identify the strengths of the relationship and experienced confiding, affection, and love making as rare or nonexistent. They felt that these aspects of the relationship had been wanting even during courtship.

The First Session

Therapist: You know, I am beginning to get a feel for your lives, but the piece that's missing for me is that you're both sitting here, very considerate of each other, and being very calm and reasonable. I'm having a hard time imagining you in a fight (*smiles*). Obviously it doesn't look like this. Could you tell me what it does look like? What happens?

Mark: It's a power struggle. That's the whole thing. We were both extremely independent individuals when we got married. I'm being asked to not move any more . . . give up my career, to change my work ethic—I work long hours, that's just me.

T: O.K. So the issue of moving is part of a larger issue about control and priorities—you were both very independent—used to running your own lives . . .

M: Absolutely.

Prue: I don't know, Mark. I guess what I'm looking for is stability. . . . I moved a lot as a child and I don't like that lifestyle. It just petrifies me to think of leaving again and being so isolated . . .

T: I understand. (*To Prue*). So what I hear you telling me is that you have an incredible amount of resentment at the loss of control over your life, you have a lot of resentment about that, and you have felt isolated and alone in this relationship.

P: Yes, I do—resentful.

T: When you feel really resentful, how does Mark know it? How do you put it out to him? How does it work?

P: It festers, it might come out like, ". . . I had to give up my job and it's *all* because of you . . . I throw out something like that.

T: And then what would happen?

M: Well, then I bring up things like, well *you* haven't really established a career. I say, let's have a long-range plan, I don't like moving either.

T: So when you start to fight, the sense I'm getting is: (*to Prue*) you say to him: "How could you do this to me?" . . . and you (*to Mark*) try to remain logical, saying "Well now, let's have a look at this, and discuss it rationally." That's the way it would go?

M: Yes, but a lot more heated.

T: (*To Prue*) Did you ever tell Mark about how incredibly angry you are that you got married, and instead of getting what you hoped for, what you experienced was isolation, helplessness, and resentment?

P: Well, I've said I resent my life, incredibly, he gets defensive, and it's like who's gonna get the last word in . . .

T: So it gets down to who's going to win, is that it? (*Couple nod*) (*Pause*) I'm hearing about power and control and the fact that you were both independent . . . and that you got together in difficult circumstances, I'm interested in the closeness between you; have you (*to Prue*) ever talked to Mark about what happens to you when you start to feel alone and isolated? Do you think he really understands what it's like for you?

The focus is not on the moving issue but on the control and closeness aspects of the relationship reflected in the way the issue is handled.

P: I don't know if he does.

T: Could you do something for me right now . . . could you turn your chair toward him . . . could you try to help him understand right now (*voice drops, pace slows, therapist leans toward Prue*) . . . what the experience of isolation has been like for you in this marriage . . . because I have the feeling it's been incredibly painful for you.

P: (*Dissolves into tears—sobs*) I remember when my father used to come home and sit at the kitchen table and say, "We're moving" (*pause—sob*), it didn't really matter what it did to my mother or us children, then you tell me that we have to move, it just makes me feel really sad, I have to give up all of my friends and my family and my life, I know that in your heart that you felt it was best, the only way our relationship was going to survive, but it didn't matter to you when I said, "It makes me sad, it makes me depressed, my self-esteem goes down, it takes a lot of energy and I can't do it over and over, I'm going to be miserable and I'm going to resent it . . . like I resented my father for doing that, I don't live for your career.

T: You felt that it didn't matter to Mark that you were so sad.

P: He was so busy—so businesslike.

T: Okay. Can you tell me what it's like to live with a husband who is so busy?

P: It's very hard on me, it hurts.

T: Can you tell him (*motions toward husband*).

P: Well, when the baby was born, she was a very colicky baby, you had that special job, working all those extra hours, and then you started French class, I was stuck in the house all by myself.

T: Can you tell him, "You weren't there for me—I was alone" (*very softly*).

P: No, you weren't there for me. Nobody was there for me. I was having a hard time with a crying baby and no support. You didn't understand that, you would go and do something by yourself . . . I felt trapped and lonesome and frustrated, and you were gone, you had all this freedom. . . .

T: What I hear you saying to Mark is not only were you trapped and overwhelmed, but you felt alone, deserted, he wasn't coming close and taking care of you, you couldn't rely on him, to respond, he was off doing his own thing—that's how *you* experienced it. I understand, Mark that you probably didn't intend this or see it this way.

P: Yes, he could have taken French at another time, he wouldn't miss a French class . . . and that was hard on me, but the baby and I didn't count.

T: And you still feel that you don't count, right?

P: Yes. I don't feel I have a say in my life at all; you say you're thinking of the good of all of us, but I don't see it that way.

T: Mark, what's happening to you when your wife is saying this?

M: (*Very calm*) First of all, there's the French class, I asked if you had a problem with this initially, and you said it was fine, and then it became difficult as things went on, and I resisted quitting the class . . . I felt committed to it . . .

T: Can I just stop you for just a second? I want to go back just one step.

Therapist refocuses process.

M: Yes.

T: What happens to you inside, what do you feel when Prue tells you that the way she experiences this relationship is that she feels lonely and helpless . . . and that she doesn't count, what happens inside of you when she's telling you this?

Therapist focuses on emotional experience underlying Mark's detached stance.

M: To a certain degree I look inside and say well, maybe I let her down . . . but there were reasons for it.

T: How does it feel to say, "I let her down"?

M: It doesn't make me feel great (*he squirms in his chair*).

T: So it feels uncomfortable, for you?

M: Absolutely. I don't like it.

T: (*Quietly, slowly*) Have you told her, "I let you down, I feel very uncomfortable, it's very hard for me. . . ."

M: No, I deal with it by asking myself, "Well, what did you do?" Then rationalizing it (*squirms again, looks down*).

T: Right. So . . . it seems that there are all kinds of incredibly strong feelings here that don't get shared, what gets talked about is issues and reasons and who is to blame, and it's like something gets missed all the time.

M: Yeah, I say "I'm sorry," but perhaps the way it comes out is in the middle of the issues that are being discussed, and then I start to rationalize . . . that's the way I cope . . . because I pride myself on being able to do a job . . . regardless of . . . it's my role . . . and I pride myself on being able to fulfill that.

T: So wait a minute . . . so what you're telling me is that, you see this in the same terms as your job, that this is your role . . . to be a good husband . . .

M: No, but, yes, that's what I said. (*Laughs*).

T: (*Chuckles*) So what you hear is that she says you've done a bad job being her husband, you've failed, you let her down.

M: Right. Well, I mean . . . it's what I've accepted as my responsibility. The question that I ask myself is, "Is it for Prue personally or is it for my wife? Do you know what I'm getting at? (*To therapist*)

T: I think so. So how does it feel to know that you let Prue down? That Prue's been *disappointed* . . . she hasn't got what she needed from you.

M: That's difficult, when things get tough I see her as my wife, not Prue.

T: How are you feeling right now?

M: Very uncomfortable. Because of that.

T: (*Long pause*) I may be wrong but what I'm picking up from you is incredible sadness. Is that right?

Therapist interprets underlying feeling.

M: Ah-ha.

T: But you don't get to share that sadness with your wife.

M: (*Tears*) I don't allow myself to, no.

T: (*Leans down to Mark, lowers voice*) You don't let yourself share that? You hold it back, keep it inside (*pause*) (*he nods*). What's striking me is that you don't get to comfort each other in this relationship. You don't show her your sadness and how awful it feels when she says, "You weren't there for me."

M: We don't confide in one another. We said that to each other yesterday . . . we don't tell each other because we're afraid . . . she's told me things that I throw back at her, and I do the same . . .

T: You're too scared to be vulnerable with each other?

M: Yeah, when we show weakness it only means we lose the next fight.

P: Well, when the baby was born you saw me at my lowest . . . I was so unhappy and sad . . . I couldn't have been any more vulnerable.

M: (*Very softly*) At the time there was nothing I could do about moving.

P: (*Sharply*) I know that!

T: When you share your feelings, Prue, then you, Mark, feel like you have to solve the problem. Is that it? That's what is expected of a good husband?

M: Absolutely.

T: (*To Mark*) I'm not sure she's asking you to solve a problem.

P: (*Crying*) I tell you and I feel so lousy and I don't feel any better telling you, I know you can't change the job right then.

T: What do you want from him when you're hurting, Prue? Do you know what you need?

P: I need to know he's listening (*cries*).

T: That he cares? That he's there—that he'll come close and comfort you? Yes? (*She nods*) But somehow that doesn't happen—and you feel even more alone and Mark, you feel like you've failed and kind of distance yourself trying to find reasons for what has happened. (*Mark nods*)

Therapist identifies cycle.

M: And then I end up feeling like there is nothing I can do, so . . .

T: So then what? You go away? And feel like a failure?

M: I guess—yeah—I do.

T: (*To Prue*) And you feel alone and deserted?

P: Yes.

T: (*To Mark*) What is happening to you right now, Mark? You look very uncomfortable.

M: I don't know what I can do. . . . caring about my "wife," about Prue, I don't know what to do about that.

T: Well, my sense is you guys didn't have much time to get to know each other . . . to learn to trust each other and learn about closeness. So perhaps you know about your roles but not much about each other.

M: One of my major concerns is the lack of commitment in our relationship, not just by me, definitely by both. We don't quarrel and sit down and come to a solution . . . we say: "I'm leaving, I don't need this . . . I'm getting out of here."

T: I guess if you say that enough times, you don't know what you have here (*gesturing between the two of them*). So fights end in declarations of independence, do they—and separateness—distance?

M: Yes, I'd like to look at this lack of commitment, we got married because I had to leave (*turns to Prue*). I can't be your sole support but I want to be depended on.

P: (*Sharply*) You needed to feel that my life revolved around yours.

M: No! No, listen . . .

T: So there's an issue here of being needed and . . .

M: (*To therapist*) Does she need me, not as a husband, as me?

T: You're not sure about that (*softly*), about how much you count, and that hurts.

M: No (*tears*)—I don't count (*cries*).

P: I need you but I don't put all my eggs in one basket, that's just not me, that's just the way it is.

Therapist notes that this may be her working model, re depending on others.

T: (*To Mark*) That's part of your pain in this relationship. You're not sure how much you, Mark, are really essential and necessary to Prue, you don't know that . . .

M: As far as I'm concerned it's nonexistent.

T: (*Pause*) That must feel very scary. To be in a relationship with someone . . . who you think doesn't need you, so they could walk out any time must be very scary.

M: Yeah, it is.

P: Well—I am here—I feel responsible that we don't have a lot of closeness, like love making, for example, in our relationship, I don't want it to go any further, but I have a difficult time putting things aside and responding.

T: You're saying you feel responsible that you and Mark aren't making love right now?

P: Yes, and I'd like to be able to be close.

T: O.K. So I'm starting to get a sense that it's difficult for you two to be close and you both feel insecure in this relationship, not sure the other person is going to be there—or that you're really special to each other. Sounds like you try to express your hurt, Prue—and it gets all mixed up with anger—and Mark, you try to stay calm and solve the problem but inside you feel like you have failed Prue and you get scared you'll lose the relationship—so you either stay distant or blow up—then Prue feels even more deserted and upset—it's kind of like a dance that keeps going and keeps you both hurting and fighting and makes it difficult to trust each other. Does that fit for you?

M: Yes, it does.

P: Ah-ha, yes.

T: So that's what we are going to deal with in therapy. I appreciate your openness and your willingness to answer questions that I ask you . . . which at times can be very painful . . . is there anything you'd like to say to me before we stop?

After this session the key moments in therapy were as follows: the therapist in EFT usually tries to mobilize the withdrawer first, since without this engagement is impossible and the other partner will resist changing from his or her rigid self-protective position. Thus, the first session focused more on Mark than on Prue: Mark began to acknowledge that he "turned off" Prue's distress because he saw it as a sign that he had failed in his role as husband and enhanced his fear that she was about to leave him. He acknowledged that he kept his "business suit on" and did not show her the "insecure Mark"; instead, he would "hide" and appear to be rational and in control. Prue turned to her parents rather than Mark for support and agreed that she refused to trust Mark and was too angry to hear him. In session 5, with the therapist's help, Mark began to explore and express his insecurity, his panic, and his fear of her anger. Prue at first refused to believe him and was disoriented; however, she then began to own her own rage, her "sore places," and her desire to keep her "guns blazing" to keep these wounds from being touched. They dialogued about his response to her pain and her need for comfort and holding rather than detached problem solving from him. He became more and more accessible in the sessions, sharing how criticized and small he felt and how on guard and withdrawn he had become, for example, finding logical reasons to sleep alone. Prue began to believe in this new version of Mark; she said it was "like he's taken his suit off." At the same time she felt sad that she had "closed so many doors." He asked for affirmation and affection. The climate of the relationship had now changed, "the doors are opening a little, there is more safety." In session 12 Mark asserted that he wanted to stop "tiptoeing" and obsessing about avoiding Prue's anger. They reprocessed key incidents and fights where she had walked out and he had experienced that she had ended the relationship. He stated that he was tired of hiding and wanted Prue to give him a chance and look at the extent of her own anger (steps 6 and 7). The therapist then shifted the main focus to Prue (who was still in step 4). Prue began to access her fear of trusting Mark, her fear of rejection, "I'll invest and then I'll be found wanting." The therapist helped Mark to let go of reasoning her out of her fear and to ask Prue to "let him in," which she agreed she had never done. Sessions 14 and 15 contained softening change events that have been associated in EFT with positive outcomes (Johnson & Greenberg, 1988).

A softening is defined as a previously hostile/critical spouse asking a newly accessible partner for what he or she needs from a position of vulnerability. Here the therapist focused on Prue's sensitivity to abandonment by Mark and the desperation underlying her anger. The process focused on her fear of trusting Mark and her resistance to needing him. She experienced her fear and her certainty that if she allowed herself to really need him, he would reject her, since even she "hated" that "needy childish part" of herself. The therapist enabled Mark to stay accessible and responsive and constantly structured for Prue the task of reaching for him. He reassured and accepted her and she was finally able to ask for comfort and reassurance. The next sessions involved her reprocessing her fear of his disapproval and a solidifying of the emotional engagement between the partners (steps 6 and 7 for Prue). The change in positions was then consolidated; he being more assertive and accessible and she being less aggressive and more vulnerable. They were now able to discuss in an open, trusting manner issues such as moving in a manner that reinforced their closeness. The problem still existed but its impact on the relationship was different. At the end of treatment the partners scored 100 (M) and 110 (F) on the DAS.

FOLLOW-UP

At the 9 month follow-up, the couple scored 110 (M) and 118 (F) on the DAS. These scores suggest that this couple's relationship continued to improve after treatment termination. At follow-up, the couple's score (114) was very close to the mean for happily married couples (114.9) on this measure (Spanier, 1976).

EDITORS' QUESTIONS

Q: How did you arrive at the idea of using four sessions for the initial assessment? This seems like a lot of time to spend in a diagnostic phase. How do you justify using this much time up front?

A: In EFT assessment does not imply that treatment has not begun. The EFT therapist is constantly tracking and assessing the process of interaction and the moment-to-moment experience of the partners. The designation of four sessions (two conjoint and one with each partner) as assessment is meant to imply that at the end of four sessions, the therapist usually has a clear understanding of the interaction and each partner's position in and experience of this interaction, a therapeutic alliance with each partner, and a plan of intervention. The first four sessions set the stage for the main therapeutic interventions. In the case of Mark and Prue, for example, by the end of session 4 the therapist had a clear picture of each partner's moves in the relationship dance and how such moves maintained the couple's distress. The therapist had also identified the vulnerabilities underlying each partner's position. At this point it was clear that Mark and Prue were suitable for EFT and that the usual form of therapy should be followed, with Mark's withdrawal being the primary focus for the first few sessions. Two conjoint sessions are also necessary to obtain the information that forms the basis for intervention. In these two sessions the therapist asks both partners how they view the problem, probes for their underlying primary emotions, asks about attachment histories and the history of the relationship, delineates prototypical problematic situations, observes present interaction patterns, experiments with each partner's responsiveness to interventions, builds an alliance, and sets a clear agenda for therapy.

Q: What do you say to couples who, after the initial four-session evaluation, are not deemed appropriate for your method of treatment? Do you refer them elsewhere? What criteria do you use to decide to whom you will offer treatment?

A: If, at the end of session 4, the couple are not deemed appropriate for EFT, the therapist presents them with a diagnostic picture of their relationship, discusses treatment goals, and gives a rationale for referral to a different kind of intervention. Couples are not offered EFT if the partners' agendas for therapy are incompatible; for example, if one partner is desperately trying to cement the relationship while another has already separated, or if violence is part of the interaction pattern. At this point, the therapist might also share certain concerns or reservations concerning the couple's difficulties or apparent blocks to engagement in the therapy process. For example, the therapist might validate how hard it is for the couple to begin to trust each other and question whether they are both motivated to attempt this risky and difficult task. If there are no contraindications and no apparent prohibitive blocks to treatment, the couple are offered a set of EFT sessions. The minimum number of sessions offered is 12; the maximum is set at 20.

Q: How do you determine how many sessions to offer the couple? Are these sessions planned in advance on a weekly basis or spaced out over time?

A: The couple is offered 20 sessions but if the problems are obviously resolved treatment may terminate earlier. Occasionally additional sessions may be considered in order to complete the therapy process. Generally, sessions are planned for once a week, with longer spaces between sessions toward the end of treatment. For example, Mark and Prue came to therapy once a week until session 16. The sessions were then scheduled 3 weeks apart.

Q: Your goals for therapy seem to be framed in terms of emotional exploration and expression of feelings between members of the couple rather than in behavioral terms. How do you know that it is time to terminate treatment? What behavioral indices do you use to mark improvement or change? What changes are you looking for in the emotional realm?

A: It is time to terminate treatment when the partners are able to unlatch from their negative interaction patterns and sustain emotional engagement in the session. The positions each partner takes shift toward accessibility and responsiveness, and each is able to risk expressing vulnerability and asserting boundaries. For example, it was clear that Mark and Prue were ready to end therapy when Mark was able to express his fears and make demands rather than withdraw, and Prue was able to confront her fear of rejection and unwillingness to trust and ask for her needs to be met from a position of vulnerability. Both partners were able to reprocess and communicate their primary underlying emotions. For example, Prue was able to experience her sense of unworthiness and terror of Mark's judgment and to acknowledge that in her fear she often shut him out. This evoked caring and compassion from Mark. This experience and presentation of self was clearly very different from the beginning of therapy. Once a couple can initiate such positive cycles, trust grows and the therapist becomes unnecessary.

Q: When you say, "The problem still existed but its impact on the relationship was different" (p. 218), what do you mean?

A: The issue of Mark's career requiring mobility was still a reality. However, the way the couple interacted around this issue was different. They were now united in the face of a common problem. It no longer divided them and evoked negative cycles and compelling distressing emotions. They were able to openly share their fears and concerns, listen to each other, and in fact agree on guidelines as to how to approach the next move. When couples feel safe and connected in the relationship they usually prove to be skilled problem solvers.

Q: Do you ever suggest that couples continue in treatment on a longer-term basis? And if so, what criteria do you use in determining this?

A: The structuring of therapy has to be somewhat tailored to the needs of the specific couple, so it is possible that some couples may need more than 20 sessions to complete the therapy process. However, we view marital therapy as essentially short term. In our experience if a couple have not responded in the first 10 sessions, there is usually a specific issue that has to be addressed. One partner may, for example, explicitly refuse to consider trusting the other and request a distant, parallel type of relationship. Longer-term individual therapy may also be necessary to address specific individual issues that block progress in marital therapy. Incest survivors often have profound difficulty trusting attachment figures and this, in our experience, is best worked through using a combination of marital therapy and longer-term individual therapy (Johnson, 1989). It is also possible that couples may complete the therapy process and return at a later date for help with a particular crisis or problematic issue.

Q: How do scores on the DAS shift as a function of EFT? What type of couples is EFT best for? For whom is it a bad choice? This couple's emotions are fairly close to the surface, what if the members of a couple are very emotionally stilted and distant?

A: DAS scores shift in EFT because the couple are able to engage emotionally, build trust and intimacy, and create positive cycles that allow attachment needs to be met. In addition, the self-reinforcing negative patterns that foster hostility and alienation are modified. This then results in improved marital satisfaction and more positive affect. The couples who do well in EFT show at least a minimal level of basic trust and goodwill, can learn to take some responsibility for their part in the creation of relationship cycles, and have an investment in maintaining the relationship. Couples who show little progress in EFT tend to contain one partner who is rigidly unable to shift his or her position or reprocess key emotional responses. No matter what the partner does in the sessions, he or she is unable to tolerate closeness. The issue of EFT's being suitable for partners who are distant or emotionally stilted seems to be largely one of therapist competence. It is difficult to work with two determinedly disengaged partners, but such couples rarely seem to request marital therapy. EFT can be a powerful intervention with one emotionally stilted partner because, once engaged, the process of discovering one's emotional life is often empowering and enriching. The therapist begins by validating the partner's inhibition and/or lack of awareness of his or her emotions, and is then able to facilitate such a partner's experiencing new aspects of him- or herself. For example, a partner who recognized that he was always "numb" emotionally was able to access the sadness that he felt when relating to others. This sadness and the anger that followed were more powerful for him in redefining the relationship, precisely because they were newly experienced and expressed.

Q: Do you ever give homework assignments or tasks to the couples with whom you work?

A: EFT attempts to create change during the treatment session that then generalizes to other contexts as opposed to creating change by giving the couple tasks to complete at home. However, the EFT therapist will request that the partners observe and note aspects of their relationship and be able to comment on these aspects in the next session. A withdrawn partner might be asked to notice how and when he or she withdraws and what he or she experiences at that time. The other partner might be asked to observe his or her response to the withdrawal. At the later stages of therapy, couples may be asked to attempt at home some behaviors already enacted in the session, such as expressing fear to the partner when it occurs during interactions.

Q: How did you become a brief therarpist?

JOHNSON: I was trained originally as a Rogerian/gestalt individual therapist, and being by nature an intense and impatient person, I became dissatisfied with long-term more diffuse therapeutic interventions. I then had the opportunity to receive training in family therapy and noticed how powerful interactions between intimates could be and how these interactions intensified the therapy process. After this, I took a position where I was expected to see many couples, on the hour, almost every hour. My survival instincts, skills, and biases combined to compel me to learn to produce results in a specific time frame. Conducting research projects with limited resources and coordinating a hospital clinic also taught me that if you have a focus and a road map, therapy can be likened to a freeway rather than a circuitous country amble. As the road map became more articulated, the journey became more fascinating and more fun, and now I'm hooked.

GREENBURG: Initially I worked with couples by attempting to facilitate greater self-exploration within each person and communication between them, but I began to see that this was not enough with some couples. There seemed to be interactional cycles that had a life of their own that did not yield to these interventions, so I began to pursue ways of dealing with these vicious cycles. I externed at the Mental Research Institute in San Francisco and learned its brief therapy model as well as other systemic approaches. In this process I became impressed with the possibility of changing partners' interactional positions in briefer treatment as opposed to changing character structure in longer-term treatment. Sue Johnson and I then set out to develop a brief structured treatment based on the accessing and communicating of emotional experience in a specified manner to change interactions. Our research demonstrated that couples could change in eight sessions of treatment, and this convinced me of the usefulness of brief treatment in changing interactions.

REFERENCES

Ainsworth, M. D., & Bowlby, J. (1991). An ethological approach to personality development. *American Psychologist, 46,* 333–341.

Bowlby, J. (1969). *Attachment & loss: Vol. I: Attachment.* New York: Basic Books.

Bowlby, J. (1988). *A secure base.* New York: Basic Books.

Collins, N. L., & Read, T. J. (1990). Adult attachment, working models, and relationship quality in dating couples. *Journal of Personality and Social Psychology, 58,* 644–663.

Dandeneau, M., & Johnson, S. M. (in press). Facilitating intimacy: Interventions and effects. *Journal of Marital and Family Therapy.*

Dessaules, A. (1991). *The treatment of clinical depression in the context of marital distress.* Unpublished doctoral dissertation. University of Ottawa, Ottawa.

Goldman, A., & Greenberg, L. S. (in press). A comparison of interactional systemic and emotionally-focused approaches to couples therapy. *Journal of Consulting and Clinical Psychology.*

Gottman, J. (1979). *Marital interaction: Experimental investigations.* New York: Academic Press.

Gottman, J. (1991). Predicting the longitudinal course of marriages. *Journal of Marital and Family Therapy, 17,* 3–7.

Gottman, J. M., & Krokoff, L. J. (1989). Marital interaction and satisfaction: A longitudinal view. *Journal of Consulting and Clinical Psychology, 57,* 47–52.

Gottman, J. M., & Levenson, R. W. (1986). Assessing the role of emotion in marriage. *Behavioral Assessment, 8,* 31–48.

Greenberg, L. S., & Johnson, S. M. (1986). Affect in marital therapy. *Journal of Marital and Family Therapy, 12,* 1–10.

Greenberg, L. S., & Johnson, S. M. (1986b). When to evoke emotion and why: Process diagnosis in couples therapy. *Journal of Marital and Family Therapy, 12,* 19–23.

Greenberg, L. S., & Johnson, S. M. (1988). *Emotionally focused therapy for couples.* New York: Guilford Press.

Greenberg, L. S., & Johnson, S. M. (1990). Emotional change processes in couples therapy. In E. Blechman (Ed.), *Emotions and the family: For better or worse* (pp. 137–158). Hillsdale, NJ: Erlbaum Press.

Greenberg, L. S., & Safran, J. D. (1989). Emotion in psychotherapy. *American Psychologist, 44,* 19–29.

James, P. S. (1991). Effects of a communication training component added to an emotionally focused couples therapy. *Journal of Marital and Family Therapy, 17,* 263–276.

Johnson, S. M. (1986). Bonds or bargains: Relationship paradigms and their significance for marital therapy. *Journal of Marital and Family Therapy, 12,* 259–267.

Johnson, S. M. (1989). Integrating marital and individual therapy for incest survivors. *Psychotherapy: Theory, Research and Practice, 26,* 96–103.

Johnson, S. M., & Greenberg, L. S. (1985). Differential effects of experiential and problem solving interventions in resolving marital conflict. *Journal of Consulting and Clinical Psychology, 53,* 175–184.

Johnson, S. M., & Greenberg, L. (1985b). Emotionally focused couples therapy: An outcome study. *Journal of Marital and Family Therapy, 11,* 313–317.

Johnson, S. M., & Greenberg, L. S. (1987). Emotionally focused marital therapy: An overview. *Psychotherapy: Theory, Research and Practice, 24,* 552–560.

Johnson, S. M., & Greenberg, L. S. (1988). Relating process to outcome in marital therapy. *Journal of Marital and Family Therapy, 14,* 175–183.

Johnson, S. M., & Greenberg, L. S. (1991). "There are more things in heaven and earth than are dreamed of in BMT": A reply to Jacobson. *American Journal of Family Psychology, 4,* 407–415.

Napier, A. Y. (1978). The rejection–intrusion pattern: A central family dynamic. *Journal of Marriage and Family Counseling, 4,* 5–12.

Perls, F., Hefferline, R., & Goodman, P. (1951). *Gestalt therapy.* New York: Julian Press.

Rogers, C. R. (1951). *Client-centered therapy.* Boston: Houghton Mifflin.

Shaver, P., Hazen, C., & Bradshaw, D. (1988). Love as attachment. In R. J. Sternberg & M. L. Barnes (Eds.), *The psychology of love* (pp. 68–99). New Haven: Yale Press.

Spanier, G. (1976). Measuring dyadic adjustment. *Journal of Marriage and the Family, 38,* 15–28.

C H A P T E R 1 1

A Cognitive–Behavioral Model of Marital Dysfunction and Marital Therapy

DONALD H. BAUCOM
NORMAN EPSTEIN
ROBERT CARELS

Research on marital dysfunction has indicated that the experiences of distressed spouses are marked by (1) the exchange of negative behaviors (e.g., criticism), (2) negative and extreme cognitions (e.g., viewing one's partner as having undesirable and unchangeable traits), and (3) negative affect (e.g., anger and depression) (Baucom & Epstein, 1990). The cognitive–behavioral model that underlies our work with distressed couples focuses on both the internal processes (cognitions and affective responses) of each spouse and the patterns of behavioral interactions between the two partners. The cognitive–behavioral marital therapist seeks to identify and intervene with the complex reciprocal interplay of cognitive, affective, and behavioral responses that results in the development of marital conflict and dissatisfaction (Baucom & Epstein, 1990). It is assumed that the behaviors exchanged between spouses are both the causes and the results of internal cognitive and affective responses of each individual. Thus, whereas one partner's rude behavior may elicit a pessimistic view of the relationship's future and a depressed mood in the other partner, the latter person's hopeless cognitive appraisal may in turn lead him or her to behave in an avoidant way, thereby escalating the alienation between the spouses.

The theoretical bases of cognitive–behavioral marital therapy are social learning theory (Bandura, 1977) and social exchange theory (Thibaut & Kelley, 1959). Both of these theories emphasize the reciprocal influences between an individual's behavior and his or her environment. Central concepts in social learning theory are that (1) behavior is controlled by its consequences (operant conditioning) as well as by antecedent discriminative stimuli signaling the existence of particular reinforcement contingencies, (2) much human behavior is learned through imitation of models, and (3) cognitive processes often mediate the learning and performance of behavior. Social exchange theory focuses on how social relationships such as marriage involve an economic exchange of "goods" between the parties. In this view, satisfaction with one's relationship is a function of the ratio of benefits to costs that one experiences in the exchange.

Based on social learning and behavior exchange concepts, the cognitive–behavioral model views problems in a couple's relationship as due to a combination of effects from each individual's learning history and from the pattern of interactions that the couple has developed together through a trial-and-error process. Consequently, it is important to understand the behavioral skills and habits, the cognitions about intimate relationships, and the pattern of emotional responses that each partner has brought to the current marriage, as well as the here-and-now responses of the couple. Knowledge of response patterns rooted in the past is less important as a source of insight per se than as a means for assessing the breadth and strength of learned responses that may require modification in therapy. Therefore, assessment covers both historical material (e.g., family of origin, past romantic relationships, and development of the current relationship) and the couple's current interaction patterns, but therapeutic interventions are focused primarily on altering the couple's present cognitive, affective, and behavioral responses to each other. It is assumed that dysfunctional responses were learned in the past (both outside and within the current relationship), but that they can be altered through a relearning process in the present.

Cognitive–behavioral marital therapy emphasizes an educational, skill-building approach, in which the couple is assisted in identifying and modifying cognitive, affective, and behavioral responses that contribute to conflict and distress. Clients are viewed as "stuck" in dissatisfying patterns because they are not aware of or skilled in more constructive ways of interacting. For the most part, client resistance to therapeutic interventions tends to be seen as due to discomfort with the nature or implications of the therapist's methods (e.g., fear that the planned changes will leave one open to being hurt again by the partner), rather than to a conscious or unconscious desire to sabotage progress. Consequently, the therapist attempts to anticipate concerns about change and to help couples plan a progression of changes that takes their sources of reluctance into account. The cognitive—behavioral therapist is open and straightforward in his or her approach, explaining to the couple the conceptualization of their problems within the theoretical model and describing how the interventions are designed to address those problems. Thus, the therapeutic relationship emphasizes active collaboration between the therapist and clients.

The behaviors of interest in a cognitive—behavioral model of marital interaction have been divided into two major categories: communication behavior and noncommunication behavior. Communication behavior includes both verbal and nonverbal messages used to exchange information. Communication problems (e.g., frequent arguments and misunderstandings) are the most frequent presenting complaints of maritally distressed couples (Geiss & O'Leary, 1981). Clear and effective communication is essential for resolving conflicts, as well as for facilitating mutual understanding and intimacy (Baucom & Adams, 1987). A cognitive—behavioral model of marital interaction proposes that members of distressed couples commonly exhibit low rates of positive, constructive communication, due either to skill deficits or to deficits in the *performance* of skills that they have in their behavioral repertoire.

Noncommunication behavior includes a wide variety of actions performed on a daily basis, which reflect the spouses' enactment of their varied roles within their relationship; for example, how marital finances are handled and how household tasks are distributed and carried out. Although such behaviors may convey messages from one partner to the other (e.g., concerning the spouses' attitudes about each other's relative value or power in the marriage), noncommunication behaviors generally are not explicitly intended to exchange information the way that communication behaviors do. Research studies have supported the theoretical prediction that frequencies of pleasing and displeasing noncommunication behaviors are associated with spouses' levels of marital satisfaction (see Baucom & Epstein, 1990, for a review).

Baucom, Epstein, Sayers, and Sher (1989) described five types of cognitions that can influence marital problems, and these tend to be the major foci of cognitive restructuring efforts in therapy. The five types of cognitions identified in this taxonomy include (1) partners' selective attention concerning those events occurring in their relationship that they notice, (2) their attributions or explanations for why the events they notice occur, (3) their expectancies or predictions about the probabilities that particular events will occur in the future, (4) their assumptions about the characteristics of spouses and intimate relationships, and (5) their standards about the characteristics that spouses and relationships "should" have. For example, there is considerable research evidence that distressed spouses are more likely than nondistressed spouses to attribute their partner's negative behaviors to stable, undesirable traits. Most research to date has focused on the association between attributions and marital distress, although initial studies with the other four types of cognitions have found results consistent with the basic cognitive–behavioral theoretical model (Baucom & Epstein, 1990; Bradbury & Fincham, 1990; Thompson & Snyder, 1986). Cognitive–behavioral marital therapists generally assume that partners' cognitions (of all five types) have the potential to be either inaccurate or extreme, and that people typically do not question their own spontaneous "automatic thoughts" (Beck, Rush, Shaw, & Emery, 1979). Consequently, such cognitive distortions can elicit dysfunctional behaviors (e.g., verbal attack and withdrawal) and emotions (e.g., rage and depression) toward the spouse.

Although affects such as anger, depression, anxiety, and jealousy have primary status in the cognitive–behavioral model, along with cognitions and behaviors, in practice the cognitive–behavioral therapist most commonly focuses on cognitive and behavioral interventions for modifying spouses' dysfunctional affective responses (Lazarus, 1985). For example, when a spouse's strong anger appears to be biasing his or her perception, such that the partner's positive behaviors are not noticed (or are perceived as negative), this process of "sentiment override" (Weiss, 1980) often is treated with cognitive restructuring procedures aimed at moderating the strength and pervasiveness of the anger. The cognitive restructuring may focus on how the individual's anger stems from attributing the partner's negative behavior to unchangeable traits or malicious intentions, or it may be designed to moderate an extreme standard such as "My partner should sense and meet all of my needs without my having to say anything."

The following case demonstrates many of the issues and constructs relevant to viewing marital discord from a cognitive–behavioral perspective.

CASE ILLUSTRATION

Bob and Ann are a couple in their mid-twenties. They are both well educated, physically attractive, establishing successful careers, and demonstrate strong social skills. They had been married for less than a year when they first contacted the therapist (Baucom), and to the outside world they appeared to be a young, happy, successful couple. They had recently begun marital therapy with a therapist in another part of the country and were referred by that therapist when they moved due to a career opportunity for Bob. In an initial telephone conversation, Ann clarified that they really had only one specific problem: they rarely had sex because Bob no longer initiated sex and typically refused her overtures. According to Ann, they had a great deal of fun being together and engaged in many gratifying leisure and social activities. However, within one year of marriage, their sex life was almost nonexistent because Bob had a problem that she said neither of them understood. Both partners were eager to begin treatment and improve this aspect of their lives.

Based on the initial telephone contact, the therapist had reason to believe that Ann viewed the marriage in a certain way and had a specific goal: with this one exception, she considered all aspects of their interaction to be very satisfactory, and she wanted Bob's problem eliminated. Whereas the existence of an isolated sexual concern was viewed by the therapist as possible, a cognitive–behavioral approach to marital discord assumes that many behaviors, particularly significant behaviors such as sexual interaction, have a great deal of meaning to both partners and often are related to other aspects of marital functioning. That is, behaviors do not occur in isolation from other behaviors, as well as cognitions and affect, and they develop as a result of a learning history. Consequently, the therapist was interested in knowing what other aspects of individual and/or couple functioning were important in the development and maintenance of their sexual concerns. Identification of such factors requires taking a history of the couple's relationship as well as gathering some information about individual histories to the extent that the latter are relevant to the current relationship concerns.

Although not always true, often when a couple presents with a single concern, this concern is actually only part of a more general pattern of maladaptive functioning. However, for numerous reasons (e.g., selective attention), the couple does not see the broader pattern and selectively focuses on one domain in which it is expressed. Consequently, it was critical for the therapist to obtain a broad picture of the couple's relationship concerns and strengths, and to evaluate whether there were other aspects of relationship functioning that formed a broader pattern of interaction with sexual concerns as one specific component. There was also the possibility that other areas of distress not focal to sexual functioning might be illuminated. At that point, the couple and therapist would negotiate whether such aspects of relationship functioning would become foci of therapy.

In addition to evaluating historical material and current relationship concerns and strengths, the therapist wanted to assess the couple's communication patterns. As noted above, frequently communication is problematic among distressed couples, and in the current situation, it was important to assess for at least two reasons. First, many couples have difficulties discussing problem areas in their marriage, and this is particularly true for highly charged and sensitive areas such as sexual functioning. For the couple to improve their sexual functioning, it would be important for them to be able to discuss this issue. Second, sexual behavior can be one way of nonverbally demonstrating or not demonstrating care and concern for the partner and the relationship. The therapist wanted to evaluate whether the couple's verbal communication patterns paralleled or more generally reflected the ways that the couple interacted with each other sexually. That is, the therapist wanted to evaluate whether communication and sexual behavior formed part of a *pattern* of relationship interaction as discussed above.

Consequently, the three elements of the initial sessions would include (1) a relationship and relevant personal histories; (2) a discussion of relationship concerns and strengths, including a clarification of sexual functioning; and (3) an assessment of the couple's communication. Whereas the therapist had some initial ideas based on the telephone call with Ann, he recognized that Bob might see the relationship very differently, or that both Ann and Bob might be focusing on only a small portion of their relationship (selective attention). In order to obtain a broader perspective on the couple's concerns prior to the first meeting, the therapist mailed two sets of questionnaires to the couple for them to complete and return prior to the first session. These measures, the Dyadic Adjustment Scale (DAS) (Spanier, 1976) and the Areas-of-Change Questionnaire (AC) (Weiss, Hops, & Patterson, 1973), would help identify more specific areas of relationship concern (finances, leisuretime, etc.) for each spouse.

The First Session

The session began with introductions, and the therapist explained that the first two sessions would be spent evaluating the couple's relationship. After that information was obtained, he would provide feedback to the couple, based on a cognitive–behavioral framework, regarding his understanding of their concerns and would obtain the couple's response. Then the therapist would recommend a treatment plan based on the conceptualization that had been offered.

Relationship History

After this introduction, the therapist began obtaining a relationship history from the couple. Baucom and Epstein (1990) provide a detailed description of the information typically included in such a history. The following excerpt comes from the couple's description of their dating period.

Bob: We really had a lot of fun during the year that we dated before we decided to get married. We did lots of things together; we camped and hiked and biked, a lot of outdoor stuff like that. We became best friends pretty fast.

Therapist: It sounds like it was a special time. How would you describe the emotional climate of your relationship? I mean, was it romantic or pretty low key or stormy or what?

Ann: I guess I'd say it was mainly fun; we've always enjoyed being together and doing things. It has never been that romantic; we really are more like best friends. We got along great with each other, and we really never have argued very much.

T: Well, what did happen when you disagreed with each other? How was that expressed, and how did you handle it?

A: The same way we handle it now. Bob doesn't say much of anything, and I tell him exactly what I think. He always stays very polite and usually agrees with what I want. But then he doesn't follow through with it, and that makes me furious.

T: Bob, what is your view on how you and Ann handled negative feelings and disagreements?

B: Ahhh, I guess that's pretty much what happened. I found out pretty early on that Ann's really opinionated, and it doesn't do any good to discuss things with her. You're not going to change her mind, and I never have liked conflict anyway. I think it is important to try to get along with people.

A: Now, that's from his family. The whole crew avoids dealing with anything. It's clear that they get upset with each other, but nobody ever says anything directly. They smile and are polite, but then they end up stabbing you in the back or making you feel guilty or frustrating you.

The therapist had at least two goals. First, he wanted to understand the role of affection and romance in the couple's relationship history. Was romance a significant part of their early relationship? Can their current sexual concerns be understood in terms of their early relationship history? At this point, the therapist had not asked about their early sexual relationship per se, but more generally he wanted to understand how the couple viewed the romantic aspects of their relationship historically. From the above statements along with other information provided in the interview, the therapist gleaned that the couple had had a sexual relationship early within their relationship, but even then it felt somewhat strained because they did not feel a great deal of emotional intimacy with each other. Throughout the interview, they continued to describe each other as good friends who enjoy each other's company and have similar interests, but placed little emphasis on being mates who are united emotionally. Consequently, the therapist hypothesized that one component of their current sexual concerns resulted from a lack of emotional intimacy, and that the husband was maintaining a distance from his wife through avoiding sex.

Second, the therapist was interested in how the couple handled conflict, because anger and frustration can lead to withholding in many contexts in a marriage. He began to see a picture of a couple in which the wife expressed her negative feelings and preferences strongly and directly, whereas the husband withheld his feelings and views for several reasons. First, Bob noted that he believed it would do no good to disagree with his wife's strongly held views; she would not yield or compromise. Second, he liked to get along with people, and that meant avoiding negatives. Third, he had found a less distressing way to express his negative feelings; he simply would agree and then ignore his agreements. Again, the therapist wondered if this pattern was related to the couple's sexual concerns. Perhaps Bob was angry with Ann for demanding that her preferences be accepted, and his sexual withdrawal was a way of expressing negative feelings and not complying.

Ann's final statement suggested that Bob's discomfort with discussing negative feelings was not specific to their relationship but may have been learned in his family. The therapist used this opportunity to explore some of Bob's personal history.

T: Bob, would you agree that that is the way your family handles conflict and negative feelings?

B: You mean, are they polite? Yes, they are very polite, and no, we don't like to argue and disagree with each other. But Ann's family is just as extreme in the other direction. You say one small thing that they disagree with, and they blast you away right on the spot.

T: So, you two come from very different backgrounds in terms of how disagreements and negative feelings are handled. And for each of you, it seems that the other's family is pretty extreme in the opposite direction. I'd like to get a sense of what each of you thinks about disagreeing. Bob, what is your view of whether it is okay for two married people to disagree with each other?

B: Well, of course, it's O.K. to disagree, if the issue is really important and it has to be dealt with. But I think it is much more important to try to overlook things and get along with people. And I'm very good at that; I can get along with almost anybody.

T: Under what conditions do you think people should avoid disagreeing with each other?

B: Well, to be honest, I think people should avoid disagreeing unless it is absolutely necessary.

T: Ann, what about you? What are your beliefs about disagreement?

A: I really don't understand how Bob can say that. To me, it is very natural that people disagree with each other, and when you do, you tell them. You shouldn't have to keep it in. It doesn't mean I don't like you because I disagree with you.

The above discussion provided some information on two fronts. The therapist learned that Bob's avoidance of negative feelings was not specific to the current relationship. It was typical of his family's style of interacting and not simply a reaction to their current relationship problems; therefore, helping Bob to express negative feelings would likely involve more than simply altering some facet of the couple's relationship that made it difficult for him to express his feelings. In addition, the therapist investigated the couple's standards for expressing negative emotions. Although neither person's perspective would likely be viewed as irrational, the two views were clearly in different directions and could lead to problems for the couple. The therapist concluded that he would need to confront Bob's belief that people should avoid disagreements; otherwise, teaching him to express negative feelings to Ann would result in the violation of his own standards for interpersonal interaction. Similarly, Ann was ready to express disagreement openly on almost any occasion. Such a style could result in an unpleasant environment, particularly for Bob who grew up in an emotionally unexpressive environment. Thus, Ann's behavior could likely make it more difficult for Bob to share his feelings for fear of being overwhelmed by Ann.

T: Thanks, that's very clear. Let's go back to your history. You mentioned that you didn't see your relationship as particularly romantic. How did you express your affection and good feelings toward each other while you were dating?

B: I don't think we meant we weren't affectionate. We just didn't have this dreamy romance. We would tell each other we love each other, and we had an active sex life with both of us initiating sex. It was pretty good.

A: Yeah, it was pretty good, but it had some weird parts about it. Even when we made love, we didn't kiss and we still don't. About the only time we kiss is a quick peck when we are headed off to work.

T: What is it about kissing that feels uncomfortable to each of you?

B: It just feels too strong. Sort of like scratching your fingernails on a blackboard. I know that that sounds strange. We can have intercourse, but kissing seems too strong. It's something about just having somebody right in your face. It doesn't give you any room.

A: I guess that's one place that we agree. It feels uncomfortable to have this long passionate kiss. I just want to back up.

T: Did you express affection to each other in other ways before you got married?

A: Well, we'd hold hands some, and we used to wrestle in a playful way. But most of the affection and sex dropped out after we got engaged, before we even got married.

T: What is your understanding about what changed?

B: Before we got engaged, it was just fun. We were just enjoying ourselves as two people in love. But we got engaged, and everything seemed serious. It was hard to relax with each other, and we just stopped having sex.

A: Well, that is sort of what happened. To me, it seemed like you really withdrew. You quit initiating sex and usually weren't interested when I suggested it. I don't know if you realized you had made a mistake getting engaged or what. It seemed like suddenly you didn't find me appealing any more. It makes me feel so terrible and unappealing. This is not what I planned for my first year of marriage.

B: That's not it at all. I didn't make a mistake; I want to be married to you. And I do find you appealing. I've told you there are plenty of times that I want to make love, but something happens in my head, and I don't follow through with it. When we do make love, I really enjoy it although I don't feel as close to you as I would like.

The therapist wanted to explore how the couple had expressed their affection with each other during courtship. This led the couple to describe the beginning of their sexual problems. The finding that their problems began when they became engaged raised the question in the therapist's mind of whether commitment was involved in their current problems. If Bob was being honest, he finds Ann sexually appealing, but something happens to deter the process. The therapist believed that it was critical to find out what Bob was thinking when he became aroused but did not initiate.

T: Bob, you said that something happens in your head at those times. What thoughts go through your mind when you are sexually aroused but do not initiate or respond to Ann?

B: As I've told Ann, it's not clear to me, either. I lay there and say, "Nope, I can't do it." But I don't know where that comes from.

T: O.K., I understand, it's not clear what thoughts you are having. How are you feeling at those times? What emotions do you experience?

B: I know this sounds weird, but I'm afraid that I'm going to get hurt. I feel too vulnerable, and I just can't put myself in that position. But that doesn't make any sense because I know that Ann will never hurt me.

T: Well, sometimes those feelings aren't just based on the present. They may be related to what has happened to people in the past. Are there some times in the past when you felt really hurt or very vulnerable?

As is common with many clients, initially Bob was not able to clearly identify the thoughts that he was having during those occasions. However, when he was asked to describe his "feelings" or emotions, his response revealed not only his affect (fear) but also some cognitive content (perceived vulnerability) associated with it. The therapist used this as another opportunity to clarify whether the current sexual problems were focal to the current relationship or whether Bob's role in the current problems was related to his past. Bob proceeded to describe three situations from the past that were related to hurt and vulnerability. First, prior to his relationship with Ann, he had had two serious heterosexual relationships. In both of those instances, the women had terminated the relationship with Bob, and he had been very hurt. Bob recalled for the first time during the current interview that he had told himself that he would never let another woman hurt him again. Second, he told of being somewhat small for his age when growing up and being picked on by bullies. He believed that showing his fears made him vulnerable and that bullies picked on him because they knew he was afraid. Third, Bob currently was a successful businessman. He had been taught and had personally experienced that he should never show weakness or be vulnerable in a business setting.

As a result of these experiences, Bob had taught himself to always appear to be strong, competent, and in control and never to make himself vulnerable. The therapist conjectured that as long as Bob and Ann were involved in a more casual relationship, he did not feel at risk. However, once they had made a lifelong commitment to each other, Bob believed that Ann was in a much more powerful position to harm him. Sex perhaps was a focal point for Bob's vulnerability because of the strong, intense feelings he experienced at those times. Thus, his reluctance to become involved in sex with Ann stemmed not from a lack of sexual desire but from a fear of being hurt at a very vulnerable time.

Unfortunately, Ann's own feelings of rejection, her style of expressing her thoughts and feelings strongly, and her frustration with Bob who seemed to be withholding led her to behave in ways that confirmed Bob's fears. That is, Ann made it clear to Bob that she could not continue in the marriage indefinitely if this problem was not alleviated. She also questioned whether Bob was gay and had feigned his initial sexual attraction for her.

The therapist continued obtaining the couple's history. During the year since they had been married, they had enjoyed numerous leisure and social activities together. However at present, they demonstrated almost no physical affection for each other, and they had not made love for several months. Fortunately, they were seeking treatment somewhat early, and their negative feelings that had focused on their sexual relationship had not generalized to other aspects of their relationship. They both still felt a great deal of love for each other, and other than in the sexual area, most of their interactions were what they described as smooth and pleasant.

Current Relationship Strengths and Concerns

A discussion of current relationship problems and strengths was structured in the following way. In order to minimize disagreement and arguments between the spouses, the therapist spoke to each spouse to clarify that person's concerns while the partner listened quietly. The rationale to the couple and more detailed instructions are provided in Baucom and Epstein (1990). Specific problem areas were gleaned from the inventories that the couple completed ahead of time. These detailed inventories help to insure that the couple did not focus only on the one or two most notable complaints in their relationship.

The excerpt below with Ann was typical of her concerns and demonstrated a broad pattern of behavior that she perceived in their relationship, although she had not recognized the similarity among her concerns.

T: Ann, you mentioned that you would like Bob to start interesting conversations with you more often. Would you clarify what your concerns are.

A: Well, I feel like I have all the responsibility for our conversations. If I don't find something for us to talk about, we just sit there quietly. Once I decide what to talk about, Bob takes part and seems interested, and we enjoy the conversation. But I get tired of always being in charge. I'd like to be able to relax and have him be responsible for what we talk about. Bob is extremely intelligent; he has an interesting job, and he keeps up with what goes on in the world. There really is a lot he could start a conversation about.

T: So, the quality of your conversations is good. You just want Bob to initiate them, so you don't feel it is totally your responsibility.

A: Exactly.

T: Fine. You also mentioned that you would like for Bob to engage in more social activities with you. What were you thinking?

A: It isn't that I want him to do more with me. We really do a lot together. It's just that I'd like for him to come up with some of the ideas of what we do on the weekends. He is very amenable to what I suggest, but he just waits for me to come up with the ideas. It is a lot of work being the social chairman.

T: It seems like you want Bob to initiate more in a lot of areas— conversations, activities that you both engage in, and sex. Is that one theme for the concerns that you have?

A: Well, I guess so when you put it that way. But I had never related the sexual problem to conversations and weekends. I just saw Bob as having some sort of sexual hangup, probably based on his past. Do you really think all of this goes together in some way?

T: I'm not really certain, but it does strike me that you have described a number of areas where you say you would like Bob to initiate things. If you initiate them and they get started, then you both seem to enjoy them. But your concern is that Bob doesn't initiate.

The therapist and Ann continued to discuss her concerns, but the most important theme seemed to be the one expressed above. Ann wanted Bob to take more "responsibility" for the relationship, not just to join in but to initiate. As Bob explains below, he has assumed the role in his relationship with Ann that he typically assumes in relationships.

T: Bob, you mentioned on your forms that you would like for Ann to help less often in planning the free time that you share. Could you explain?

B: I guess it's the same thing you were talking about with Ann. I feel really mixed about it. She typically plans all of our weekends. I've always just gone along with what other people want to do, and I enjoy it typically. I'm pretty flexible. But I would like to plan things some times, and Ann has also told me lots of times that she gets tired of planning all our free time.

T: Do you ever do that? Do you ever suggest ideas?

B: Oh, I have some, but it almost never works out. Ann doesn't seem to like the movies I suggest, or she is too tired for biking when I bring it up. You know, I told you, she has really strong opinions about things. And I . . . she, when she doesn't want to do something, she says so. So it's pretty hard.

And I don't want to be defensive, but it is the same way with conversations. She usually doesn't like the topics that I bring up when I bring them up. For example, we had gone to visit the relatives this past week, and we had a 7-hour trip back alone in the car, just the two of us. While I was driving, Ann told me to come up with some things to talk about, so I tried. Three times I came up with something for us to discuss, but each time she didn't like it for one reason or another. I'm not saying it was her fault; maybe my ideas were boring or stupid, but any way she didn't like them. So I

just sat there quietly, feeling stupid, and trying to think of something to say but knowing she wouldn't like it. Then she got mad
because she thought I wasn't trying.

*Both Bob and Ann had elaborated on a major theme in their relationship. Ann is
generally much more expressive than Bob, and has assumed the role of "social
chairperson" for the couple. They both would like for Bob to assume more of an
initiating role in the relationship, but when they try, it does not work well. Ann expresses
feelings of dissatisfaction, and Bob then withdraws. Although not likely her intent, the
impact of Ann's behavior is that Bob feels punished when he does attempt to initiate
interactions between them.*

*In focusing on relationship strengths, both Bob and Ann commented on how well
matched they were for each other in many ways. They both shared a love of the outdoors
and a commitment to the environment; their political views were the same, and they
shared many common values. They also really enjoyed doing things together, socializing
with friends, or being alone with each other.*

Communication

The therapist wanted to evaluate the couple's ability to communicate in
two major ways: (1) to problem solve or resolve a conflict; and (2) to
share both positive and negative feelings with each other. Therefore, the
therapist asked the couple to have several conversations with each other
while he observed. Again, specific instructions for this portion of the
assessment are presented in Baucom and Epstein (1990).

During the problem-solving interaction, the couple demonstrated a
number of communication strengths and weaknesses. They were very
effective in selecting a topic, staying focused on it, and reaching a
solution. As might be expected, Ann took the lead in offering suggestions, although Bob did offer ideas. Bob rather quickly accepted Ann's
proposed solution, and they both seemed genuinely satisfied with it.

The therapist asked the couple to have three conversations in
which they shared feelings with each other. First, he asked them to
discuss something that they had enjoyed recently, and to share their
feelings with each other. The couple had noted throughout the interview
how much they enjoyed their activities with each other. The therapist
believed that this would be a relatively nonthreatening set of feelings for
the couple to discuss. As expected, the couple was quite adept at
expressing their feelings in this domain. They openly discussed their
feelings of excitement and joy and the fun they had with each other.

Second, the therapist asked the couple to discuss some recent
situation in which they had felt close and tender toward each other.
Based on previous portions of the interview, the therapist believed that

intimacy was uncomfortable for the couple, and he wanted to observe whether they were able to discuss more intimate, and perhaps vulnerable, feelings. Not only Bob, but also Ann, had difficulty with this request. They spent most of the interaction describing the situation but avoided expressing actual feelings. After this pattern was clear, the therapist prompted them to express the feelings they had for each other during that occasion, in order to see if they could comply with more structure. Again, the couple avoided sharing tender feelings and started to joke with each other.

Third, the therapist asked the couple to describe a situation in which they were upset or had negative feelings toward each other recently and to share those feelings with each other. Ann expressed her feelings rather forcefully in a way that led to Bob's withdrawing and becoming somewhat quiet. Bob expressed no negative feelings toward Ann. Once this pattern was apparent, the therapist intervened. He asked Bob to share his feelings with Ann. Bob demonstrated difficulty sharing his negative emotions in two ways. First, he used many qualifiers, stating that he was "slightly" or "a little bit" upset. Second, he had great deal of difficulty differentiating specific negative affective states. He described his feelings only as "unhappy," "displeased," or "upset"—all rather general terms.

The assessment of communication suggested several patterns to the therapist. During the problem-solving interaction, the couple demonstrated a form of interaction that they had previously described in many ways. The couple quickly adopted what Ann wanted. They demonstrated an interesting pattern of expression of emotion. One of their fortes as a couple is having a good time together, and they were both comfortable discussing these fun times and expressing their enjoyment. However, both spouses were uncomfortable when asked to share intimate, tender feelings with each other. Thus, there were some aspects of positive emotions that they could share with little difficulty, but more intimate, positive feelings seemed much more uncomfortable. Whereas Bob and Ann showed similar patterns of expression for positive feelings, they differed greatly in terms of negative feelings. Ann attacked and Bob withdrew. Even when encouraged by the therapist to express his negative feelings, Bob seemed uncomfortable and uncertain what his emotions were except to describe them at a mild, global level.

CASE CONCEPTUALIZATION

The above evaluation was conducted over the first two sessions with the couple. Based on the information provided by the couple, the therapist derived the following understanding of their relationship which he shared with the couple during the second session. Although the couple initially presented with an isolated complaint of infrequent sex, the therapist believed that this was part of a broader set of dysfunctional patterns within the relationship that needed to be addressed. The therapist considered it important to share the major points of his case conceptualization with the couple, but he couched his feedback in terms that would be unlikely to be especially threatening to either spouse. The cognitive–behavioral marital therapist shares information with clients in a collaborative manner; however, he or she recognizes that directly confronting clients' core cognitions about themselves and their marriages can elicit significant anxiety that could impede therapy. Consequently, the following are descriptions of how the therapist conceptualized Bob and Ann's problems, as well as session excerpts that illustrate how the therapist introduced those concepts to the couple.

First, the assessment suggested that the couple had developed a relationship that embodied a strong friendship, emphasizing considerable satisfaction with joint activities. However, their level of emotional intimacy had not paralleled the growth of their friendship, and their infrequent sexual activity was a reflection of their discomfort with intimacy. The discomfort with intimacy was demonstrated in at least two other ways during the assessment. First, the couple was very uncomfortable sharing tender feelings with each other. Second, although other interpretations might be possible, both persons' discomfort with kissing each other seemed to result from a fear of being too close. Whereas both Bob and Ann demonstrated these discomforts, Bob seemed more uncomfortable with closeness; therefore he made efforts to avoid sex with Ann. For Bob, intimacy (both sexual and otherwise) meant vulnerability and the potential for hurt. Several experiences during Bob's youth and young adulthood had contributed to this perspective. As a result, he had developed the expectancy that being close to a woman increased the probability of being hurt, and he developed the standard that one should never show weakness or make oneself vulnerable. Within their own relationship, Ann's expression of her opinions and negative feelings in a somewhat punishing way confirmed Bob's belief that he needed to be cautious in making himself vulnerable to her. The therapist was uncertain how Ann would respond if Bob became more comfortable with intimacy because both partners had demonstrated a fear of closeness. Therefore, it was difficult to predict whether she would withdraw in some way or would be pleased with their increased closeness and greater frequency of sex. The therapist discussed these concepts with the couple as follows.

T: From the information you have provided, it seems clear that your relationship includes a strong friendship, in which you both get a great deal of enjoyment out of sharing interests and activities. That is a real plus, which, as you know, not all couples have. However, you also have described some discomfort in getting close to each other, both sexually and in sharing tender feelings with each other. There are a lot of possible reasons why members of couples find it difficult to be intimate in those ways; for example, Bob, you told me about some experiences you had while growing up which made you cautious about being vulnerable and possibly getting hurt. Often experiences like those have a lasting impact, so it will be important for us to explore whether events that occur in your relationship with Ann bring up old memories and responses. Ann, because you described some discomfort with certain aspects of closeness too, it also will be important for us to examine the way you view and respond to those situations. Mostly, we'll look at the types of closeness that lead to discomfort *in the present* and focus on the ways that you think about those situations which produces the discomfort.

Note that the therapist did not introduce the idea that Ann's style of expressing her negative feelings may confirm Bob's fear of being vulnerable with her. At this early stage of therapy, the therapist wanted to avoid any suggestion that one partner's problematic responses were caused by the other's behavior. Although the concepts of reciprocity and mutual causality would be stressed as the couple became engaged in therapy and comfortable with the impartial stance of the therapist, initially the therapist considered it important to counteract the distressed couple's tendency to attribute blame to one another.

In addition to a discomfort with intimacy, the couple demonstrated a second major pattern. Ann not only typically initiated sex when it did occur, she also initiated most activities for the couple as well. Both spouses wanted to change this pattern, although with some ambivalence. Bob had learned to get along with people by doing what they wanted to do, and he viewed himself as flexible with many interests. He also expressed that it was easier not to make the effort to start conversations or suggest activities. At the same time, the therapist wondered whether Bob was not somewhat frustrated by almost always going along with what Ann wanted (and other people). Although not certain, the therapist believed that a component of Bob's not initiating sex or responding to Ann's overtures was a way of not complying with what Bob knew Ann wanted, a domain in which he could passively say "No," even though his own sexual needs were unmet in the process. Ann wanted Bob to initiate in many domains, but she often was dissatisfied with the ways that he initiated. Unfortunately, her responses to Bob on those occasions were negative, discouraging him from initiating. The therapist's initial feedback to the couple about this pattern included the following comments.

T: Both of you have described how Ann usually initiates sex and other activities that the two of you share. Bob, although you said that you are pretty easygoing and are used to going along with other people's ideas, it seems to me that at times you might find it frustrating not to get Ann and other people to do things your way.

B: Most of the time it really doesn't matter all that much to me, but to be honest, sometimes I wish people would go out of their way to ask what I'd like.

A: Bob, you know that I've wanted you to initiate things more.

T: Well, even though both of you would like Bob to feel comfortable taking the initiative more, you both also have gotten pretty used to the pattern where Ann initiates and Bob complies, disagrees, or just does nothing. Patterns like that may be uncomfortable in some ways, but they also can develop into habits over time. In fact, both of you might even find it a bit strange if suddenly Bob took the initiative in sex and other things, because you have come to expect life to go along in certain ways. Ann, you have even expressed some dissatisfaction with the particular ways that Bob has initiated activities on those occasions when he has done so. It seems that this isn't just a simple matter of Bob's deciding to initiate more. The two of you have some different standards about what kinds of "initiating behavior" are appropriate, so we will have to examine how you can reconcile your different beliefs.

As suggested above, another component of Bob's not initiating sex might have been a passive–aggressive response in which he withheld from Ann, thus expressing his anger at Ann for pushing for what she wanted. More broadly, the therapist was concerned with the way that both partners dealt with anger and other negative feelings and the interaction of their two styles. Bob avoided dealing with negative feelings at almost all costs, and as a result he had difficulty differentiating and labeling his feelings to himself, as well as difficulty expressing them to Ann. Ann was not hostile in the expression of her negative feelings, but she seemed to make little effort to be tactful or consider the impact of her expressions on Bob. Bob experienced Ann's expression of negative feelings as somewhat painful, which confirmed the value of avoiding negative feelings. Both of these styles of expression reflected the partners' standards for how people should deal with negative feelings; these standards clearly conflicted with each other and contributed to the couple's different ways of expressing negative affect. The therapist's feedback to the couple included the following comments.

T: Based on what you have told me, and on my observation of your communication here in my office, it appears that the two of you have different styles of expressing negative emotions such as anger, with Bob trying to avoid focusing on such feelings and Ann speaking openly about hers. Each of you seems uncomfortable with the other's style, and so far you have not found a way to mesh the two styles. Again, this may be due partly to each one of you having developed habitual ways of dealing with emotions, going way back to your experiences growing up in your families. On the other hand, your different styles of expressing negative feelings also seem to reflect different beliefs or standards about how people "should" express such feelings. Any work that we do together on your communication patterns needs to take into account the differences in your beliefs about expressing emotions.

　　It can be tempting to view one's own way of dealing with emotions as "right" and the other person's way as "wrong." For example, Ann, you seem to get frustrated with Bob's lack of expressiveness, and in return you choose to hold back little in expressing anger to him. Bob, based on your discussions with Ann and from other things that you told me, it is my impression that you are uncomfortable with Ann's tendency not to censor her negative feelings, and the more she does it, the more you keep your defenses up and avoid expressing feelings. So, it becomes a cycle in which each person's communication is influenced by what he or she doesn't like about the other person's way of communicating. Looking for an answer as to whose way of communicating is "right" is likely to be a lot less productive than finding a pattern of communicating that is comfortable and palatable for both of you.

It was important to take into account the couple's perspective on why they were experiencing difficulties in the sexual aspect of their relationship. Ann entered the session attributing the difficulty to Bob as an individual, with little awareness of how couples issues might be contributing to their problems. Bob viewed himself as the cause of their sexual difficulty but had little understanding of the basis for "his problem." The above interpretations from the therapist were intended to cast the sexual problems in a broader context. Some of Bob's concerns about vulnerability and discomfort with intimacy, his general difficulty initiating activities in interpersonal contexts, and his discomfort with negative feelings were not ignored. However, the ways that Ann contributed to their relationship patterns and how the two spouses' styles interacted to create the current problem also were emphasized.

TREATMENT PLAN

Ann and Bob understood and accepted the conceptualization that the therapist offered. Based on this conceptualization, a multifaceted treatment plan was devised centered around the cognitive, behavioral, and affective components of (1) intimacy and vulnerability, (2) initiation, (3) expression of feelings, and (4) problem solving that included respect for both persons' needs and desires. This treatment plan was presented to the couple during the later part of the second session. The treatment plan would officially begin with the third session, although the conceptualization and explanation of the treatment plan that were presented to the couple were intended to initiate cognitive changes immediately in the couple's understanding of their relationship problems.

With regard to intimacy, several interventions were employed. First, it was critical to deal with the couple's cognitions concerning intimacy and whether they felt it was worth being vulnerable in order to develop greater intimacy. This was accomplished by having a conversation with the couple in which they considered the pros and cons of making themselves vulnerable for the sake of intimacy. This was especially difficult for Bob to evaluate, given that he had been hurt in two previous relationships by females, and Ann had clarified that she would not maintain their relationship if they did not succeed in improving their sexual functioning.

Following these discussions, the couple decided that increased intimacy was a goal that they desired and that they were willing to take a risk to achieve the goal. The therapist then employed several behavioral strategies. Intimacy was approached from both a physical and a psychological perspective. To assist the couple in becoming comfortable with each other's body and relaxing with each other, they were instructed in how to employ sensate focus exercises (Kaplan, 1974). Given Bob's reluctance to initiate, he was asked to initiate many of these activities. A specific aspect of physical affection that the couple wanted to address was their difficulty with kissing each other. They clarified that they believed that kissing should be a nonverbal form of communication in which an individual expressed feelings for the partner; however, they found little of this communication in their infrequent kissing. Given the couple's enjoyment of playful activity, the therapist and couple devised a game entitled "Read My Lips" in which they would take turns on a daily basis kissing each other and the partner would attempt to label the emotion that the other was expressing nonverbally through the kiss. The couple also had some difficulty discussing sex, and again the therapist relied on the couple's playfulness to increase their comfort in this domain. Bob and Ann clarified that they enjoyed playing scrabble with each other; therefore, the therapist helped them devise a version of the game called "sex scrabble" in which any word they came up with in the game had to have some sexual connotation. The couple found both of these "games" to be enjoyable and easy ways to introduce them to areas that previously had created anxiety for them. Whereas neither of these specific activities has ever been reported as a cognitive–behavioral intervention, they are consistent with a behavioral philosophy of devising specific behavioral assignments to meet a particular couple's needs in a nonthreatening way.

Sharing with each other and becoming more intimate in nonsexual ways also was critical. Consequently, the therapist taught the couple communication skills in emotional expressiveness to assist in sharing feelings (Baucom & Epstein, 1990; Guerney, 1977). In order to help the couple deal with issues of increasing intimacy that involved taking greater risks with each other, the therapist provided a list of 100 topics that the couple might discuss with each other that focused on them as individuals and as a couple. The couple rated each item from 1 to 100 in terms of how much intimacy would be involved in discussing the topic together, in essence creating a hierarchy of intimate conversations. The couple was then instructed to discuss a topic each night using the skills they had been taught, working their way up the hierarchy.

The topic of initiation also was discussed with the couple, and their cognitions were examined. The pros and cons of always and never initiating activities in an intimate relationship were evaluated. Bob came to recognize that in relationships, going along with other people's desires can seem cooperative but has at least two negative consequences. First, one's own needs are ignored, and, second, the other person can become resentful for "doing all the work." Ann came to realize that always initiating meant you get to do what you want to do, but the other person can feel ignored and become resentful, plus it is tiring to always be in charge. Consequently, the couple decided that they would like to strive toward a better balance of initiation in their relationship, although it would be difficult, given their well-ingrained pattern. Therefore, on many of the assignments that were given to the couple, the couple agreed that Bob would initiate at least half of them (e.g., coming up with weekend plans). On some occasions, the couple worked out a schedule for initiating the activity, believing the structure would assist them in changing the pattern of Ann's quickly taking charge.

Included among the initiation activities was Bob's initiating sexual overtures. This was phased into treatment as the couple became more comfortable with physical affection through the activities described above and after they felt closer to each other as a result of their communication exercises.

As noted above, the couple needed assistance with the expression of feelings. Bob and Ann needed to be able to share thoughts and emotions with each other verbally so that they would feel closer to each other. In addition, expressing negative feelings adaptively would help Bob avoid indirect expression of his feelings through withholding. The couple's standards for expressing negative feelings were clarified, challenged, and moderated such that they came to value the importance of sharing negative feelings with each other in a tactful way. (See Baucom & Epstein, 1990, pp. 320–339, for a discussion of details about how to challenge standards.) Because expressing negative feelings as well as "tender" positive feelings was more difficult for this couple, first they were instructed to share positive feelings that involved fun, joy, and so on. As noted above, Bob initially had difficulty labeling his feelings, so a list of feeling words was given to the couple to use as they practiced this exercise.

Finally, the treatment plan included explicit attention to the couple's problem-solving strategies because of their tendency to focus on Ann's suggestions and preferences. This component was scheduled for the latter part of treatment, after the couple had mastered the other communication skills described earlier. The work on this couple's problem-solving skills would include encouraging Bob to share his preferences and needs and encouraging Ann to compromise and not disagree in a punitive way.

FOLLOW-UP

Bob and Ann have been in therapy for several months, and they are making a number of positive changes. They have become adept at expressing positive and negative emotions, and they can discuss topics on their intimacy hierarchy list that have a maximum intimacy rating of 100. They also are much more comfortable with each other physically. They enjoy caressing each other and are somewhat comfortable with kissing, although continued progress in this latter area is still needed. They have sex once or twice a week, and Bob initiates sex the majority of the time (Specific frequencies and proportion of Bob's initiation were not goals of therapy. The therapist hoped both persons would feel comfortable initiating their sexual interaction but without any intent that Bob would necessarily initiate sex the majority of the time.) Bob initiates a great number of activities in their relationship, and both he and Ann seem comfortable with him in this role. Bob in particular seems to feel good about the changes that he has made. At present, problem solving has not been instituted with the couple, but their cooperative attitudes and good feelings about the changes that they have already made bode well for this intervention.

However, the interventions are not without complication. Most important, Ann has become less interested in sex in recent weeks, to a degree that concerns both she and Bob. The bases for this shift are unclear, but the therapist and couple have discussed two possibilities. First, Ann describes that she experienced so many sexual rejections from Bob prior to therapy that she was hurt a great deal. In order to protect herself and minimize her pain, she attempted to convince herself that sex was not important to her and that she did not really care about that aspect of their relationship. She tried, and may have succeeded in cutting off her feelings as a form of self-protection. Second, Bob's changes and willingness to disclose, make himself vulnerable, and initiate are a significant shift for the relationship. It may be that Bob is now interacting with Ann in a way that creates more intimacy than she is comfortable with; it is also Ann who continues to feel some discomfort with their kissing. Thus, Ann's decreased interest in sex may be her attempt to maintain the distance she feels she needs. Clearly, further exploration of this area is needed, but it will not be surprising if the couple experiences some discomfort as they attempt to find a level of intimacy that is comfortable for both persons.

SUMMARY

The above case illustrates important aspects of cognitive–behavioral marital therapy that often are misunderstood. First, cognitive–behavioral marital therapy is at times interpreted as demonstrating an interest only in the present and only in the couple's interaction pattern. To the contrary, a cognitive–behavioral approach recognizes that current relationship discord can result from a multitude of factors. Each individual's experiences, learning history, and individual style often are important factors in current relationship functioning. In addition, the manner in which the two persons have learned to interact with each other is typically of great importance. Thus, both individual and relationship factors should be explored in understanding the couple's current functioning. In a related vein, the cognitive–behavioral marital therapist is interested in current functioning in the relationship, but in order to place that functioning in a meaningful context, understanding relationship and individual historical factors is critical. Historical factors can be of great importance in designing interventions, particularly cognitive interventions in which the spouses are asked to rethink their beliefs, many of which began developing prior to the current relationship. Consequently, although the primary focus of intervention is on attempting to alter the current relationship, historical features of the individuals and the couple are not ignored.

Second, this case demonstrates how cognitive–behavioral marital therapy involves a conceptualization of the couple and a uniquely designed set of interventions based on that couple's specific needs, strengths, and weaknesses. Given that cognitive–behavioral marital therapy involves a number of specific interventions, some therapists assume that the intervention involves a set of routinely applied techniques. Such is not the case. As is illustrated in the above treatment plan, the interventions employed, the ways that these techniques are adapted, and the sequence of interventions are a function of the particular couple. In fact, the therapist developed specific behavioral interventions just for this couple. Consequently, developing a clearly delineated, individualized treatment plan based on the cognitive, behavioral, and affective factors impacting each spouse and the couple is the goal of the cognitive–behavioral marital therapist.

EDITOR'S QUESTIONS

Q: How does cognitive–behavioral marital therapy differ from other behavioral marital therapies? What does the "cognitive" piece offer that is not found in other behavioral therapies?

A: Traditional forms of behavioral marital therapy (e.g., Jacobson & Margolin, 1979; Stuart, 1980) have taken into account spouses' perceptions of each other's behavior, but they have focused primarily on the overt behaviors exchanged by couples. Based on concepts such as reinforcement and reciprocity of behavior exchanges, which were derived from social learning and social exchange theories, behavioral marital therapists have worked to reduce a couple's distress by increasing exchanges of positive behaviors and decreasing exchanges of aversive behaviors. Behavioral contracting and training in communication and problem solving skills are the interventions most commonly used to alter behavioral patterns, and results of treatment outcome studies have provided considerable evidence that such behavioral interventions have a favorable impact on spouses' levels of marital distress (see Baucom & Epstein, 1990, for a review).

Nevertheless, research studies (e.g., Jacobson et al., 1984) also have confirmed therapists' clinical impressions that pure behavioral interventions do not address all of the issues contributing to marital distress, leaving a notable proportion of couples distressed after treatment. Cognitive–behavioral marital therapy gives equal weight to spouses' behaviors and the subjective ways in which spouses perceive and interpret each other's behavior (Baucom & Epstein, 1990; Epstein & Baucom, 1989). As described in the beginning of this chapter, an individual's satisfaction or distress with his or her intimate relationship is likely to depend on the particular meanings attached to the events that occur in the relationship. Earlier approaches to behavioral marital therapy did not devote much attention to cognitive factors, but the integration of cognition into behavioral marital therapy is becoming common practice.

Q: A significant investment of time and effort, on the part of both the therapist and the couple, seems to go into the assessment phase. Are there any ways to shorten or streamline this process and still get the needed information on which to plan your interventions? How did you arrive at the idea of a two-session evaluation process? Are there ever times you might begin to intervene in the initial session?

A: As is the tradition in behavioral marital therapy, treatment is focused on altering specific problematic aspects of marital interaction identified through systematic assessment. Although we have found that a fairly comprehensive assessment of behavioral, cognitive, and affective components of a couple's interaction takes about two sessions, even within the first session the therapist is likely to identify a variety of targets for intervention. For example (as was the case with Ann and Bob), the therapist commonly will identify some problematic patterns in a couple's communication during the first session. The couple can be given feedback and instruction in more constructive communication at that point. Given how distressed and hopeless many couples are when they start marital therapy, any interventions that can begin to reduce aversive behavior exchanges may give the spouses some hope that therapy will help them. However, even when the therapist uses assessment data to plan interventions for the initial sessions, he or she still expects to continue the assessment process. In fact, the cognitive–behavioral marital therapist assumes that new information concerning spouses' behaviors, cognitions, and emotions will surface throughout therapy and will continue to shape the course of treatment.

Q: Part of your assessment process involves looking for ways to expand the couple's complaint and relate it to other relationship issues. How do you handle situations in which the couple continues to see their problem in a very focused way and are not amenable to your explanations? How are goals for treatment "negotiated" between the therapist and client?

A: Although the therapist strives for a collaborative relationship with clients, at times the concept that a specific presenting problem reflects wider relationship issues can be threatening to the clients' long-standing assumptions and standards concerning their relationship and themselves as individuals. The cognitive–behavioral therapist assumes that people are more likely to change their core beliefs when they are faced with consistent evidence that challenges those beliefs. Consequently, when the couple rejects the therapist's conceptualization, rather than attempting to impose the therapist's view on the clients, the therapist is likely to suggest to the couple that they proceed with treatment according to the couple's assumptions about the scope of their problem. If the presenting problem is indeed tied to broader issues, it is likely that interventions focused on the presenting problem will have limited effects. We often have found that when a couple becomes "stuck" in their attempts to alter an overly restricted treatment target (e.g., Ann and Bob's problem with initiation of sex), the necessity of examining other factors that are "getting in the way" becomes much more clear to them. At such a point, many couples are more open to the therapist's suggestion that they collaborate on experimenting with interventions with other relationship issues.

Q: The couple you present is relatively bright and articulate. How do you work with couples who don't understand your attempts at "explanation"? Can you work with those couples who do not see the connection between the presenting complaint and other relationship issues? What types of couples do best with this approach, and which ones are most problematic?

A: As we noted previously, for some couples the realization that presenting problems are tied to other relationship issues develops with time, as direct efforts to resolve the presenting complaints are impeded by cognitive, behavioral, and emotional responses to the specific interventions. Also with clients who are less bright and articulate, the therapist has considerable leeway in the complexity with which basic concepts are explained to couples. For example, the central concept that one's emotional and behavioral responses to a partner's behavior depend on how one interprets the partner's behavior can be presented in simple terms. Use of examples of cognitive mediation from the couple's own reports of situations that have upset them is a powerful way of conveying principles of cognitive–behavioral marital therapy. Thus, we have found that adjusting the way that explanations are presented permits use of the cognitive–behavioral approach with quite varied intellectual and linguistic abilities.

On the other hand, spouses who enter therapy heavily invested in proving that they are "right" and that their partners are "wrong" commonly have difficulty accepting the basic premise that problems are affected by the responses of both partners, as well as the goal of working collaboratively with their partner and the therapist to effect change. Such spouses may be just as likely to have difficulty engaging in other forms of marital therapy. Nevertheless, research studies have indicated that the quality of a couple's communication when they enter therapy is not predictive of how well they respond to treatment (cf. Baucom & Epstein, 1990). Therapists need to be cautious in prejudging clients' potential for response to therapy.

Some research studies have indicated that behaviorally oriented marital therapy is more effective with younger couples than with older couples, whereas other studies have found no association between client age and response to therapy (see Baucom & Epstein, 1990, for a review). Combined with the other research results and clinical observations noted above, these results suggest few limitations for the application of cognitive–behavioral marital therapy with distressed couples. Of course, research on cognitive–behavioral marital therapy is only in the initial stages, and future studies may identify specific limitations of the approach. In the meantime, therapists need to assess the match between interventions and client needs on a case-by-case basis.

Q: Some approaches bypass "understanding" and more immediately pursue the idea of creating change in the system. How important is it in your approach for the couple to "understand" *why* they are experiencing their current difficulties?

A: Although changes in a couple's behavioral interactions, instituted through a variety of interventions (including paradoxical and other forms of directives), have the potential to be self-sustaining, cognitive–behavioral marital therapists emphasize building clients' skills in identifying and modifying cognitive and behavioral factors that are producing difficulties in their relationships. The goal of such an educational approach is to develop skills that clients can apply to their own problems in the present and future. Thus, if clients are to learn skills that they can apply without the assistance of a therapist, they need to gain insight into the specific factors contributing to their problems, as well as the specific steps needed to change problematic marital interaction. Cognitive–behavioral marital therapists assume that insight is essential, but that it is effective only if it guides active use of skills for solving relationship problems.

Q: How much longer do you think you will be seeing this couple? Would that represent an average course of treatment? How long does treatment usually last? Are couples seen on a weekly basis or "intermittently" (e.g., every 2 to 3 weeks)? Are sessions 50 minutes long?

A: It is likely that the couple will be seen for approximately 6 months. Although most published studies evaluating the effectiveness of behavioral and cognitive-behavioral marital therapies report treatments lasting about 3 months, that particular length of treatment typically has been dictated by methodological issues and constraints. In clinical practice, some couples are seen for as little as a month or so, whereas others may be seen for up to a year, or longer, depending on the breadth and severity of their problems. In our experience, the average course of therapy for a clinically distressed couple is 6 months of weekly 50- to 60-minute sessions. As a couple moves toward termination, we commonly taper off sessions by scheduling them less frequently.

Q: How do you determine when it is time to terminate treatment? What indices do you use to evaluate treatment success?

A: Criteria for termination include modification of the presenting problems, increases in spouses' subjective satisfaction with their relationship, and evidence that the couple have mastered skills for solving problems in the future. These indices would indicate the development of a more satisfying relationship. However, not all couples who seek marital therapy decide to continue their marriage. As a result of treatment, some couples decide that they do not wish to continue the relationship. Such a decision is not viewed as a treatment failure. In these instances, the criteria for termination include whether the decision seems to be well thought through and is not based on major distortions in perception or reasoning. As is true of the approach overall, the therapist considers the decision concerning termination to be based on a collaborative evaluation of progress conducted by the therapist and couple.

Q: How did you become a brief therapist?

BAUCOM: The roots of my interest in brief marital therapy can be traced to my graduate school days in the early 1970s. At that time, there were no well-controlled outcome studies investigating the effectiveness of marital therapy. One of my fellow graduate students, Neil Jacobson, decided to undertake such an investigation for his doctoral dissertation. Jacobson, another student, and I were the therapists in that first large, well-controlled outcome study of marital therapy in the United States, based on time-limited behavioral marital therapy. Not only was I intrigued by the work with couples, but the results spoke for themselves; this brief therapy was effective in helping distressed couples. Almost immediately, I began to conduct treatment outcome studies, exploring different parameters of brief therapy with couples. I have continued those efforts empirically and in my own clinical practice up to the present. My model for brief marital therapy has expanded over the years to include a focus on cognitive variables, but my commitment to assisting couples in the minimal amount of time possible using empirically validated strategies has been the guiding principle behind my professional work.

EPSTEIN: I first became involved in brief therapy during my graduate training in clinical psychology at UCLA. My internship emphasized crisis intervention. It became clear to me that rapid intervention focusing on clients' coping skills and their perceptions of themselves, their interpersonal relationships, and the world could lead to fundamental shifts in functioning and the potential to generalize well beyond the crisis at hand. Furthermore, as a staff member at the Center for Cognitive Therapy in Philadelphia, I was able to view the effectiveness of brief therapy firsthand. My work as a psychotherapy researcher has also reinforced my belief that brief therapy can lead to rapid and significant change.

CARELS: I am a clinical psychology graduate student at the University of North Carolina at Chapel Hill. It is my impression that brief marital cognitive behavioral therapy is an approach with both clinical and empirical support.

REFERENCES

Bandura, A. (1977). Social learning theory. Englewood Cliffs, NJ: Prentice-Hall.

Baucom, D. H., & Adams, A. (1987). Assessing communication in marital interaction. In K. D. O'Leary (Ed.), Assessment of marital discord (pp. 139–182). Hillsdale, NJ: Lawrence Erlbaum.

Baucom, D. H., & Epstein, N. (1990). Cognitive–behavioral marital therapy. New York: Brunner/Mazel.

Baucom, D. H., Epstein, N., Sayers, S., & Sher, T. G. (1989). The role of cognitions in marital relationships: Definitional, methodological, and conceptual issues. Journal of Consulting and Clinical Psychology, 57, 31–38.

Beck, A. T., Rush, A. J., Shaw, B. F., & Emery, G. (1979). Cognitive therapy of depression. New York: Guilford Press.

Bradbury, T. N., & Fincham, F. D. (1990). Attributions in marriage: Review and critique. Psychological Bulletin, 107, 3–33.

Epstein, N., & Baucom, D. H. (1989). Cognitive–behavioral marital therapy. In

A. Freeman, K. M. Simon, L. E. Beutler, & H. Arkowitz (Eds.), *Comprehensive handbook of cognitive therapy* (pp. 491–513). New York: Plenum Press.

Geiss, S. K., & O'Leary, K. D. (1981). Therapist ratings of frequency and severity of marital problems: Implications for research. *Journal of Marital and Family Therapy*, 7, 515–520.

Guerney, B. G., Jr. (1977). *Relationship enhancement*. San Francisco: Jossey-Bass.

Jacobson, N. S., Follette, W. C., Revenstorf, D., Baucom, D. H., Hahlweg, K., & Margolin, G. (1984). Variability in outcome and clinical significance of behavioral marital therapy: A reanalysis of outcome data. *Journal of Consulting and Clinical Psychology*, 52, 497–504.

Jacobson, N. S., & Margolin, G. (1979). *Marital therapy: Strategies based on social learning and behavior exchange principles*. New York: Brunner/Mazel.

Kaplan, H. S. (1974). *The new sex therapy: Active treatment of sexual dysfunctions*. New York: Brunner/Mazel.

Lazarus, A. A. (1985). *Marital myths*. San Luis Obispo, CA: Impact.

Spanier, G. B. (1976). Measuring dyadic adjustment: New scales for assessing the quality of marriage and similar dyads. *Journal of Marriage and the Family*, 38, 15–28.

Stuart, R. B. (1980). *Helping couples change: A social learning approach to marital therapy*. New York: Guilford Press.

Thibaut, J. W., & Kelley, H. H. (1959). *The social psychology of groups*. New York: Wiley.

Thompson, J. S., & Snyder, D. K. (1986). Attribution theory in intimate relationships: A methodological review. *American Journal of Family Therapy*, 14, 123–138.

Weiss, R. L. (1980). Strategic behavioral marital therapy: Toward a model for assessment and intervention. In J. P. Vincent (Ed.), *Advances in family intervention, assessment and theory* (Vol. 1, pp. 229–271). Greenwich, CT: JAI Press.

Weiss, R. L., Hops, H., & Patterson, G. R. (1973). A framework for conceptualizing marital conflict, a technology for altering it, some data for evaluating it. In L. A. Hamerlynck, L. C. Handy, & E. J. Mash (Eds.), *Behavior change: Methodology, concepts and practice* (pp. 309–342). Champaign, IL: Research Press.

Reflecting Conversations in the Initial Consultation

JUDY DAVIDSON*
WILLIAM D. LAX

Therapists and theoreticians in the field of family therapy have recognized the role and importance of the initial interview in therapy.[1] This initial consultation often sets the tone in which therapy will continue, and the outcome of therapy is often directly related to how this initial session is conducted. A variety of theoretical perspectives and approaches to the initial session have been described, including defining problems distinctly at the outset of therapy (Haley, 1976), formulating and revising goals and hypotheses (Selvini-Palazzoli, Boscolo, Cecchin, & Prata, 1980; Weber, McKeever, & McDaniel, 1985), joining the family system (Minuchin, 1974), encouraging the therapist to be active and directive in the session, and being thoroughly prepared prior to the interview (Bryant, 1984).

This chapter discusses the conceptualization and use of the "reflecting process" (see Andersen, 1987, 1991; Davidson, Lax, Lussardi, Miller, & Ratheau, 1988) in an initial consultation. This model allows the therapist and clients to collaboratively develop multiple ideas about therapy at the beginning of treatment.

THEORETICAL FRAMEWORK

Since 1985, the staff at Brattleboro Family Institute has been utilizing the reflecting process as the primary conceptual framework for their clinical work. This model follows some of the basic approaches and

*The authors are listed alphabetically, with authorship equally shared.

assumptions introduced by the Milan Associates (see Boscolo, Cecchin, Hoffman, & Penn, 1988; Selvini-Palazzoli et al., 1980) and has been expanded through the influence of ideas from literary criticism, philosophy, social constructionism, and radical constructivism (see Andersen, 1987, 1991; Hoffman, 1990, 1991; Derrida, 1976, 1978, 1986; Gergen, 1985; Lax, 1992; Rorty, 1979, 1991; von Glasersfeld, 1984). The model focuses on several theoretical concepts and practical applications which include a lateral relationship between clients and therapist, the distinctions between "talking" and "listening" positions, therapy as "conversation" (see also Anderson & Goolishian, 1988), an emphasis on the meanings that people ascribe to their world, and the role and value of narrative in therapy (see Sarbin, 1986).

Given this framework, we make several assumptions. We believe that families/social systems come to therapy with a story or multiple pictures of their situation. These narratives may be formally expressed or not, but they contain a description of a problem. They are not fixed premises, but are developed in the context of another person or persons. The story that the therapist "hears" is one developed in the context of that clinical interaction. Narratives are embedded in myriad meaning systems carried by the individual members. The therapist enters the interview, as best as he or she can, without any fixed or predetermined story or hypothesis about the content of the problem description. He or she attempts to form an understanding of the family's picture(s) and embedded meanings through conversation, and, through questions and reflections, it is hoped, generates a new one that is not too different but different enough to make a difference (see Penn, 1982, 1985; Tomm, 1987). Through this process of asking questions and offering reflections, new ideas can fold over one another, potentially leading to a new view or story of the situation. If, at the end of the session, the clients' picture has changed in any way and/or a different solution, besides therapy, has become apparent to them, it needs to be examined. Perhaps they have developed a different enough narrative about their situation that does not contain a problem description and future therapy may not be desired or indicated. Thus the conclusion of an interview is very similar to its beginning. Clients are consulted about their ideas about future meetings, what might be talked about, who might be invited, and how we might talk (Andersen, 1991).

THE FIRST INTERVIEW

Format

Our initial interview makes several departures from established formats (see Lax, 1991). Attention is given to the context of the meeting rather than immediately discussing the content or problem and to the format of the meeting. When working with a team, we have a presession meeting and do not talk about content in terms of formulating a hypothesis but consider the information we have obtained over the telephone from the client only in terms of what format might be most useful given their concerns and which of us will be the interviewer. For example, if a family calls and says that they have been investigated for issues of sexual abuse by the state and are very upset about all the spying on them and invasion of their privacy, we might suggest that we have two people in the room with them rather than have a team observing from behind the mirror. Even though they could meet the team beforehand and will see them during the interview, this may parallel their experiences outside the therapy context too much. We would discuss these ideas with them and let them decide what they would like at the beginning of our first meeting.

Asking Questions

The interview usually begins with a discussion of their ideas about coming to therapy (Andersen, 1987; Hoffman, 1988). The therapist asks questions about the context of this particular meeting, such as the following: "How did the idea to come to therapy come about? Who had that idea first? Who agreed the most/least with it? If you had that idea in the past, how do explain that you did not come in then?" This process allows us to engage in conversation with the clients, attending to their agendas and not imposing any predetermined ideas, formulas, or hypotheses upon them. Starting in this manner, at this semantic/meaning level, we are also interrupting the expected process and marking this meeting, from the very start, as different from their usual ways of addressing and thinking about their situation. This view allows the therapist to more fully understand how the stated problem(s) are nested within the clients' larger meaning system, their ideas about therapy itself, and the context of this particular meeting.

As the interview progresses around the history of the idea of coming to therapy, the conversation moves naturally to a discussion of the problems as defined by the clients. Problems are addressed when they arise in the interview and are not ignored. However, our primary focus is on the meanings people ascribe to "problematic" behaviors and the language they use in this description.

The interview proceeds only as quickly as the participants can go, neither too slowly nor too fast for them to remain connected. Throughout the interview attention is given to who can be talking with whom, about what, and how. Our intention is to maintain the therapeutic conversation and not continue in a manner that is too different from the client's style, pace, or willingness to proceed. If the conversation were to be either too similar or too different from their usual mode of interaction and understanding, the conversation might come to a halt.

When a new topic or idea is raised by the clients, questions are first asked "about talking about" the topic rather than the issues themselves. When ideas are considered by the team or therapist(s), they can be "put on the table" to be considered by the other participants by stating them in front of the clients. New ideas can continually be introduced from this position, and this process allows both clients and therapist to determine what ideas and questions can and cannot be considered. For example, in a situation where someone raises drinking, we might first ask, "What would it be like if we were to discuss drinking now? If we were, who would have the most difficulty/ease discussing this? How do you explain that this would be difficult for him or her? With whom, if anyone, would he or she have an easier time discussing this issue?" (see Lussardi & Miller, 1991).

The therapist may even have specific suggestions or ideas for the client. These too can be introduced *as an idea* either during the interview or later as reflections. While the "ideal" position of the therapist is for him or her to maintain a position of equanimity and curiosity to all people and ideas, sometimes he or she has strong feelings and thoughts. These can be introduced to the clients from a perspective of "I have some thoughts now about your situation that may even seem somewhat biased. What would it be like if I were to share them with you?" The conversation can proceed *talking about talking about* these ideas with the therapist as an active participant with one outcome being the discussion of his or her thoughts. The therapist can utilize his or her expertise while maintaining a lateral position with the client. When working in this collaborative model, the therapist is fully considered a member of the therapeutic system. Therefore, the therapist's ideas "count" and can be expressed.

We pay particular attention to clients' usual and unusual patterns of behavior and thinking. Hence, in the interview we will ask if what they are doing/thinking/feeling is usual or unusual for them. We will often ask both process and content questions in this style. For example, when a couple is fighting in the room, we may ask if this fighting is usual or unusual for them. This process often places them in a different position to their "fighting" discourse and allows them to comment on the interaction. It also informs us as therapists about how they relate to one another. In terms of content, we may ask this same couple to tell us what they usually fight and do not fight about. Again, they are *talking about* the fighting and giving us information while not being lost in their usual way of interacting.

REFLECTIONS

Central to the reflecting process are ideas concerning the listening and talking positions (see Andersen, 1991). When one is in a talking mode, one is in a different position or discourse than when one is in a listening position. It is believed that it is very important to allow clients to be in a listening position when reflections are offered. They are then better able to hear what is being said without any feelings of a need to respond. They can also listen to all the reflections without responding to each one, allowing them to experience their own gestalt of the reflections, forming their own notions of what is relevant to them and what is not.

Our initial consultation usually lasts about 1½ hours. At some point in the interview, usually after 40 to 60 minutes, the conversation will reach a natural pausing point or conclusion. When working with a team observing from behind a one-way mirror, team members can exchange places with the therapist and clients and offer their reflections. In the absence of a mirror, the team members may be in the room with the client system, maintaining an imaginary boundary between themselves and the clients. With only two therapists, both may wish to be in the room, taking turns being the interviewer and the "observer" at different times during the interview. They can also choose to have fixed roles, with one member consistently being the interviewer and the other being a "reflector."

Reflections follow some general guidelines (see Andersen, 1987, 1991; Lax, 1989). These center on presenting comments within a positive or logical framework as opposed to a negative one; moving from an either/or position to a both/and or neither/nor position; presenting a "smorgasbord of ideas" versus correct "interpretations"; and offering ideas not as rigid explanations but as tentative thoughts.

Comments and questions may also be raised which the therapist did not or contextually could not say in the interview. These can include comments on "difficult" topics, such as alcohol/substance abuse, suspected incest or violence, and an individual team member's subjective ideas or concerns that were not raised or addressed during the interview. The team can introduce these issues in the presence of the family, allowing these ideas to be present in the room as a potential part of the ongoing conversation. The family and therapist then have the possibility of addressing them in ways that they had not been able to prior to this moment.

Following ideas from literary criticism and deconstruction, new ideas are introduced both in the reflections and in the therapist's questions and comments, often from a perspective of what is opposite or different from what the clients present (Derrida, 1976, 1978; see also Lax, 1992). We intend to create a difference between two perspectives similar to Derrida's ideas of *différance* in which there is a tension between the two perspectives. This tension creates the potential for a new understanding to emerge. This new understanding/narrative is not a duality or either/or between words and meanings but a shift, at a minimum, to a both/and position. With this interplay of what is said and what is not said by the clients, and what is presented by the reflections, there is always the potential of another position or perspective to emerge. It is this other position for which Derrida further suggests we continually look: a description that is even outside of the both/and perspective. For Derrida, another view is already there for us, and we should always attempt to deconstruct our world as we know it, looking for the unexpected that might replace that view.

COMMENTS ON THE REFLECTIONS

After the reflections, the therapist and clients switch back to their original places and the therapist usually asks questions such as: "Did you have any thoughts or ideas while you were watching and listening and what ideas seem to make sense to you? Was there anything that they should not have talked about or you disagree with? Was there anything else that they should have included?" The first two questions are generally asked to determine what "fit" for the clients. The last question is particularly important because the clients may have begun to develop a new story or picture of their situation and are generating new solutions that were not thought of prior to the interview. This question gives them the opportunity to explore these solutions with the therapist. After the clients have fully responded, the therapist can introduce ideas of his or her own.

CASE ILLUSTRATION

This is the first couples session of a family with whom the therapist (Davidson) had been working. The family consisted of Hank, age 43, Mary, 36, and two natural children, Sandy, 15, Darren, 14, and Andy, a profoundly retarded, multihandicapped 10-year-old boy whom they had adopted. Hank was a worker in a local factory; Mary had been a foster mother for many years and now was taking courses at a local community college. After 5 months of family sessions, Mary had called Judy asking if she would be willing to see her and Hank for some couples therapy around their sexual relationship. Mary also asked if it would be possible to have a male cotherapist.

In our private practice, we often have families make this kind of request. Sometimes couples do not seem to feel safe bringing up painful marital issues until they get to know the therapist better. In other situations, the marital issues become primary in the family therapy, and the couple wish to address them without the children present. Generally we do not see this as an abrupt shift in roles for the therapist and we try not to make rigid distinctions between individual, couples, and family therapy. Since we view therapy as a conversation, we are open to the idea that sometimes the conversation might include different members of the system. However, whenever a change in participants is suggested, we will always ask each family member what he or she thinks of the idea and what it would mean to him or her if there were such a change. When considering a shift such as the one above, we ask ourselves whether it would affect our role in the therapy sessions, such as interfering with our ability to ask questions or hearing the ideas and concerns of all family members. In this case, when the idea for couples therapy was introduced in the family session, the children were in favor of the idea of the parents meeting without them and hoped that it would lead to Hank's "speaking up more," even if this meant more open conflict between the parents.

Judy felt by adding a male therapist her position as the family therapist would be maintained. As is usual, she did not share much background information with the cotherapist (Lax) before the session except for the presenting request for "couples therapy around their sexual relationship."

The First Session

Judy: (*To Bill*) Hank was telling me that Mary had "cold feet" so he had to bring her down early so she wouldn't back out. That's why they were in the waiting room 10 minutes early. (*Everyone laughs*) (*to couple*) This is a big step. . . . Bill and I were talking a few minutes ago about what would be the best way to start, how I might fill Bill in on my past work with your family, and about your reasons for wanting couples therapy now. We had the idea to just have a conversation in front of you. That would be a way for me to give Bill my ideas and you can correct me if you want to add something different. Does that feel like a good way to start?

Bill: (*To Judy*) Or, if you want to talk to them about it, I can eavesdrop or however you all want to do it.

J: (*To the couple*) What would be more comfortable?

Mary: (*Laughs nervously*) Why don't you two just talk together!

Judy then summarized her work with the family. She had started meeting with them after the couple's 15-year-old daughter had returned home after living in a group home for a year. This daughter, Sandy, had been sexually abused as a young child and had become increasingly depressed and suicidal at the age of 13. Following a 3-month hospitalization and numerous other crises, she refused to attend school and was eventually placed in the group home. At about the same time that Sandy was hospitalized, Mary started to have flashbacks to her own severe sexual abuse as a child. She was hospitalized briefly for severe panic attacks and suicidal thoughts and had been in intensive individual therapy ever since. Remembering her abuse stirred up sexual issues for her, and she and Hank had not had sex for a long time. Judy mentioned how much she has enjoyed working with this family and described the kinds of issues they have been talking about as they adjusted to having Sandy rejoin the family. At this point, Bill and Judy began to talk between themselves about Judy's summary.

B: Was it Mary's idea for couples therapy? Did that come from her therapist or was it something she had been thinking about on her own?

J: That is a good question. I think the idea for couples therapy may have come from Mary, but it was Mary's therapist's idea to have a male cotherapist because of Mary's issues around trusting men. The therapist may also have thought it would be good for Hank to have another man present, but that is just my idea. When I asked Hank in the family session if he agreed with the plan for couples therapy, he said he did. Hank's role in the family is often to be agreeable. He is the peacekeeper.

B: I was wondering actually about the cold feet.

J: (*Nods*) Uh huh.

B: It sounded like it was Mary's idea to come, but she is the one with the cold feet. What is your understanding of that?

J: I don't know. I think that would be a good question to ask Mary (*laughter from the couple*)! (*To Mary*) Maybe the cold feet would be the best place to start and then we could find out what you think about what I told Bill about your reasons for wanting therapy. Can you tell me a little bit about the cold feet and what that would be about?

M: I don't know exactly. It is generally increasing anxiety. I think some of it is because Bill is here and . . . (*long pause*)

J: And do you know what that has to do with in terms of Bill? I mean, is it just this guy sitting here . . . (*everybody laughs*).

M: I don't even know this man (*laughs*)!

J: . . . or is it because he is a man?

M: That he is a man, I guess.

J: Uh huh. What does that mean in terms of your feeling Okay?

M: I don't know, I guess. I guess I need about two more women sitting over here. (*She points to a space next to her*)

J: In order to feel OK about what?

M: In order to feel OK about two men sitting over there! And that is the only way I can explain it.

J: If there were two women over here and just the two of them over there, how would it feel different than with just the two of us here?

M: I would feel safer, I guess.

J: I guess I am wondering, given that you feel that way, how did you even get to the point of deciding to come in? What kind of a process did you go through to get you to this point?

M: (*Sighs*) Well, I think I know that I really want to do this and that it is really important and I haven't been having a lot of real anxiety or panic attacks in a long time and then the closer I got to the time for this [meeting], the more anxious I felt and it is almost like the best thing to do is to just come in and do it rather than just run away from it and then it would just be an issue forever.

J: And have you ever been in this kind of therapy with a male and female therapist before?

M: No.

J: Have you ever been in a therapy situation with a male therapist?

M: (*Laughs*) No!

J: And did you have any idea about what any of us could do to make it a safer place for you? Would it be best if Bill just sat down over there and kept his mouth shut? (*Mary laughs*) Would you like a chance to ask him some questions so you would get a chance to know him? Do you have any sense of what would make the process go at a comfortable pace for you?

M: (*Shakes head*) No. I didn't think about that, I guess. Well . . . I know that for him just to sit there and say nothing is going to be kind of threatening because then I am not going to have any idea what is

going on over there. I don't have any particular questions or anything like that.

B: (*Smiles*) So, I had better say something soon. (*everyone laughs*)

M: Well . . . well, voices are important to me, so the tone of people's
voices is very important, so, yeah, it would be threatening if anyone
sat in a room and never said anything. Then I would have no idea
what was going on.

B: And is that usual? Like for the tone of voice and how people sit and
how people are? Is that usual for you to think about that for women
as well as for men?

M: Oh, for everybody.

B: I guess I was also wondering as you were saying that . . . I was kind
of taken with this idea of just "come here and do it." Is that a usual
or unusual way of your facing uncomfortable, anxiety-producing
situations?

M: It's kind of common except for when I first got out of the hospital
and I started dealing with the panics. They were so bad . . . these
issues were so bad that I couldn't even go in the grocery store or
anything for a while, especially by myself. I couldn't even drive
myself places.

*Mary and Hank describe several intense panic attacks from the past and how she coped.
Bill comments on how hard she worked to overcome them, ending with, "It sounds like
there were a whole lot of successes."*

B: (*To Judy*) I am also wondering about the difficulty that Mary talked
to you about that had them consider marital therapy.

J: Uh huh.

B: (*To the couple*) It sounds like the difficulty that you described to Judy
was one about the amount of sex you were having, and I am
wondering what it would be like to even talk about that with a man
here?

M: (*Looks at Judy and laughs nervously*)

B: Is that even possible at this point? To even talk about that with
someone. Is it possible to "just dive" into it with them, as you said?

M: (*Pause*) I don't know. I think so. That is one of the main reasons that
we are here. I guess I believe it is at least possible or I wouldn't be here
at all. I don't think it is going to be easy, but it is at least possible.

B: (*To Mary*) Do you think it will be easier for Hank than for you?

M: (*Laughs*) No, not necessarily.

Hank: (*Smiles*)

B: If you hadn't called Mary, would Hank have called? Would he have said, "Judy, we need to have a look at this?" Or is he so agreeable that he would have just gone along with this for another while?

M: No.

H: For me it was just kind of sitting back and thinking, "In her own time, when everything is ready, it will all eventually come back." That is the way I felt and, you know, "No big hurry." Myself, I have thought . . . I have doubts that when we get going again, when we get back into sex, it is it going to send her back into a flashback and put us back 2 years to where we are starting all over again and so that is why I am just sitting there.

B: (*To Hank*) So, there might be a concern on your part about going too fast?

H: Yeah, in a way. I see things between us better now, and I don't know how she looks at it. I guess if we go back 1½ or 2 years to when she first got out of the hospital, she couldn't go upstairs and sleep with me. She would sleep on the couch sometimes. Eventually she would come to bed, and she would have to roll the other way. She couldn't face me. Now she has gotten to where she can face me. We can hug each other and once and a while she will just reach down and give me a little play or touch me a little bit and then it just stops. So, to me, I can see a gradual coming back.

B: (*Interrupts*) Let me just interrupt for just a second. You are concerned about going too fast, but you are sort of moving right along, and I am wondering, what do you think Mary's speed is about talking about this stuff? She doesn't have her two women here with her sort of backing her up! She only has Judy (*everyone laughs*)! What do you think her comfort level is about your diving right in? You are already talking about her reaching down and stuff like that. What is your guess?

H: That is a good question. I never really stopped to think about it.

(*Mary is wiping tears from her eyes and Judy gets up to get her some Kleenex*).

H: (*Glances at Mary*) Yeah, it could get her nerved up.

B: Can you tell when she is nervous?

H: (*Looks at Mary crying*) Yeah, yeah. Sometimes not. It is not quite that obvious. (*Looks at Mary again and laughs nervously*) I guess I did go sort of fast.

B: That is not a scold. I am just wondering if you can read Mary in terms of her tears. What is your guess about what those tears might be about?

H: I guess I don't really understand at this point. Probably some anxiety or maybe I went too fast or . . . (*shakes his head*).

B: (*To Hank*) If this were to happen at home, how would you find out? What would you do if Mary started to tear up about something at home?

H: Sit back and wait for her to tell me.

B: (*To Mary*) Is that the usual way Mary? (*She nods*).

Bill and Judy then have a conversation in front of the couple. Bill asks Judy if she knows what Mary's tears are about, and Judy says that she is not sure. She knows Mary well as a parent but she doesn't know that much about her as a woman or about the struggles she has gone through as a survivor of sexual abuse. Bill then explores if Judy thinks Hank knows about Mary's struggles as a "survivor" of sexual abuse. Judy explains that it has been hard for them as a couple to talk about the abuse. Hank was raised in a family where no one talked about feelings so he is just learning how to do this. Mary has been trying to teach him, but this has been very painful for her when she has so many strong feelings about the abuse and he does not say much. It has often been easier for her to talk with women.

B: (*To Hank*) What do you think about what Judy has been saying?

H: Oh, yeah. She hit it right on the head. Mary is always trying to get me to talk more, or she wants to explain more. I guess I listen a little bit and then at some point I don't understand or (*sigh*) it kind of just goes over.

B: Yeah, so you sort of listen and . . .

H: Well, I don't even listen that good because . . . once she tried to explain something to me that was a hard situation for her. But I tried to find a little bit of light to the hard situation, something that was good when I really should have just sat still and been quiet. As a rule, I have a hard time just sitting still.

B: Is it hard for you to watch her in so much in pain?

H: Sometimes, yes. Sometimes more than others. I guess yeah.

The focus of the interview had been on the history of the idea of coming to therapy until Hank jumped into a specific content issue, their sexual relations. We usually do not interrupt clients when they are talking. However, since a conversation can only proceed as fast as the participants involved, it was important to make sure that Mary was still able to be a part of the conversation. Hank had gone too fast for her, and it was important to go at a pace that was manageable for both of them. Mary had said earlier that she thought that they could "possibly" talk about sex, but was clearly not ready yet.

The conversation then moved to trying to understand what is usual and unusual for them in their interactions around talking about difficult topics, including when Mary is feeling sad. We continue the conversation with an exploration of Hank's understanding of Mary's ways of talking with her women friends. He responds saying, "I think she is more detailed with them, because they understand better than I do." We specifically then describe our thoughts to them in a reflection so that they can comment on our ideas and determine the direction of the conversation.

J: *(To Bill)* I guess I was interested in how we got to this point in the conversation. At first you were talking about how comfortable they were in talking about sex and what was the right pace to go. Then Mary got teary and you went on to talk about talking in general, not just about sex, but about how they communicate and on what level. And the conversation just moved in that way. But there is a part of me that just wants to check in with Mary about her tears and about what their different ideas are about how we can proceed to talk about something that is very difficult like sexuality, especially with you, a male therapist, present, and all the safety issues that that raises for Mary. So I'm wanting to think about some overall ideas about how we can proceed to do this in a way that is comfortable for both of them and about whether this is a good place for us to begin?

B: Yeah, I'm sort of wanting to know what Mary's thoughts are about me. In some ways I have been very bold by asking lots of questions, and I would like to check in with her, like, "How am I doing?"

J: *(Laughing)* I think that might be a good idea, kind of wanting to know from her, "Is the anxiety down, even a little bit, at this point?"

B: Yeah, and are we going too fast, because I am asking some very specific types of questions.

(Bill and Judy turn to Mary)

M: *(Laughs)* I'm okay *(turns to Bill)*. You're okay. Your voice is okay. I guess where you and Hank were talking, what you were talking about was really the best place to start, because that is really where I feel a lot of the issue is, that I would really like to be able to talk to Hank more and he just . . . he says, if he can't fix it, then he just doesn't want to hear about it. And, sometimes things happen to people that, you know, there really isn't anything positive about it. I mean you can look forever and there is nothing positive to be said about some things. But he searches and searches for it, for something positive about something that is so horrible that it can't possibly be positive. I do feel that we, like we are very separate in many ways and my life is just so far apart from Hank's. I mean, we share news, we do things together, we raise kids together, but I don't feel I can talk to him much about anything.

J: What's your understanding, Mary, of Hank's belief that that if he can't fix it, he doesn't want to hear it? Do you know what that is about?

M: Yes, I mean, I understand, that it's hard not to be able to fix things and make things better. I mean, I like to fix things too whenever I can (*laughs*), but it is like . . . (*pause*). last week I was having a real hard time and I was crying a lot for a day or so, so I cried part of the night and Hank put his arms around me and I just cried and cried and the next morning he says, "I wasn't very helpful." I said, "Yes, yes, you were." He said, "No I wasn't because you didn't stop crying."

J: How do you explain that he doesn't quite get it that he really is taking care of you when he is just there?

M: I don't know. I have never figured that out. (*Laughs*) It's like he just doesn't believe me. Almost like he figures it has to be something else. It can't be this simple. There has to be something else. I don't know.

J: You mean, that it wasn't enough that he was just there and holding you?

M: Yeah.

J: Do you feel like there is any change at all in the last two years in terms of Hank's ability to hear the question? Even if you haven't convinced him yet that it is enough, has there at least been some change in the conversation?

M: (*Laughs*) He at least lets me cry now. He lets me cry in the same room as he is. That's an improvement.

H: (*Chuckles*)

M: Yes, there have been changes.

Mary presents a very fixed story about Hank's not wanting to hear her if he cannot fix it. Judy intentionally asks about any changes in his ability to hear over the past 2 years to explore the possibility of exceptions to this picture of Hank. Judy is also now following Mary in what she is able to talk about in the session, furthering the conversation.

J: (*To Hank*) How do you explain that Mary is really trying to tell you over and over again that it is really exactly what she needs for you to just hold her and somehow it doesn't seem like you get it?

H: (*Sighs*) Yeah, I don't know. It is hard for me to get in touch with feelings sometimes. I don't really think about it. I guess like she says, I try to find a way to get something positive, to show something positive quick. Whereas in a case like this, you are not going to get anything positive for a long period of time, which, I guess I am learning more or less bit by bit. But to me, as a kid, I was brought up not to really show emotions or cry or anything. When you fall down and get hurt, then my father would say, "Are you all right? Well you're not bleeding, right? Then there's no reason to be crying then." And that is the way I was brought up, so I guess for me it is a hard bridge to cross and as for that remark that "if I can't fix it I don't want to hear it," yeah, I did say that a few years ago, but I find myself doing a little better at it now. Probably not as fast as I should though.

Hank has the idea that he has changed over the past few years and that there have been improvements in his ability to tolerate Mary's feelings. He also begins to provide a context for his "lack" of ability to express feelings.

Bill then has a long conversation with Hank about his father and Hank's ideas about why his father seemed "cold." Bill also asks about Hank's relationship with his mother. Bill wonders, if Hank's father were alive now, what kind of advice might he give Hank about how to deal with Mary. Hank also describes how he has taken on more household responsibilities (e.g., he pays all the bills now) since Mary was hospitalized.

Mary has been silent, in a "listening" position to Bill's and Hank's conversation. Judy now asks her to reflect on that conversation.

J: (*To Mary*) I am sitting here feeling curious wondering what it has been like for you to hear Hank talk so much.

M: (*Giggles*) It is really different. I don't think he's talked this much at one time probably over the course of 3 days. It takes him 3 days to say that many words usually.

J: How do you explain that? How do you make sense out of the fact that he is talking so much?

M: I have no idea, because he doesn't talk to me.

H: Oh, I don't talk a lot. A lot of the time I get home, I am tired. I have been working a lot lately. As for what is making me talk more, I don't know. (*Shrugs his shoulders*) We are at a point where we are trying to head in a new direction and this is just another step to go through it to work on it.

J: Uh huh. For you, it almost sounds like you are seeing signs of hope that you and Mary are moving in a new direction.

In this model, the therapist may often choose to have a longer conversation with one member of the family. This allows the other members to be in an observing position, which often allows them to take in new information. With this couple, Bill's conversation with Hank introduced a different picture of Hank as a man capable of talking about feelings and relationships.

One of the things we try to do in sessions is to underline any differences that we think might indicate a positive change and would thus produce a sense of hope. Judy's questions to Mary highlight Hank's talking and result in Hank's description that they are "heading in a new direction."

At this point we had been talking for about 1 hour and 15 minutes. We had to finish the session and talk about whether we would meet again and how. We do not start therapy with a preconceived idea about what the length of therapy ought to be. We are likely to end each session with questions like, "How was this session for you? Was there anything we didn't talk about that we should have? What's the next step? Would you like to meet again? When should we meet?" In this way, the client is truly in charge of the content, pace, and length of the therapy.

J: I guess I am wondering how you both feel about this as a start. Is this a conversation you would like to continue? Because I know, Mary, you decided to "just dive in and let's do it," and I am wondering whether this feels like a safe enough place for you to continue talking together?

M: (*Looks at Hank and then at her feet*)

H: (*Looks at Mary*) Do you want me to go first?

M: (*Laughs nervously*)

H: I think it is something I want to do. I feel comfortable.

J: (*To Mary*) What about you?

M: (*Sighs*) Yeah.

J: Are you okay?

M: (*Laughs*) I'm okay . . .

J: Do you think you feel comfortable enough to be able to say if you don't feel comfortable? Like at those times when you feel like you need two women in the corner? Or if something was happening that was making you feel too anxious? Could you say, "I'm really feeling upset," so that we could pay attention to that?

M: I guess I need to work on that some more. The problem is a lot of the times I don't really know until it is too late that I am getting to that point and then I am already ready to fall apart. I guess one of the things that surprised me was that Bill recognized I was getting uncomfortable before I really had thought about it in those concrete terms, that I was uncomfortable. Something was going on, but I was somewhere else I guess, and then I heard Bill say that maybe I was uncomfortable and it was like "Whew!" so I don't know. I hope I can get to that point where I can recognize that soon enough to say something.

J: Is that what the tears were about? That Bill recognized that you were uncomfortable before you did?

M: (*Nods*) Yeah.

B: (*Turns to Hank*) That is also something that you recognized once it was commented on as well. It was a matter of giving it a label and then "Oh, yeah." It is sort of like working on a piece of machinery and you don't see what is wrong and then somebody else says, "what about that?" and you say, "Of course."

The fact that Bill was able to anticipate Mary's feelings had a major impact on the therapy. Mary started out the session believing that she needed "two women" in her corner in order to feel safe talking with two men. By the end, she has the new experience of feeling understood by a man even before she herself was aware of her feelings. Bill's comments to Hank are another example of positively describing Hank's behavior, again underlining his potential ability to become perceptive in the way that Mary has experienced Bill.

The issue whether it is safe to trust men and whether men can be supportive of women turned out to be very significant in light of Mary's history of sexual abuse. In the beginning of the next session, we focused on the couple's beliefs about why it was hard for Hank to listen and talk with Mary about painful feelings. We explored in greater detail the lessons Hank had learned from his father about how a man deals with feelings and in our reflections, questioned whether it would be possible for him to remain loyal to his father if he were to experience and express feelings more. By the third session, Hank was talking about incidents in which he became "choked up" and our reflections focused on whether there were risks to Hank if he were to become overwhelmed by feelings. Hank acknowledged he sometimes tuned out feelings when he did become overwhelmed. We then commented on how Mary had survived the sexual abuse by dissociating and disconnecting from feelings and, because this couple's belief was that they were very different, we used our reflections to describe how we saw a similarity in how they both coped with painful, powerful feelings. In our reflections, we wondered about whether, when they had first married, both had been "fuzzy about feelings" and that they had had a pact to protect each other by not bringing up difficult feelings. They agreed with this idea. Mary said she used to know about feelings "in her head but not in her gut." It wasn't until her severe depression lifted a year ago that she began to "feel" feelings.

At the fifth session, a crisis arose when their 15-year-old daughter was forced to engage in some sexual activity by a friend of her brother. Mary came in furious at Hank, saying he was again trying to find something good about this incident whereas for her, it threw her back into flashbacks of her own abuse. Her story was that he was not willing to hear how awful she thought this incident was and that he just did not want to "put up with my crying." Because Mary was so upset, we decided on a format of Judy's interviewing Mary while Hank and Bill listened behind the one-way mirror and then us switching places with Mary and Judy listening to Bill and Hank.[2] In her conversation with Judy, Mary described how severely depressed she had been over the weekend and how she had dissociated to the extent that she "didn't know if she was ever going to come back!" She described how Hank had tried to help her by giving her space and doing extra chores when what she most needed was to hear his voice and to have a human connection. Hank, in his talk with Bill, emphasized how scared he was that Mary might actually kill herself and how he was trying to look on "the bright side" to keep her alive and his fear that something he could say might throw her into deeper despair. Bill explored with Hank whether he also "got down," and how he coped and whether he could let Mary know more what he was feeling. Bill emphasized how responsible Hank felt for Mary's well-being but commented that what Mary most seemed to need from him was a sense that "he understood," that he accepted how awful she felt.

Both Mary and Hank liked this format. Hank said listening to Mary "gave me something to go on," and Mary felt surprised again at how Hank could put his feelings into words.

As Hank became more expressive and spontaneous, Mary began to acknowledge that it was not what Hank did or did not do that threatened her, but rather that sometimes she hated all men because of the past abuse. Our reflections then focused on how she could separate out Hank from all the men who abused her in the past. We wondered about what it would be like for her to tell Hank the details of the past abuse. What did she want him to know? What was she afraid would happen if she were to tell him? Was Hank anxious about hearing the details?

Because of Mary's anxieties about talking about the abuse in a positive way and in front of Hank, we again used the format of Mary and Judy's talking about the details of the abuse with Hank and Bill watching and listening behind the one-way mirror. Mary haltingly related a very painful account about how her uncle had abused her when she was very young. After Bill and Hank switched positions with Judy and Mary, Hank expressed his reactions to this new information and expressed his fear that something he would say might throw Mary back into a flashback. Bill emphasized that it was not Hank that Mary was angry with but the ghosts of other men.

In the next session, Mary mentioned that she had written something in her journal after the last session that she thought was interesting. She had written that "mostly I ignore Bill's presence in the sessions even though he says important things." This made her realize that, as a way of coping with the abuse, she generally treats all men like ghosts. "I see them and hear them, but mostly I walk right through them." She has noticed though that lately Hank has become more real, more important to her. "I'm letting his kindness filter in." Many of our questions and reflections in this session focused on what would happen if Hank slowly became even more important to her? What were the risks and benefits? How would this affect their sexual relationship? What would happen if this change led to all men becoming more real, including the ghosts of the past? Mary was able to acknowledge how scary it was to allow herself to feel positively toward Hank. This was a theme that continued to be discussed in the remaining sessions as Hank became more involved with both her and the children and she became more able to see and acknowledge his changes. She described feeling very connected to Hank, wondering if she were falling in love with him for the first time. Eventually, we moved to talking about their sexual relationship and how they could begin to work on this, in what ways, and at what pace. After a total of nine sessions, they came and told us, with much laughter, that they didn't need to continue because they had successfully made love at "2:00 A.M. on August 3rd!" All other parts of their relationship were working well too. We met with this couple a total of nine sessions over a period of 4½ months.

FOLLOW-UP

Because Judy was continuing to see the family for monthly checkups, she received some immediate feedback on the results of couples therapy from Hank's and Mary's son. Darren came into the next family session with a list of ways his parents had changed and with a grin announced that his parents "were kissing and hugging more," both seemed happier, and were more "fun." "Dad even asked Mom to go out four-wheeling to catch fireflies!"

Seven months after termination, Mary sent us a letter when she was settling their bill. She wrote, "Your group is proof that family therapy can be helpful. The most dramatic difference in our experience with you and those whom we had seen before lay in the degree of validity each person was offered. Couple sessions were invaluable. My first experience in recognizing the male as even remotely competent!''

EDITORS' QUESTIONS

Q: My sense of the Milan team is that they do a lot of behind-the-scenes hypothesizing while you seem to avoid this practice. In what ways is your approach influenced by the Milan Associates?

A: In the early 1980s, we were very much influenced by the Milan Associates. Our clinical and training teams used the format of the five-part interview, and we were guided by their principles of hypothesizing, circularity, and neutrality. Some of their ideas and techniques continue to influence us, for example, their use of circular questions and their inclusion of the therapist/observer as part of the therapeutic system. We especially appreciate their emphasis on positive or logical connotation (i.e., understanding how the problem behavior makes sense within the context of the family's situation) because this enables us to avoid a blaming position with the family. In addition, we agree with their position that the therapist's job is not to discover "the truth" but rather to discover what fits and is useful for the family and will help them get unstuck.

Q: I am impressed with your sensitivity to the client's position, needs, and wishes. Your approach is very respectful of the client. How did your work evolve in this direction? How did you create a team atmosphere in which these values were nurtured and developed?

A: Our work together at Brattleboro Family Institute has always been based on a collaborative, nonhierarchical model and has been our approach to all our interactions. We run the business in this manner as well as the clinical work. Around 1984, we were becoming uncomfortable with some of the more strategic practices of the early Milan-style teams that led to the feeling that the family was the enemy whose resistance had to be overcome by the cleverness of the team. Interventions were delivered and the therapist made a hasty exit without permitting any feedback from the family. At times, we were disconcerted by some of the negative, disrespectful comments that were made about the family behind the one-way mirror. We wondered if the negative energy being generated by these comments could be communicated to the family in subtle ways. We felt disrespectful of one another when we had to reduce the ideas of the team's discussion to one or two comprehensive "interventions." While we did not believe that we were "experts," our interactions with the clients implied that position. In 1985, we met Tom Andersen, MD, from Norway, who introduced us to the "reflecting team." We immediately saw this as a way to resolve our dilemmas and to include the family as true collaborators in the therapy. We utilized a no-talking rule behind the mirror to ensure that therapists would neither eliminate some ideas in conversations behind the mirror nor strongly influence others. Rather, *all* ideas would be respected and presented to the family, and the family would decide what was useful. The family became the experts on what was a "fit" for them. We, as a team, began to feel like collaborators again, with each of us having different expertise.

What helped us also, as a team, foster this respect for the client was our belief that there is not one "truth" but rather a multitude of different realities resulting from each individual's experience. This meant that we had to respect the client's view as equally as valid, within its context, as our own. In addition, in a very practical way, we tried to help ourselves and our trainees understand the experience of families by using role plays so that we could experience firsthand the family's position, first as they talked about their problems and then as they listened to the therapists talk about them (see Davidson & Lussardi, 1991).

Q: Can you explain in more detail your comment that "our primary emphasis is on the meanings people ascribe to problematic behavior" rather than on the problems themselves? How does this distinction relate to what has been referred to as "postmodern" thinking in systemic therapy?

A: Postmodernism stresses the idea that the "self" is conceived not as a reified entity but as a narrative. If anything, self is viewed as an ever-changing process of relationships in contexts (see Gergen, 1991). Narratives or stories add a sense of coherence to lived experience through which we create meaning in our lives. These stories are recursively related to our world: We experience our world based on our narratives and construct our narratives in light of our interactional experiences with others. We believe that clients who come to us have constructed stories about themselves and others that somehow limit them in developing new ideas or approaches regarding their life situations and problems.

It is our belief that our actions are guided by our thoughts and intentions (see Bruner, 1990). As we are able to help people alter the narratives they have about themselves in the world, their behavioral interactions with others will also be different.

Throughout our work, we do not "know" what a client's new story might or should be, nor do we believe that one story is better than another. This process is consistent with postmodern thinking in that it stresses the lateral arrangement between client and therapist, and, as stated above, we maintain a respect for multiple perspectives versus a "truth."

Q: Would you comment further on the idea that the therapeutic conversation "might come to a halt . . . if the conversation were too similar or too different from the couple's usual mode of interaction and understanding"?

A: Andersen (1991) addresses this most appropriately in his description of three kinds of differences, including ones too small or too big to make a distinction. Our job as therapists is to stay connected with our clients and introduce differences that are discrepantly different from theirs (but not too different). It is through this process that new narratives can be developed. When we are engaged with clients and are beginning to introduce ideas or questions that are out of their range of interactional or cognitive repertoire, the interaction usually breaks down. We know when this is happening: we feel disconnected from them, our minds wander thinking about other unrelated subjects (like lunch or our next client), or we merely "space out" for a few minutes. On the other hand, the conversation may also come to a halt when it is finished. A "gestalt" may be closed with a new figure or narrative developed for the client(s).

The conversation might also come to a halt if there were topics that either member of the couple might not want to speak about. These may occur when there is a secret or there are contextual constraints, such as in situations of violence where one member fears that what is said will have serious repercussions after the meeting.

Q: Many of us have learned that for therapy to be effective, the therapist must be clearly in charge of the process, guiding and structuring the action. How can the therapist "utilize his or her expertise while maintaining a *lateral* position to the client"?

A: In working from this perspective, there is no need to dismiss our years of training, skills, or experiences. We respectfully view different theoretical perspectives as narratives themselves, which may be useful to call on with some clients. Rather than think that we know what is best for our clients (which is impossible), we find that it is most useful to share our ideas (and theories) with them. We will utilize our expertise by offering it to them in the form of questions, ideas, and suggestions, seeing what they think might be best for them (see Lax, 1992). At times when we have a strong idea, such as thinking that a specific treatment modality like inpatient hospitalization might be useful or feeling that someone is being treated unjustly as in cases of violence or abuse, we share our thoughts with them, asking perhaps some of the following questions: What is it like for you to hear us suggest/state these ideas? What do you think of these ideas? Might they be altered in any way? What would it be like for you if we were to hold this position throughout our work with you or you were to try any of them?

By acting in this manner, we feel we are being consistent with our own ethical positions/beliefs, and the clients are more fully participants in the "intervention" components of the interview. In addition, by *talking about* the ideas and/or suggestions, we are still in the realm of meanings and are attempting to shift the narratives clients have about themselves.

Q: Cotherapy seems to be a relatively expensive model to employ at most human service agencies. How could a therapist, working solo, effectively use your model? You describe a very interesting use of the one-way mirror where one of you is behind the mirror with the husband and the other one interviews the wife. Can this technique be modified so that the average practitioner can do something similar in his or her office?

A: Since we cannot afford to see clients only as a team, we have been experimenting for several years with various ways to use this model when working solo. If we are seeing a single client, we might pause at a certain point in the interview and ask if he or she would like to hear some of the ideas and thoughts we have had while we have been talking together. We would then share these with the client and, at the end, ask for feedback from him or her on our ideas. If we wanted a little time to reflect on the session, we might excuse ourselves from the session briefly before sharing our ideas. When working with a couple or a family, particularly those who do a lot of interrupting and have trouble really listening to each other, it is very helpful for a therapist to use variations of this model. The therapist can propose having a dyadic conversation with one partner while the other partner just listens and then reflects on what is being discussed. In this situation we act as if there is a one-way mirror between the listening spouse and the others preventing communication. The therapist explains to the listening spouse some guidelines for making reflections, and at the end of the interview with the partner the therapist asks for the listening spouse's reflections. The therapist may also ask the listening spouse what it was like to be in this listening position, whether he or she has heard anything new, and so on. Finally, the partner may then be asked for comments on the reflections. With families, the therapist may converse with one member of the family in the format described above or the therapist may ask two members of the family to have a conversation while the rest of the family listens. Then the rest of the family will be asked to offer reflections. We feel this process often can help family members to have the experience of being heard and understood and can facilitate more useful conversations.

Q: It's quite impressive how you both share your thoughts and ideas in such an open manner with the couple. Are there some things that should not be discussed in front of the client?

A: If we are having any strong negative thoughts about the clients or our work, they should be discussed in private between the therapists. In addition, when either therapist has thoughts or feelings that are not a part of the therapeutic conversation (are not adding further distinctions or clarification to the ongoing conversation), they should not be discussed with them. These might include personal memories or images that pertain more directly to us than to them.

Q: Although the content being discussed in the interview was quite serious, both of you maintained a sense of humor. A significant amount of laughter seemed to go on in the session. What part does humor play in your work? Does the humor found in this interview have to do with the particular couple seen or do you often use humor in your therapy?

A: We often look for ways to introduce humor into sessions as a way of lessening anxiety and tension. If a couple or family do not respond, we will discontinue it because we assume that its use is too different from their style. This particular couple relaxed visibly with the use of humor, and it was used effectively throughout the therapy.

Q: How important is the role of the therapist in generating a sense of hope and optimism about change? How do you accomplish this in your therapy?

A: Hope is very important in therapy, and we try to develop an atmosphere of hope through our questions and reflections, particularly through logical connotations and offering different views to our clients. We find that when clients are not blamed and feel understood, that is, have "their story" reflected back to them in another form which seems to fit for them, they feel hopeful. They have come to us because they are stuck with only one version of their life, and we are offering them others. When they are able to see that there might be at least one other perspective on their life's dilemma, they feel hopeful. Optimism for change usually follows this sense of hope. When clients leave a session stating that they feel hopeful, it is a strong indication that they are beginning to entertain a new description of their situation. The actions that follow are often directed by this hope and new story.

Q: How did you become a brief therapist?

DAVIDSON: You are curious about how I became a brief therapist and I have to smile because, sometimes, I do work with clients over a long period of time! My overall goal, as a therapist, is to help clients grow or change in ways that are useful to them. I don't think of therapy in terms of permanent "cure" but rather in developmental terms. I'm interested in helping people get "unstuck," in empowering them and helping them see their own strengths and worth. I try to respect my clients' goals for therapy and their ideas about the number and frequency of sessions. Often I see people for brief periods of therapy at various points in their life cycles. We work together on a specific issue until they feel able to move forward again.

LAX: Throughout my career, I have been most interested in the ideas about therapy, why certain models are useful and why others are not. I have never really made a strong distinction between short- and long-term therapy until recently. While I actually am a patient person (in most contexts!), I like to see "things moving along." This interest in movement parallels my own shifting theoretical perspectives, which never stay constant for too long. Currently I am most interested in the influence of postmodern thinking on the social sciences and widening my personal areas of intellectual interest.

NOTES

1. We generally consider our first meetings with clients a consultation. This consultation is usually only one meeting, but sometimes can last up to three sessions before a decision to continue therapy is made.

2. We often choose this format when a couple is having difficulty hearing each other's stories (see Miller & Lax, 1988).

REFERENCES

Andersen, T. (1987). The reflecting team: Dialogue and meta-dialogue in clinical work. *Family Process, 26,* 415–428.

Andersen, T. (Ed.). (1991). *The reflecting team: Dialogues and dialogues about dialogues.* New York: W. W. Norton.

Anderson, H., & Goolishian, H. (1988). Human systems as linguistic systems:

Preliminary and evolving ideas about the implications for clinical theory. *Family Process*, *27*, 3–12.

Boscolo, L., Cecchin, G. Hoffman, L., & Penn, P. (1987). *Milan systemic family therapy*. New York: Basic Books.

Bruner, J. (1990). *Acts of meaning*. Cambridge, MA: Harvard University Press.

Bryant, C. (1984). Working for families with dysfunctional children: An approach and structure for the first family interview. *Child and Adolescent Social Work Journal*, *1*, 102–117.

Davidson, J., Lax, W., Lussardi, D., Miller, D., & Ratheau, M. (1988). The reflecting team. *The Family Therapy Networker*, *12*, 44–46.

Davidson, J., & Lussardi, D. J. (1991). Use of the reflecting team in supervision and training. In T. Andersen (Ed.), *The reflecting team: Dialogues and dialogues about the dialogues* (pp. 143–154). New York: W. W. Norton.

Derrida, J. (1976). *Of grammatology* (G. C. Spivak, Trans.). Baltimore: Johns Hopkins.

Derrida, J. (1978). *Writing and difference* (A. Bass, Trans.). Chicago: University of Chicago Press.

Derrida, J. (1986). Différance. In M. C. Taylor (Ed.), *Deconstruction in context* (pp. 396–420). Chicago: University of Chicago Press.

Gergen, K. J. (1991). *The saturated self*. New York: Basic Books.

Gergen, K. J. (1985). The social constructionist movement in modern psychology. *American Psychologist*, *40*(3), 266–275.

Haley, J. (1976). *Problem solving therapy*. San Francisco: Jossey-Bass.

Hoffman, L. (1988). A constructivist position for family therapy. *The Irish Journal of Psychology*, *9*, 110–129.

Hoffman, L. (1990). Constructing realities: An art of lenses. *Family Process*, *29*, 1–12.

Hoffman, L. (1991). A reflexive stance for family therapy. *Journal of Strategic and Systemic Therapies*, *10*(3/4), 4–17.

Lax, W. D. (1989). Systemic family therapy with young children in the family: Use of the reflecting team. In J. J. Zilbach (Ed.), *Children in family therapy*. (pp. 55–71). New York: Haworth.

Lax, W. D. (1991). The reflecting team and the initial consultation. In T. Andersen (Ed.), *The reflecting team: Dialogues and dialogues about dialogues* (pp. 127–142). New York: W. W. Norton.

Lax, W. D. (1992). Postmodern thinking in a clinical practice. In S. McNamee & K. J. Gergen (Eds.), *Constructing therapy: Social constructionism and therapeutic process* (pp. 120–148). London: Sage.

Lussardi, D., & Miller, D. (1991). A reflecting team approach to adolescent substance abuse. In T. Todd & M. Selekman, (Eds.), *Family therapy approaches with adolescent substance abuse* (pp. 227–240). Boston: Allyn and Bacon.

Miller, D., & Lax, W. D. (1988). Interrupting deadly struggles: A reflecting team model for working with couples. *Journal of Strategic and Systemic Therapies*, *7*(3), 16–22.

Minuchin, S. (1974). *Families and family therapy.* Cambridge, MA: Harvard University Press.

Penn, P. (1982). Circular questioning. *Family Process, 21,* 267–280.

Penn, P. (1985). Feedforward: Future questions, future maps. *Family Process, 24,* 299–311.

Rorty, R. (1979). *Philosophy and the mirror of nature.* Princeton: Princeton University Press.

Rorty, R. (1991). *Objectivity, relativism, and truth. Philosophical papers. Vol. 1.* Cambridge, Eng.: Cambridge University Press.

Sarbin, T.R. (Ed.). (1986). The narrative as root metaphor in psychology. In *Narrative psychology: The storied nature of human conduct* (pp. 3–21). New York: Praeger.

Selvini-Palazzoli, M., Boscolo, L., Cecchin, G., & Prata, G. (1980). Hypothesizing–circularity–neutrality: Three guidelines for the conductor of the session. *Family Process, 19*(1), 3–12.

Tomm, K. (1987). Interventive interviewing: Part II. Reflexive questioning as a means to enabling self-healing. *Family Process, 26,* 167–183.

von Glasersfeld, E. (1984). An introduction to radical constructivism. In P. Watzlawick (Ed.), *The invented reality* (pp. 17–40). New York: W. W. Norton.

Weber, T., McKeever, J., & McDaniel, S. (1985). A beginner's guide to the problem-oriented first family interview. *Family Process, 24*(3), 357–364.

Constructing Solutions (Stories) in Brief Family Therapy

STEVEN FRIEDMAN

"Any story one may tell about anything is better understood by considering other possible ways in which it could be told."
—JEROME BRUNER (1987, p. 32)

A university commits funds to improve the quality of teaching by videotaping instructors in class and then giving them feedback on what they are doing wrong. A corporate executive decides to fire any employee who does not meet productivity standards. By removing the "bad apples," the employer hopes to solve the problem (Berwick, 1989). As a way to prepare for her next match, a tennis player watches herself (on videotape) playing well in an earlier tournament. A program is developed for teenagers who are responsible for a significant amount of graffiti on the subway cars in a major city. The program provides opportunities for these teenagers to express their artistic talents in other, more socially appropriate ways. How do the first two examples differ from the second two? And what does this have to do with psychotherapy?

Too often as psychotherapists, we spend our time looking for weaknesses and deficits rather than building on the strengths and competencies of the people with whom we work. We have been telling ourselves stories (generating narratives) that have skewed our thinking toward a disease or medical model. The alternative model outlined here presents an optimistic, future-oriented perspective in amplifying the client's capacities and strengths in moving toward change. Rather than focusing on limitations, deficits, and pathology, the author's time-effective model of family psychotherapy emphasizes possibilities, strengths, and resources (Friedman, 1989a, 1990, 1991; Friedman & Fanger, 1991).

A "wellness" model of family therapy has its roots in a strength-oriented and competency-based philosophy (e.g., Masterpaqua, 1989; Seeman, 1989). "Rather than a professionally driven therapeutic process in which the therapist is expert (and the family is viewed as 'dysfunctional' and 'resistant'), the possibility-oriented therapist sees him or herself in a *partnership* with the family in pursuing a negotiated set of achievable goals for change. A 'wellness' model assumes that family members are doing their best, but may benefit from consultation in building on already existing systemic strengths and resources" (Friedman, 1991, p. 23).

The following set of assumptions (from Friedman, 1991; Friedman & Fanger, 1991), in work with children and families, are ones that I have found helpful in generating self-narratives that orient my perspective toward health and wellness:

1. *Approach the family with an open mind*, setting aside assumptions and biases that may orient your thinking toward pathology and dysfunction. Avoid becoming enamored with others' diagnostic formulations.

2. *Respect the family system and its resources.* Assume that the family network has within it the potential to develop its own solutions with minimal facilitation by the therapist. Utilize and build on the previous successes and accomplishments of family members in supporting their capacities for change and growth and empowering them to take responsibility for making further changes. The therapist serves as a catalyst for change (Bennett, 1989; Budman & Gurman, 1988).

3. *Respect the family's original request.* Develop an alliance with the family around their desire for change. Form a partnership with family members, taking the role of consultant in helping them achieve *their* goals.

4. *Generate an optimistic and hopeful stance* regarding change (i.e., within any difficulty or dilemma is an opportunity for growth [Haley, 1973]). Assume that change is inevitable. *View time as an ally* (Hobbs, 1966).

5. *Negotiate with the family in setting limited and achievable goals.* Think small (Weick, 1984). Build on small successes. Since a small change may trigger further changes, it is important that family members notice and appreciate small changes that they have made that are in the direction of achieving their goals. As White and Epston (1990) point out, "It's never the size of the step that a person takes that counts, but it's direction" (p. 61).

6. *Avoid complex assumptions* about a situation when simple assumptions will lead more quickly to change (Friedman & Fanger, 1991). Complicated problems do not necessarily require complicated solutions (de Shazer, 1988; O'Hanlon & Wilk, 1987).

7. *Develop and nurture a constructivist philosophy* in which multiple realities are accepted (Watzlawick, 1984). Generate therapeutic conversations that provide alternative views of reality and open up (rather than close down) options for change (Andersen,1990; de Shazer, 1991; Mittelmeier & Friedman, 1991; Tomm, 1987).

Each individual creates maps or constructs through which he or she organizes data. Each construct or map provides avenues for organizing the data in unique ways but also constrains other options (Epstein & Loos, 1989). By using language creatively, it is possible to open up options and alternative views of reality that will create shifts in the meaning system that the family has developed about its predicament. "The goal of treatment . . . is to maintain a conversation until what was originally defined as a problem is no longer viewed as a problem. Therapeutic change, then, occurs when new meaning develops through linguistic interaction" (Epstein & Loos, 1989, p. 415).

8. *Use the language of possibility* to generate a hopeful, optimistic perspective about the inevitability of change. Use words constructively and in ways that support multiple options and views of reality rather than reify pathology (Anderson & Goolishian, 1988; O'Hanlon & Wilk, 1987). Avoid pejorative labels inherent in such classification systems as DSM-III-R. Since "our self-understandings are mediated through language" (White & Epston, 1990, p. 28; see also Maturana & Varela, 1987) and are "inherently negotiable and tentative" (Anderson & Goolishian, 1988, p. 381), the therapeutic process becomes one of using language to construct alternate meaning systems that liberate the client from the problem (see Friedman, 1989b for dramatic example). As Bruner (1987) points out, since clients' "autobiographical accounts [verbal self-reports] . . . [are] notably unstable . . . [they become] . . . highly susceptible to cultural, interpersonal and linguistic influences" (p. 14).

9. *Use humor, play, and metaphor* as a way to provide perspective (Barker, 1985; Friedman & Fanger, 1991). Minuchin (1984) makes the observation that "we [too often] label as deviant what is actually the creative attempt of a family . . . to develop a new shape—the shedding and becoming that precede a butterfly" (p. 20).

10. *Insist that family members be active partners* in developing solutions. Assign tasks that afford family members an opportunity to actively participate in the change process. *See clients on an intermittent basis* to allow time for implementation of tasks.

11. *Match the family's linguistic style and be sensitive to cultural norms and expectations.*

While I try to meet with as many of the people in the household as possible for the initial visit, I will usually see whomever decides to come as long as at least one parent is present. In the initial session, I find it helpful to work with a minimum of presuppositions or hypotheses about the possible etiology of the problem. As O'Hanlon and Wilk (1987) say, "every now and then . . . a hypothesis might accidentally enter the therapist's head, and the best remedy for it, is to lie down until it goes away" (p. 98). Rather than accept the illusion of an objective reality (or linear cause–effect process), I begin by simply accepting the presenting complaint and its meaning system as a "story" or narrative that the family has creatively constructed in making sense of their predicament (Bruner, 1987; Parry, 1991). I try to understand how the family makes sense of their situation and to look for openings that provide a "foot-hold" from which to build on their already demonstrated successes and strengths in empowering them to take further steps toward their goal. I maintain an optimistic set by reframing, in positive terms, both the behaviors and intent of family members. My goal in the initial interview is to join with each family member in a partnership with the goal of liberating the family from the problem as quickly as possible by moving them to view the future with a changed perspective.

Rather than contract for a series of meetings, I ask the family after each session whether and within what time frame they wish to recon-vene. If the family wishes to return for another meeting, I often ask, "Within how many weeks would you like to set the next appointment?" By leaving the client to decide about the spacing of appointments I demonstrate my respect for his or her autonomy and ability to regulate therapeutic contact. I set the expectation for a brief treatment by not agreeing to set up more than one appointment at a time.

As a part of joining with the family in the initial visit, I listen to their use of language and try to match my conversation to their rhythm and style. As I listen to their conversation, I look for places to introduce new ideas or ways of thinking about their predicament. I work the hardest at trying to notice, comment on, and amplify behaviors that lead the family away from a "problem-saturated" picture of their lives and toward a picture of life without the influence of the problem (de Shazer, 1991; White & Epston, 1990). My goal is to help the family "re-story" their experience in a way that liberates them from the problem and creates new options for change and growth.

CASE ILLUSTRATION

The Ramos family consists of the father, Manuel, the mother, Marie, and their two sons, Manuel (age 15) and Luis (age 9). The parents, from Puerto Rico, emigrated to the United States at the time they were teenagers, and speak Spanish in the home. The referral, which was initiated by the school, focused on Luis, whose behavior was characterized as "aggressive, showing poor impulse control, and poor self-esteem." The school adjustment counselor believed that "it would be beneficial for him to engage in some therapy." This is all the information I had about the family prior to my initial contact. The initial meeting was with the parents and Luis. The older son did not attend, although the mother wanted him to be there. The father decided to let him sleep in that morning rather than come to the meeting. Both parents work and arranged to take a day off to make the initial appointment.

The First Session

After making conversation for a few minutes about the weather, the parents' jobs, and the absent older brother, I formally began the interview. I begin with my typical opening question which is an attempt to move the family immediately away from a problem focus and toward a focus on goals for change.

Therapist: So, tell me a little about what you were hoping to accomplish here? What were you thinking about why it would be useful to come here?

Father: One of the main reasons we've come is because of Luis; he misbehave, he act up. . . . Sometimes when we say something to him he get angry easy . . . he acts quick. And the school sees the same problem.

T: Who does he get angry with?

F: Actually, when we say something to him, he can get angry too quick . . .

I try to redirect the father toward those times Luis's mood is seen as acceptable.

T: And sometimes his mood is fine and he will listen and there's no trouble . . .

F: Sometimes he is, but most of the time I have a lot of problem with the reactions. . . . We just switched him from one school to another because he had a lot of angry reactions with teachers.

T: (*To Luis*) What grade are you in?

Luis: The third.

When I hear that Luis has recently changed schools, I see an opportunity for framing this as a "new beginning" which does not include the problem.

T: And when was that change made in the school?

F: The change was made in the school just last week.

T: (*To Luis*) So, you're in a different school now than you were? You've been in the new school now for a week?

L: (*Nods "yes"*)

T: How was that week? Was it better?

Mother:　He like it.

T: (*To father*) What did you think?

F: He did a little better improvement there.

I immediately tune in to any mention of improvement that family members have noticed and try to support and amplify this.

T: So, have you noticed recently, some changes?

F: In school, he do a lot better. We got a note saying that he behave excellent.

T: It's just a short period of time, but it's a good start.

F: Yes.

I then ask the "miracle question" (de Shazer, 1988) as a way to help the family give me a clear and specific picture of life without the problem.

T: Tell me, if a miracle happened, you woke up in one morning and everything was the way you wanted it to be, what would things look like? What would Luis be doing? What would be happening?

F: I don't know how to explain.

T: What would be going well? How would you like things to be?

F: What I would like in the house, is for him to listen to us the way he should . . . and to do whatever he has to do in school, the right way. . . . and behave in the house. We tell him something and sometimes he listens and sometimes he doesn't. Most of the time he doesn't. He get angry.

T: And when he listens, how does he let you know that he's listening?

F: His temper is different. He's calm and does what he's told to do.

T: He's calm and pleasant and says "yes" and goes off and does it.

F: Yes. Whatever we tell him he take in the right way. But, we get to a point sometimes when we can't have both [Luis and his older brother] together. . . . They fight a lot. But 2 minutes later they're kissing each other and making up.

T: Do you get involved in that or do you let them figure it out?

F: Well, most of the time I try to stop them. I tell Manuel, leave it alone, go leave it alone. I would rather not get involved in it though . . .

T: (*To Luis*) Can you take care of yourself when your brother starts with you? Or do you need help from one of your parents?

L: I move to a different place.

T: So, if you move away you get some space from him and it's better. So that's what you do.

L: Sometimes we fight, but then he comes and says, "I'm sorry."

T: He will apologize after. Because he really loves you . . . but sometimes you get on each other's nerves or something.

I then find out that Manuel is also not doing so well in school; that he also "acts up" and gets into trouble, talks too much, and so on.

T: (*To mother*) Does he [Luis] take you seriously when you tell him to do something?

M: He doesn't listen to me.

T: Who does he listen to the most?

M: They don't listen to me. . . . (*Laughs*)

T: His dad?

M: Yes, his father.

F: Yes, that's a big problem in the house. When she say something to them, it like goes in one ear and out the other. But the only one who has a little bit control of the situation is myself. Because they know I won't take what they want to give. . . .

T: (*To mother*) What is it that your husband does that makes Luis listen to him?

M: I think when he talks loud, they listen.

F: I tell you right now why they listen to me. Cause I tell them once with my loud voice. They don't listen then I spank. I don't take no crap from them. And she [mother] is so soft.

T: So they know you [father] mean business.

F: I tell them once. If I see they pay no mind, I tell them twice. The third time they'll be no talking. I don't like to do that myself, I don't like to hit them.

T: Who does Luis spend most of his time with in the evening?

F: She work and I work. When we get home I have other things to do, so she spend time with him. I don't get to spend a lot of time with them. The only time I spend time with them is sitting in front of the TV and watching a movie or something.

The mother explains that at home she and her husband speak Spanish as does Manuel. Luis has not learned to speak Spanish, although the parents think he understands what they're saying in Spanish. In the following segment I encourage the mother to present her picture of change.

T: (*To mother*) So, how would you like things to be at home?

M: I'm not the boss at home. Nobody respect me, I think. Because of the way that I talk or something like that.

T: They don't take you seriously?

M: No, my husband is like the big man in the house. I say something, nobody respects (*Laughs*). My husband is nice person, but not when he's drinking . . . that's another thing.

The mother raises the issue of her husband's drinking.

T: Who's drinking?

M: My husband.

F: I use to drink a lot . . . on the weekends. I don't drink now. But my temper is still bad. . . . It's like the person who quits smoking, you know, I don't know how to explain it . . .

Rather than focus on the father's drinking, I choose to focus on the time he's been sober. I then question him about who decided that he should stop and finally compliment him on his successful initial efforts at sobriety.

T: How long has there been no drinking?

F: About 6 weeks.

T: How come you stopped?

F: Because I had to. . . . I was thinking it was no good. I look at this way. You spend more money drinking. . . . A lot of time when I want to say something to the kids, I can't say it when I'm drunk. Because I know it's no good example to tell them . . . I can say something and then the next day when I'm sober they will say you told me this . . . I say "hell, no," I didn't say that. And that's when the problems comes up. I also want to lose some weight, and so you've got to cut that stuff out.

T: Did a doctor tell you to stop?

F: No, I decided.

T: So, you decided to make some changes. (*To mother*) Are you happy about that?

M: Oh, yeah. I'm happy, but I see the other side too.

T: His temper is. . . . He's more irritable.

M: He's different.

T: How is he different?

M: Sometimes he's happy and sometimes he's moody.

T: (*To father*) So, you're moody too?

M: Yes, he and Luis have the same temper.

T: The two of them.

M: Yes. I think so. They're like macho man . . . like "I'm the boss" . . .

Puerto Rican families have traditionally been patriarchal (Garcia-Preto, 1982), with the husband expected to be the protector and provider for his family. In this segment, the mother is emphasizing her sense of powerlessness in the face of the "macho men" in the household.

T: (*To Luis*) So you take after your dad that way. You think you're the boss. Except you're only 9 years old . . .

M: Manuel is like that too. I told my husband I wanted him to come today too. But, my husband said no, let him sleep. Luis doing the same like Manuel. . . .

She describes her sense that the brothers talk to one another and that Luis is following in his brother's footsteps in becoming a "macho man."

T: (*To Luis*) So, you think you're a macho man, Luis?

L: I don't think I'm a macho man, it's just my attitude.

I question Luis about how he would like things to be and ask him to be specific about those changes that would tell him that things are different.

T: So, how would you like your attitude to be? Are you happy with your attitude?

L: (*Shakes head no*)

T: No, you'd like it to be different. How would you like to be, give me an example. What would you like to be doing different?

L: I would like to do better.

T: What would "better" mean, what would it look like, what would you be doing that you'd like better?

L: Listening to my parents.

T: If they asked you to do something, you'd listen. What kinds of things do they ask you to do?

L: Pick up things.

T: I see, to clean up around the house. How would you like to answer them when they ask you about that?

L: Just do it.

T: Just go off and do it. And now sometimes, you don't. You get angry, you say "no."

M: I do it because they don't.

T: (*To mother*) You end up doing it.

M: Yes

F: When we get home, they watching TV. They leave everything all over the place. It's like a tornado hit the living room. And I say, "will you clean that up" . . . forget it. It's like talking to the wall. They don't want to pay attention. Then I scream . . . grab the belt and then they get their ass together.

T: Then they get moving.

M: When they want to do something they do it . . . when they don't want forget about it . . . I try to talk . . .

T: (*To mother*) You end up doing a lot, then. You end up doing what they should be doing.

M: Yes.

T: The children have gotten the idea they don't have to help because their mother will do it. (*To mother*) You're working overtime. (*To Luis*) Your mother can't do it all. But she does a lot now . . . doesn't she? She takes care of the house . . .

The mother raises the issue of the Luis's stuttering and wonders if this is the reason he is having behavior problems. Rather than accept this hypothesis, I simply ask Luis and his parents if the stuttering has become less *of a problem over time.*

M: I don't know if the problem is that Luis stutters. (*Turns to Luis*) Does that bother you?

L: It did in first grade.

T: Do the children say anything to you in school about your stuttering?

L: No.

T: They have just accepted that that's how you talk. Has that improved over time? Is that better now, Luis's speech?

F: Yes . . . It used to be really, really bad before, but it's better now.

T: (*To father*) It sounds to me like you've begun to make some changes for yourself. And Luis, you've started a new school, and you're starting some changes, too. It's a fresh start, you know what I mean? It's a new school, new teachers. . . . Are you happy about that?

L: (*Nods yes*)

T: Luis, it sounds like you've started making some changes . . . And you were getting good progress reports in the new school?

L: Yes.

F: I asked them to write a progress note each day . . . whether poor or good or excellent and then I sign it. Then I know how he's doing. So up to this point I got pretty beautiful notes on it . . .

Again I work to emphasize difference and change from some point in the past, to the present.

T: That's a great start! Have you noticed any difference at home during this week at the new school, in Luis's behavior?

F: He's doing a little better, yeah.

The father describes how he grounded Luis for a week (about 2 weeks earlier)—not allowing Luis to go out with friends—and this made a difference.

F: Right now when he come from school, he do his homework before he goes out. I don't have to be really strong to him now. He understands. The last week I don't have to be so strong with him, like I used to be when he was at the other school.

T: It was easier this week.

F: Lighter, a little lighter.

T: Hopefully, it will get lighter and lighter. And you won't have to work so hard. (*To Luis*) The harder you work, then your dad doesn't have to work so hard. You don't want him on your back, do you?

L: (*Shakes head no*)

T: I didn't think so. (*To mother*) Somehow the kids don't take you seriously, enough. They're not respecting your voice. They think they're macho guys and their not going to listen to a woman tell them what to do, uh? (*To Luis*) You know your mother has something to say too. What she says is important. So it's important to listen to her too, not just your dad. (*To Luis*) How come you're smiling?

M: (*To Luis*) You listen to daddy, not to me.

T: Your mother has a voice too. . . . Is there someone at school who I can speak to who knows Luis?

M: The school social worker, the principal . . .

T: Please have one of them give me a call. What I suggest we do is set up a time when Manuel can come in too, so the four of you can come here.

M: Okay.

T: I think you've all made a good start for this one week. It's only a week but that's good. (*To father*) It sounds like you're in the middle of making changes for yourself. Your moods are changing, too, and you're going to have to look at that and how that affects everybody else in the family.

M: Yes (*smiling*).

T: It's certainly affecting your wife. And I'm sure it's affecting Luis, too. So they've got to see that you're going to be able to take care of yourself and deal with this calmly. It's some big changes that you're making. I'm going to take a short break right now to gather my thoughts and I'll be back in a few minutes.

I give myself permission to step out of the room for about 5 minutes at this point to gather my thoughts before concluding the interview.

I want to compliment you [the parents] on your caring and commitment to Luis in making his life better. It is impressive to see how everyone is trying to make changes in this family. You (*to father*) are making some big changes in ridding your life of alcohol so that you can be a better father to your children. You (*to mother*) are making it clear that your voice also needs to be respected in the family. And Luis, you are beginning to show how well you can do in school and in cooperating at home. This is all very impressive.

What I'd like to ask you to do is to watch for times when Luis is doing what you'd like him to do . . . when he's listening, following through, doing his homework, keeps getting good reports from school, is calm in the way you described you can be [not so emotional], those are good signs. Keep track of those. Sometimes we miss those things and get sidetracked by the times he's not cooperating. But, I'm sure Luis, that there are times when you're doing the things your parents want you to do, and they need to notice that and tell you, "That's great Luis"! Try not to get caught up in the times Luis doesn't follow through but to support the times that he does—because I know that there are many times when this happens. Also, would it be possible to keep track of the times when Luis does take you [mother] seriously in the way you'd like? Just jot down on a piece of paper what happened.

Mother indicates her willingness to try this.

I would like for us to set up another time when Manuel can join us for a meeting. What if we let about 2 weeks go by to see how things are going? (*Parents agree*) I think it was a good time to come in at this point and I will see you in 2 weeks.

In order to emphasize the points I made at the end of the session, I put my thoughts in a letter (following White & Epston, 1990) to the parents, which I mailed 4 days after our meeting.

Dear Mr and Mrs. Ramos:

I enjoyed meeting with you and your son Luis last week. I wanted to write to you so that I could summarize some of my thoughts from that meeting. After a meeting I sometimes get thoughts I wish I had shared in person, so I am writing them down.

I was very impressed with your caring and commitment to your children and making a better life for Luis and Manuel. It was very exciting to me to see how you are both making changes. You (Mr. Ramos) are working on making some big changes in ridding your life of alcohol so that you can be a better husband and father to your children. I know how difficult this process can be, and I admire your courage and strength in making this effort. By ridding your life of the influence of alcohol you are setting an important example for your sons. It is clear to me that Luis looks up to you and that you are a very important person to him. By staying calm and taking care of yourself you pro-

vide an example for him to follow. I am still puzzled by how you accomplished this. Can you let me in on your secret?

You (Mrs. Ramos) are making it clear that you also want some changes in the family. You want your voice to be respected. As the only woman in a household with 3 men, you have your work cut out for you. However, from our meeting last week I have the sense that you are already establishing your voice in new ways. I wonder how you would like to further develop your voice and what ideas you have for doing this.

I was also impressed with your son Luis who has gotten off to a very good start in his first week at the Corbin School. Luis seems like a very nice young man who you can be proud of. I know, as you do, that Luis is capable of being calm and cooperative. I know that you both have seen that side of him. I want to encourage you both to keep track of those times Luis is doing what you want him to do. You might write down all the times he cooperates in a positive manner. I would suggest that you (Mrs. Ramos) write down all the times that Luis listens to you (takes you seriously) in the way you'd like him to. I'm sure you will find many opportunities to appreciate his respect. Please let me know in what ways he shows this respect.

When we meet again I look forward to hearing about the ways you've continued to build on the changes you've already made. One note of caution. I would advise not making too many changes at once. I'll see you on [about 2 weeks later].

Sincerely . . .

The second session, held about 2 weeks later, included all four family members. When I went to the waiting room to greet the family, mother gave me a big smile. I began the session with the statement, "I hope you didn't make too many changes at once." The mother then began describing an incident in which Luis was not cooperative and his father got angry with him. I moved the focus back to "What's better . . . what has improved?" (de Shazer, 1991). Father reported that he has stopped "bribing" Luis for his cooperation by buying him things. We talk about how Luis is "testing" the father to see if he means business.

The mother then shows me Luis's notebook with the progress reports from school, which indicate that out of the last 10 school days, 7 were viewed by the teacher as "good or great days," meaning that Luis did not get into trouble for talking in class and that he completed his papers. I read the teacher's comments out loud and compliment Luis on this progress. Mother reveals that she, rather than Luis's father, is now signing the progress notebook for school, and that "Luis is listening to me now, not just his father." I compliment the mother on getting Luis to take her more seriously. I then ask the family if they received my letter and how they have continued to make changes. The father discusses his struggle to stay clean of alcohol (which he has now accomplished for over 2 months). I congratulate him on his successful efforts to stay sober and acknowledge how hard this is to do.

An incident is then described in which the father got upset with everyone in the family, stormed out of the house, but then regained his composure and returned home. The following excerpt describes this process. Instead of focusing attention on the "storming out," I emphasize, instead, the strength it took for the father to return home. I frame it as an example of the father's modeling for his sons, that "macho men have a soft side."

F: I just blew my stack . . . I had an appointment . . . and everyone take their time . . . and I don't want to be late when I have something to do. . . . I get mad . . . I just go crazy . . . I drove off, but when I got to the highway I changed my mind . . . I cooled down . . . I don't want to admit it, I was wrong but I guess . . . my attitude was showing . . .

T: That's good that you realized that, and showed Luis and Manuel you could do that.

F: That's the bottom line. . . . I was feeling lousy . . . Since I stopped drinking my temper can be pretty rough.

M: When he [husband] has a problem, we all get it. . . . [his anger]

F: I've got a lot of stuff on my mind. One day I said to my wife I'd like to have a glass of wine and a beer . . . but then I fight with myself.

The father described how previously when under stress he would drink himself into oblivion. Now he becomes more irritable and easily upset. It is also clear that his wife draws him out about his worries and serves as a good listener.

T: It's going to be rough, but you're winning. . . . I want to come back to the other situation. You left the house angry and then you came back. . . .

F: When I was driving I was thinking it was the wrong way to act. If we're going to help Luis out, I just got to do this. I saw his [Luis's] face when he saw me angry and . . . no good.

T: You wanted to show him a different picture.

F: So I tried to control myself. I was still mad but I shut up.

T: It was important that your sons see that, see you do that. Everybody can lose their cool, and that you can be strong enough to come back and say "let's start this over again" is very important. You know, last time you [mother] were saying that Luis and Manuel think they are "macho men" . . . but the kind of thing you [father] did by coming back . . . is really letting all of you know that he can say "I was wrong." You know macho men have a soft side, too. You know what I mean?

I then ask Luis what will he have to do to keep getting "great days" from the teacher. He tells me "finish my work and not talk out in class." I ask if he sees anything that might get in the way of doing this. He says "no." I then ask each family member to predict how many school days out of the next 10 do they expect Luis to have a "good or great day" on his progress note. Luis says "10." The father says "8"; the mother predicts "7" and Manuel says "5." I ask them to bring the notebook back to the next session so we can see how much progress Luis is making. I then end the session with a statement emphasizing how impressed I am with the work they're all doing. I tell the father that "the more you can keep in control the more you show your sons that they can too." And I compliment the mother on getting Luis to take her seriously and ask her to continue to notice when he does this. We schedule a third session in 3 weeks. All four family members shake my hand as they leave. Three days after this session I sent the family the following letter as a way of consolidating a new picture of this family as in a quest toward change ("becoming a butterfly") rather than languishing in a problem-saturated world.

Dear Mr. & Mrs. Ramos:

I wanted to write to you to share my thoughts after our last meeting. I continue to be impressed with the love and caring that each of you show in your own ways in helping your sons grow up right. Somehow the two of you decided to each take different roles with the children, you, Mr. Ramos being the "tough guy" and you, Mrs. Ramos being the "easy or soft one." However, I know from our past meeting that you, Mr. Ramos also have a "soft side" and that you, Mrs. Ramos can be tough-minded in your own way.

I am impressed with how each of you are trying to let your sons see more of the hidden sides of you. This was demonstrated by how you, Mr. Ramos, responded when you thought of the look on your son Luis's face and decided to return home after being so angry. It takes real strength to be able to show such caring. At the same time, I think you, Mrs. Ramos are really stronger than you let on. I admire the way you have taken responsibility around Luis' school progress report and are available as a loving wife to listen to your husband's worries.

I like your idea, Mr. Ramos, of using the money you would have spent on alcohol and spending it on records and tapes. I wonder if your love of music could somehow be helpful to you when you are starting to get "stressed-out" and upset. Let me know if you come up with any ideas about how this might work.

I think Luis has somehow gotten the mistaken notion that you, Mr. Ramos need to have someone to yell at once in awhile (you know, to "blow-off steam"). He has decided to be the person to help you do this. I don't think you need his help in this way and that you can handle your upset and stresses with the help of your wife and your music. In order to let him know that you don't need him to do this, I would suggest that you try to catch Luis doing something right and let him know that you noticed. I think your noticing the good things that Luis does will help him know that he doesn't need to worry about you anymore.

Luis is taking you, Mrs. Ramos, more seriously now. He understands that you have an important voice in the family. Please keep track of those times you notice that Luis is listening to you and what you do that makes this happen.

I can tell how hard you both are working to see that your children have a good life and a happy future. I think this may be a transition time in the life of the family as each of you make changes which will make the family stronger.

When I think of your family I think of the beautiful smiles I've seen on each of your faces and your children's faces at different points in our last meeting. Share those smiles with each other and let me know what happens.

I look forward to seeing all of you on Tuesday _____ at 6 PM and to hearing about the progress you are making. Please bring Luis' progress reports from school so I can see "firsthand" how well Luis is doing. Please feel free to share this letter with Manuel and Luis.

Sincerely . . .

At the third session, Luis brought in an award he received at school as "Student of the Month." In addition, in the 3-week interval between sessions, he received *10 out of 10* "good reports" from his teacher! Both parents were surprised and pleased with his performance. At the fourth session (3 weeks later) Luis's mother proudly presented me with Luis' report card. In addition to showing significant improvement in his academic subjects, *all* of Luis's marks for "conduct" (e.g., exhibits self-control, assumes responsibility, gets along well with peers) had gone from "minus" ("weakness") to "plus" ("strength"). Following this session, I sent the family a letter affirming Luis's improvement and change. At the fifth session (3 weeks later), the oldest son noted that he has seen changes in his father: "Instead of yelling and going out to drink, he stays there and listens to music." Although the father did drink on one occasion (and got sick to his stomach), he continued to maintain his sobriety (now over 5 months). At the fifth session, Luis was awarded a "winning against bad habits" certificate (after White & Epston, 1990, p. 200) to affirm his success in reclaiming his life from bad habits.

Besides my signature, the father witnessed the process by signing the certificate. A follow-up meeting was scheduled and then canceled when the father had to return to Puerto Rico. After not hearing from the family for over 3 months, I phoned and spoke with the father. He said that Luis finished the school year with both excellent grades and good behavior and that at home Luis's behavior was no longer seen as a problem. The father indicated that he has had some alcohol since we last met but had not been "crazy drunk" like before. The door was left open for future appointments.

SUMMARY

Since "we become the autobiographical narratives by which we 'tell about' our lives" (Bruner, 1987, p.15), therapy can best be described as a process of developing narratives or "stories" that promote healing and connection. The strengths and resources of the family serve as a foundation for the generation of new stories or alternative futures. As Friedman and Fanger (1991) point out:

> We do not want to enlarge the client's view of his "problem" by exploring it in detail, and thus intensify his distress. Nor do we believe that you need to find past causes to help clients' achieve their desired goals. We immediately direct clients' attention to future possibilities [alternative narratives] and help them shift their limiting visions to expanded views of reality that allow for new effective actions. . . . By consciously and methodically employing the language of possibility, we influence people to find options that liberate them from the problem and increase their sense of effectiveness and autonomy. (pp. 295–296)

EDITORS' QUESTIONS

Q: Do you use the letter-writing method with all your clients? It seems to me that this process would be very time-consuming. What are the benefits of writing letters to clients following therapy sessions?

A: The letter-writing approach is not one I use with all the families I see, but one method with which I have recently been experimenting. Probably because of my background in experimental psychology I tend to like to try out various approaches and observe their effectiveness. I consider my whole approach to therapy as "experimental" in the sense that I am always trying to integrate different ideas into my work. It helps keep the therapy process lively for me. My sense was that this particular family would benefit from hearing from me between sessions. The letters served to both summarize and expand on the in-the-room discussions and was a way of engaging the family in the therapy process. Letters provide a formal (more permanent) description of events and ideas and can be effective in highlighting important therapy issues. Menses (1986) discusses the usefulness of letter writing in therapy and how doing so can also help clarify the therapist's ideas and thinking. This process also allows the therapist to put forth ideas he or she may have not thought of during the session. Trying to write a letter after every session would be an impossible task for most of us. Instead, Menses suggests we consider writing a letter after the crucial initial interview, since this is where you are most likely to be introducing the family to new perspectives.

White and Epston's work (1990) has been a clear influence in my recent thinking about using a narrative model in therapy. Although the letter-writing activities with this family were time-consuming, they seemed to be a relatively effective (and time-efficient) mode of intervention.

Q: How would you have dealt with the situation if the father had been actively drinking at the time of the initial visit? What if he had been drinking heavily and refused to stop drinking?

A: I think I would have tried to engage him around the idea that his sobriety is important in order for him to be the effective parent I know he wants to be. If this didn't have any impact I would frame Luis's problematic behavior as a way for Luis to communicate his worry about his father. Some of these ideas and others are discussed in Treadway's excellent book (1989) and in Friedman and Fanger (1991, Ch. 8). It might have turned out that the father would have dropped out of treatment and that I would be left meeting with the mother and the children. If this happened I would make attempts to involve the father by possibly writing to him, summarizing our sessions, or calling him during the therapy hour to get his point of view. I would work with the mother and the children on dealing with the father's drinking and would encourage their involvement in Al-Anon and Alateen.

Q: I am intrigued by your use of the "miracle question," something that de Shazer and Berg developed. When do you use the "miracle question" and what information are you trying to elicit? Do you always ask it? How does it shape your interventions with the family?

A: I like the "miracle question" because it engages the family in a process of wondering about a future that doesn't contain the problem. It also allows the therapist to get concrete and specific information about what the goal is for treatment. In effect, you're beginning with the goal and then working backwards to achieve it. The "miracle question" has a playful quality to it yet is a very powerful intervention in that family members are engaged in a process of talking about their goals in ways that make them more possible and even inevitable. I generally use some form of the "miracle question" in all my first interviews. It not only disorients the family in a positive way, since they are expecting me to pursue them about details of the "problem," but also sets the stage, from the very beginning of treatment, toward a future orientation. Chasin, Roth, and Bograd (1989) are also using this question in a psychodramatic format with couples.

Q: When you leave the room, as you did at the end of the first session, to "gather your thoughts," where do you go and what do you do?

A: I excuse myself from the meeting and go find an empty office. I sit down with my pad and pen and outline some thoughts and ideas that I would like to feed back to the family before ending the session.

Q: Why is it that you maintain a focus on Luis as the "identifed patient" rather than on the father who's behavior more clearly impacts on all family members? Aren't you scapegoating the "victim"?

A: No, I don't see it that way at all. The parents have come to me with a specific goal in mind, to help Luis improve his behavior. I respect their request while incorporating them into the therapy process. In effect, I am dealing indirectly with the father's issues while keeping my primary focus on Luis's behavior. Therapists can become too presumptuous in deciding about what should be the primary focus of treatment rather than listening to the family's story and respecting their request. Rather than a therapy based on a formal set of diagnostic criteria (e. g., DSM-III-R), my therapy is based on the client's request. By listening to and respecting the parents' request I am able to quickly and effectively engage the family in treatment which then increases my leverage in achieving a successful outcome. I am not interested in making the father the patient or expanding the problem into a "family" one.

Q: How is it that the father, "a macho man," stayed involved in therapy throughout the process? I would have expected that he might feel uncomfortable having another man direct the process.

A: That is an interesting question and one that the mother commented on at the end of the third or fourth session. The father had left the room to accompany one of the children to a medical appointment in another part of the building. I was left with the mother to reschedule the next appointment. The mother said that she was surprised and pleased about her husband's involvement in therapy and that she "never expected that he would continue to come." What made the difference, I think, was my early and active attempts to connect with him as an important figure whose behavior directly influences his sons'. I respected his focus on Luis while gently engaging him in discussions around his own life. I tried to be sensitive to cultural norms and always framed my comments in ways that supported the importance of his role as the father in the family. This is a family with a lot of love and caring for one another.

Q: You refer to your approach as "family therapy," yet it differs considerably from such models as structural or strategic family therapy. How would you compare your approach with some of the original family therapy models?

A: My original training was in structural and strategic family therapy. My current thinking has led me away from these models. My aim is not to hypothesize about structural (hierarchical) problems in the family or to see the presenting problem as reflecting dysfunction in the marital subsystem. My work does contain elements of strategic family therapy and is influenced by the creative work of the Mental Research Institute (MRI) brief systems thinking. However, rather than seeing the presenting problem as serving some function in the family (i.e., the strategic model) or focusing on what maintains the problem (i.e., the MRI approach), I look for "exceptions" to the problem and for family strengths and successes and build my interventions around these areas.

My current work is most closely aligned with the ideas of de Shazer, O'Hanlon, and White. I avoid unnecessary hypothesizing about etiology and focus instead on generating, through a structured conversation, positive futures. The approach I use is basically a linguistic one in that I take responsibility for guiding the therapeutic conversation in ways that open up options, reframe realities, and empower family members. This model avoids attributing pathology to the system and instead joins with family members in a cooperative venture or partnership with the explicit understanding of reaching a targeted goal. Tomm (1990) has presented some useful and thought-provoking ideas that relate to ethical decision making in clinical work. He makes a strong case for using approaches that serve to increase and maximize options and therefore empower clients in contrast to those that reduce or restrain options and may end up leaving clients feeling manipulated or coerced. This is a very important issue in regard to whether the ends justify the means. My own belief is that our modes of intervention, the processes we use in therapy, need to reflect a position of "therapeutic uncertainty" (Tomm, 1990) so that we do not become too committed or wedded to the "rightness" of our methods. I see my work as evolving in this direction.

Another difference between my work and traditional family therapy models is the avoidance of seeking the "underlying meaning of people's experiences" (Parry, 1991). Too often we have tried to make psychotherapy seem more legitimate by thinking of our work as "science." By so doing we have bought into the notion that there must be some "explanation" (a deeper level) of what is happening that we can decipher and understand. By taking a narrative approach, the therapist accepts the client's presentation as a story which, in being told and retold, comes to define the client's perceptions and perspectives. This narrative is susceptible to change and modification as a function of the therapist's generating alternative stories or posing questions that "deconstruct" the narrative in such a way that the story changes. Letter writing is one way to generate alternative narratives or amplify already existing narratives that support positive futures.

Q: What is the usual number of sessions that you see families in therapy?

A: The number varies considerably. My aim is to make each session count and I don't set contracts for a specified number of meetings. For 300 families that I saw consecutively over a 3-year period, 90% were seen for 10 or fewer sessions. The average (median) number of sessions was 3.3 (range 1–20). In situations where I do see a family over an extended period of time, the meetings are scheduled on an intermittent basis (e.g., every 2–3 weeks). My work with a family is "completed" when they let me know that they are satisfied with the results of our joint efforts. However, I remain available for future "consultations" as needed and in that sense do not formally "terminate" with anyone (Budman, 1990).

Q: How did you become a brief therapist?

A: My professional career began in academia as an experimental psychologist, conducting research with infants. My research interests led me to studies of interactional behavior, initially of mothers and infants and later of whole families. Out of this research, I became interested in how to clinically intervene to create change in family systems. Career-wise I made a decision to retrain as a clinical psychologist, with an emphasis on family therapy. Early on I was influenced by the thinking of Nicholas Hobbs, a pioneer in the development of innovative ecological/systems approaches. Hobbs developed a strength-oriented, competency-based approach (Project Re-ED) which effectively utilized the resources of the child's social network in creating a context for change. From

Hobbs work I learned how small systemic interventions would create ripple effects that would lead to even more change while reducing client dependency on institutional resources.

Personally, I've always been an "efficiency freak", looking for ways to manage my activities in more time-effective ways. Transferring this thinking to my clinical work just happened naturally. I also have a strong belief in the resources and capacities of individuals to create better lives for themselves. This is something I think I got from my father who always saw possibilities and who believed that dreams and aspirations were the first step in getting there.

My goal in therapy is to generate ideas that empower clients to create more satisfying futures for themselves. My work continues to evolve as I collaborate with clients to find new pathways and increased options.

REFERENCES

Andersen, T. (1990). *The reflecting team: Dialogues and dialogues about dialogues.* United Kingdom: Borgmann.

Anderson, H., & Goolishian, H. A. (1988). Human systems as linguistic systems: Preliminary and evolving ideas about the implications for clinical theory. *Family Process, 27*, 371–393.

Barker, P. (1985). *Using metaphors in psychotherapy.* New York: Brunner/Mazel.

Bennett, M. (1989). The catalytic function in psychotherapy. *Psychiatry, 52*, 351–364.

Berwick, D. M. (1989). Continuous improvement as an ideal in health care. *New England Journal of Medicine, 320*, 53–56.

Bruner, J. (1987). Life as narrative. *Social Research, 54*, 11–32.

Budman, S. H. (1990). The myth of termination in brief therapy: Or it ain't over til it's over. In J. K. Zeig & S. G. Gilligan (Eds.), *Brief therapy: Myths, methods, and metaphors* (pp. 206–218). New York: Brunner/Mazel.

Budman, S., & Gurman, A. (1988). *Theory and practice of brief therapy.* New York: Guilford Press.

Chasin, R., Roth, S. A., & Bograd, M. (1989). Action methods in systemic therapy: Dramatizing ideal futures and reformed pasts with couples. *Family Process, 28*, 121–136.

de Shazer, S. (1988). *Clues: Investigating solutions in brief therapy.* New York: W. W. Norton.

de Shazer, S. (1991). *Putting difference to work.* New York: W. W. Norton.

Epstein, E. S., & Loos, V. E. (1989). Some irreverent thoughts on the limits of family therapy: Toward a language based explanation of human systems. *Journal of Family Psychology, 2*, 405–421.

Friedman, S. (1989a). Child mental health in an HMO: A family systems approach. *HMO Practice, 3*, 52–59.

Friedman, S. (1989b). Strategic reframing in a case of "delusional jealousy." *Journal of Strategic and Systemic Therapies, 8,* 1–4.

Friedman, S. (1990). Towards a model of time-effective family psychotherapy: A view from a health maintenance organization. *Journal of Family Psychotherapy, 1*(2), 1–28.

Friedman, S. (1991). Toward a "wellness" model of time-effective family psychotherapy. *The Family Psychologist, 7*(2), 23–24.

Friedman, S. & Fanger, M. T. (1991). *Expanding therapeutic possibilities: Getting results in brief psychotherapy.* New York: Lexington Books/Macmillan.

Garcia-Preto, N. (1982). Puerto Rican families. In M. McGoldrick, J. K. Pearce & J. Giordano (Eds.), *Ethnicity and family therapy* (pp. 164–186). New York: Guilford Press.

Haley, J. (1973). *Uncommon therapy: The psychiatric techniques of Milton H. Erickson, MD.* New York: W. W. Norton.

Hobbs, N. (1966). Helping disturbed children: Psychological and ecological strategies. *American Psychologist, 21,* 1105–1115.

Masterpaqua, F. (1989). A competence paradigm for psychological practice. *American Psychologist, 44,* 1366–1371.

Maturana, H. R., & Varela, F. J. (1987). *The tree of knowledge.* Boston: Shambala.

Menses, G. (1986). Therapondulitis and theraspondence: The art of therapeutic letter writing. *Family Therapy Case Studies, 1*(1), 61–64.

Minuchin, S. (1984). *Family kaleidoscope.* Cambridge, MA: Harvard University Press.

Mittelmeier, C., & Friedman, S. (1991). The Rashomon effect: A study in constructivist conversation. *Family Therapy, 18*(1), 17–36.

O'Hanlon, W., & Wilk, J. (1987). *Shifting contexts: The generation of effective psychotherapy.* New York: Guilford Press.

Parry, A. (1991). A universe of stories. *Family Process, 30,* 37–54.

Seeman, J. (1989). Toward a model of positive health. *American Psychologist, 44,* 1099–1109.

Tomm, K. (1987). Interventive interviewing: Part II. Reflexive questioning as as means to enable self-healing. *Family Process, 26,* 167–183.

Tomm, K. (1990, June). *Ethical postures that orient one's clinical decision-making.* Paper presented at the American Family Therapy Association Conference, Philadelphia, PA.

Treadway, D. (1989). *Before it's too late: Working with substance abuse in the family.* New York: W. W. Norton.

Watzlawick, P. (Ed.). (1984). *The invented reality.* New York: W. W. Norton.

Weick, K. E. (1984). Small wins: Redefining the scale of social problems. *American Psychologist, 39,* 40–49.

White, M., & Epston, D. (1990). *Narrative means to therapeutic ends.* New York: W. W. Norton.

Brief Therapy— MRI Style

JOHN H. WEAKLAND
RICHARD FISCH

How one conducts treatment—and evaluates its outcome—depends to a large extent on one's general view of the nature of problems and their resolution. Therefore, any attempt to convey an understanding of the handling of a specific case treated in psychotherapy, in addition to a description (or better, exemplification) of case specifics and their discussion, also must describe the model of therapy within which the therapist is operating, or, at least, believes he or she is operating.

In the present case, this is likely to involve certain difficulties, and we think it may be helpful to start by giving fair warning of these. First, although we have been working on and using this model for more than 20 years at the Brief Therapy Center of the Mental Research Institute, Palo Alto, CA (MRI) (Fisch, Weakland, & Segal, 1982; Watzlawick, Weakland, & Fisch, 1974; Weakland, Fisch, Watzlawick, & Bodin, 1974), and have taught it widely, it is quite different from the psychodynamic approach that is still the prevailing model in psychotherapy generally and probably even in brief treatment. Moreover, it is different in some basic respects even from conventional family therapy, out of which it grew. Second, the model itself (though not necessarily its application) is very brief and simple. Perhaps this should not be a cause of difficulty—indeed, in scientific work generally, theoretical simplicity is considered a highly desirable aim. Yet, it appears that the world of human problems commonly is assumed to be unavoidably complex, so that people have difficulty believing that a simple model could be relevant and effective. We can only report that a number of people who have read our publications and then come to see our actual practice say, with some surprise, "You really do what you say you do!" and that it seems to work.

In common with the general orientation of family therapy, our center views problems as interactional—that is, not as something residing within a particular individual, but as an aspect or a resultant of interaction between individuals in a family or in some other system of social interaction and communication. Consonant with this, we view problems as behavioral in nature—that is, as consisting of some persisting behavior by the identified patient which is stimulated and shaped by behaviors of other persons involved, or sometimes by other behavior of the patient himself. We see problem resolution, accordingly, as requiring behavioral changes by those involved in the system of interaction, and the essential business of the therapist as the promotion of such change, which the members of the system have not been able to accomplish on their own.

We differ from many family therapists, however, in our focus of inquiry and intervention, our means of promoting change, and our goal and evaluation of treatment. In large part, these differences may be seen as related to our pursuing the interactional view of problems further than is commonly done, both in concept and in practice. To start with, we concentrate on the presenting problem and behaviors that are directly related to this, much more than is usual. Correspondingly, not only do we avoid looking behind or beneath the "symptom" as is emphasized in dynamic psychotherapy, we also avoid looking around it broadly as in much of family therapy. Our aim is to narrow, rather than expand, the treatment field.

More broadly, this focus on the presenting complaint has increasingly led us away from the dichotomous conceptual framework of "pathology" versus "normality"—with its implication that there is only one right way for an individual or a family to function. Instead, our view of problems and treatment is essentially complaint based. Likewise, our goal of treatment and the basis of its evaluation are resolution of the original complaint. This, after all, is the basis of entering into therapy in the first place.

Since we also take the concept of interaction more seriously than many do, we believe it is possible to bring about whatever change is needed to resolve a problem in a system through promoting change in any one member, with the expectation that this will, in turn, promote change in other members. The immediate consequence of this view is that instead of seeing all members of a family routinely, we concentrate our treatment attention and effort on whomever seems most concerned to see change happen—not necessarily the identified patient—or the one who possesses the greatest leverage in the system. That is, who we see directly in treatment, as well as the nature of our inquiries and interventions, is a matter of strategic choice.

Now, to be more specific: If one really focuses on behavior, any problem of the kind people bring to therapists may be defined as consisting of (1) some observable behavior, which (2) is characterized as undesirable (deviant, difficult, distressing, dangerous) either by its performer or by some other concerned person, but which (3) persists despite efforts to alter or get rid of it, therefore (4) the concerned person seeks professional help. Accordingly, our treatment begins by inquiring *who* is doing *what* that is seen as a problem, *who* sees it as a problem, and *how* is this behavior seen as a problem. (We may also inquire, especially with long-standing problems, just what provoked the client to call requesting help at this particular time.) Throughout this inquiry—and in subsequent inquiries equally—our aim is to get as clear and specific a description as possible—who is, observably, doing and saying what. That is, we see the behavior of concern as itself the problem, not as just "the tip of the iceberg," another sign or symptom of some more fundamental inner or deeper state, or even, necessarily, a manifestation of some deep and pervasive disarray in the system of interaction.

On this basis, we next inquire not about the nature of interaction as a whole in the family, but about the behavior most immediately related to the problem behavior, namely, what is being said and done to try to handle (prevent, resolve) the problem by the identified patient and/or any others concerned with it.

Both a general viewpoint and concrete experience underlie this concentration of attention. The interactional view of problems implies a cybernetic rather than a linear concept of causation. Therefore, with this view, it is not the origin of a problem but its persistence that is central for understanding and treatment: What unwitting behaviors function to maintain or reinforce the problem behavior, even though this is defined as undesired or undesirable? Ironically, in our clinical experience it appears over and over that some aspect of people's attempts to control or eliminate the problem—though these attempts are usually well intentioned and seemingly logical ("common sense")—constitutes the reinforcing behavior: "The 'solution' is the problem" (Watzlawick et al., 1974).

In other words, problems consist basically of vicious circles, involving a positive feedback loop between some behavior labeled "wrong" and inappropriate (i.e., ineffective) efforts to get rid of it. Several features of our approach follow from this view. Our general treatment aim is to interrupt the vicious circle maintaining behavior. Accordingly—except in a limited number of cases where the problem behavior can appropriately be redefined as "no problem" or "just one of life's difficulties"—our specific interventions aim primarily at interdicting continuation of the misguided "solution" behavior. Since one cannot just cease any given behavior, such interventions often involve the prescription of some new alternative behavior, but the crucial element remains stopping the performance of the attempted solution. An apparently small change in this respect can be strategic; it may initiate a reversal in the feedback loop, leading to further positive change.

In making such interventions, we do not try to bring about overall revision of the client's intellectual understandings or behavioral patterns. Our concept of a problem is that it is a limited behavioral issue in which someone is "stuck"—although its effects may have spread widely. Our corresponding aim is to help clients get "unstuck" so they can get on with the daily business of life as they see fit. A problem may be solved by behavioral changes—ceasing the attempted solution—or sometimes by a reevaluation of the original focus of complaint as "no problem," just one of life's daily difficulties. In promoting either sort of change expeditiously we "speak the client's language," and avoid argument, as much as possible, although our questions and suggestions imply a behavioral and interactional view of life with a strongly pragmatic orientation. Such interventions mainly involve suggestions for behavioral changes in the real world outside the therapy room. Usually, however, these are not direct prescriptions but depend on reframing the problem situation, avoiding argument, and utilizing the clients' own preexisting ideas about people and problems—speaking the client's "language"—so as to make different problem-handling behavior appear logical and appropriate to them. Since our aim is specific behavioral change rather than intellectual understanding (which may produce no change in actual daily behavior), we do not devote much effort to clarifying and discussing the overall interactional system to those involved. However, behavioral change may lead to new views; also, our mode of inquiry and intervention may promote a pragmatic and behavioral view by implication.

CASE ILLUSTRATION

The case presented is typical of our work in most respects: It closely follows the model sketched above; the problem is similar to many encountered in our practice; the family is self-referred (although we do get some referrals from physicians or other therapists); and there was no intake procedure beyond filling out a simple demographic information form, since we believe that information gathering is itself a basic aspect of treatment. In one respect, however, this case was not typical, but in a way that helps to underline a major emphasis of our usual procedure. Ordinarily, we would conduct the initial interview with that member of the family we regard as the main complainant. Most often this is the person making the telephone call asking for help. We can confirm this by asking how motivated the other members of the family are: "How eager to come for therapy?" If it is reported that any one or more are "eager," we include them in that first session. In this particular case the caller, the identified patient's mother, said she would be quite glad to come in as soon as possible. Unfortunately, she added that she was about to go away for a 2-week business trip but asked if we would go ahead and see her 19-year-old son about whom she was concerned. She indicated that he was "interested" in coming in, but it seemed to us that his motivation was questionable. Ordinarily, we would have waited until his mother returned from her trip and have seen her first, alone. As it happened, we were about to do a workshop and were counting on this case for a live demonstration of interviewing methods. We therefore decided to go ahead for the sake of the workshop and see the son first, despite our misgivings about his motivation. As it turned out, he was rather passive about his problem—"I get into fights"—and apparently more concerned about his mother's nagging than any consequences stemming from his fighting (e.g., a broken arm).

The identified patient, Bob, had a 21-year-old sister, Jean; his mother was 47 and divorced. In the first session with Bob, he explained that his currently broken arm was actually a refracture of a broken arm that had occurred during a previous fight and had not healed sufficiently before this last fight. He also mentioned that he had recently gotten arrested simply by "loudmouthing" police when they came to investigate a complaint about the behavior of some of his friends. He said he himself had not committed any offense, nor was he under investigation, but his verbal abuse and aggression were such that police felt it necessary to take him into custody. His stance throughout this interview confirmed our prior view that he was not a serious "customer" for treatment.

The following interview with his mother, Nancy, was for us, then, the beginning of treatment, and thus we consider it the initial interview since it is more representative of our approach. We have not included, in the transcribed excerpts given here, our usual orienting the client to the features of the Brief Therapy Center such as our audio and videotaping, observation of treatment by other members of the team, the schedule of our follow-up interview, fees, and the like.

The First Session

Therapist (Fisch): What's the problem?

We want to convey to clients that the counseling will be a problem-solving venture. We usually do this by starting right off with, "What's the problem?" or "What's the trouble that brings you in?")

Nancy: Well, I don't know what the problem is, but the reason he's here is he's angry. . . .

T: What I mean by What's the problem?"—I don't mean anything profound by it and I don't mean the whys and wherefores, but just that, assuming you are coming in because you are concerned about him, my lead question would be, "What reason do you have to be concerned . . . what's the trouble?"

It is not unusual for a client to interpret the question as asking for "why" there is a problem or what the underlying reason is for the problem. In those cases we will explain to indicate we are asking for the client's complaint, that is, what is the behavior she is concerned about.

N: Well, he has been arrested twice. He did nothing wrong except he couldn't control his temper. He really didn't break the law but he kept hassling the policeman. He hassles me all the time. He used to be delightful and fun and laughing. Now I'm with him 2 minutes and I'm ready to scream. He's just angry. He gets into fights . . . that's not like him. I guess you know he's broken his arm five times now, three of them fighting. He's going to kill somebody or get killed. I . . . he's just not a happy kid. He's miserable and he's making me miserable.

T: Can you give me an example of that or how would that go? . . .

As can be seen, Nancy describes the problem in general and vague terms and we need to have the complaint described in specific and tangible terms. The most frequent way we do this is by asking for an example since this tends to direct the response toward descriptive terms.

N: Well, recently . . .

T: . . . where he was fine, and then he starts to change in his behavior?

N: Okay. Monday he came home from the hospital and he was fine and we discussed all this and he was so relieved and delighted and he was pleasant and helpful, and we'd laugh, and I said, "Bob, I haven't seen you laugh in so long." Everything was going great. I left for Boston

Tuesday morning and I called in Tuesday night. First thing he says is, "Jean isn't home. She hasn't been around. Nobody's cooked my dinner, nobody's . . ." I said, "Bob, wait a minute. I'm in Boston . . . I can't, I can't do anything about this." And I said, "Talk to your sister," and he knew where she was "and ask her, if you need something, if she could come home. Call me back." This is in Boston. "Jean won't come home!" "Well, you're mobile; you can take care of your problems and . . ." He called me seven times that night complaining. Finally, I said to him, "Bob, you're out of control again. You're, you're. . . . All this good behavior is gone. You're right back to where you were." And then his sister called me there and said, "Mom, he's calmed down, he's okay now." I . . . but . . . he's 19 and he called me that many times. . . ? And I don't deal with with it well. I just think, why can't he appreciate that I can't do this? (*Long pause*)

T: That's in part because the reasonableness doesn't work.

Usually, after a client has given a sufficiently clear presentation of the complaint, we will ask, "How do you try to deal with it?" In this case, she has included her attempts to deal with Bob's demandingness, and the therapist decided to intervene by reframing her efforts at exhorting Bob to calm down as being "reasonable." Choosing such a reframe has two advantages: (1) it is noncritical of her, and (2) if the client accepts that being "reasonable" doesn't work, she is in a better position to accept a suggestion to handle things in a "nonreasonable" or "unpredictable" (i.e., very different) way.

N: I always lose. I always give in first. I always back down. I can't deal with the high velocity thing. I've never liked it. I back off . . . and he knows that.

Her response indicates that she has accepted the reframe, at least to the extent of agreeing that her customary attempts don't work.

T: When you get angry, what kind of thing would you be saying?

Again, another attempt to have the client be more specific and descriptive.

N: I would be trying to make him hear what he is saying to me; "Now, Bob, why are reacting like this? Why are you doing this to me?"

Summarizing excerpts from that session, the following information is pertinent to our approach:

1. The mother is the complainant, certainly the principal complainant.

2. Her complaint is that Bob fails to exert restraint on his impulses, resulting in frequent fights and arrests outside the home and infantile demandingness at home.
3. She has attempted to deal with with this problem by pointing out his unreasonable stance and exhorting him to modify his demands. In particular, when she feels it neccessary to deny his demand—"No"—she attempts to get him to acknowledge the "correctness" of her decision.

We next include an excerpted transcript of the second session with Nancy to illustrate how this information is utilized in the treatment. The reader will see that it takes up where the previous session left off.

The Second Session

T: The way you've tried dealing with Bob normally, is to try to be reasonable?

This is not intended to elicit information so much as to confirm that the client has still accepted the reframe described in the first session. This is important before going ahead with any other agenda since acceptance can provide for a time-saving shift or step in treatment, the building block, so to speak, for a specific suggestion later. The suggestion will offer an alternative way of dealing with Bob's demandingness, a way that will interdict her more customary and counterproductive method.

N: Uh huh, and I give in a lot. That's also a way of dealing with it.
T: Okay, but that's in part because the reasonableness doesn't work. He needs to come to terms . . .
N: Yes.
T: . . . He needs to grow up.
N: And he knows that too.
T: Well, he knows and he doesn't know it.
N: I think he knows the difference . . . and what it's going to entail.
T: And I'm saying that, in particular, I think a good part of your helping him would be avoiding, as much as you can, legitimizing his stuff, his comments when he's coming on abrasively, rudely, demanding, being unrealistic about it.

The therapist is deliberately being general and vague. While Nancy's previous responses indicate she has accepted the idea that her being "reasonable" doesn't work, the therapist is not certain enough that she is ready to accept a specific suggestion and he is using these general comments to see how she responds to them. We would prefer to make the error of taking unnecessary time—"playing out the line" than risk the alternative error of making specific suggestions too precipitously. That latter error invites the client to discount the suggestion and, thereby, diminish the therapist's credibility. This can cost far more time in treatment.

N: I do what?

The client appears to be asking for specific instruction but without indicating her position on the previous remarks. Because of that, the therapist continues with noncommittal statements.

T: Well, if you're not going to be reasonable, then, I guess, it would be some form or forms of being nonreasonable. It would be any form that, mainly, would convey, without argument, there's no room for discussion on this. This is not a legitimate thing to discuss, anymore than what should you pack to go to Mars. That would be in general. Let me show you how tricky it is because to say, "Look, there's no point in discussing this," is to be reasonable.

N: Yes . . . "And why can't we discuss it? And just give me three reasons why we can't discuss this."

T: Right.

N: "Well . . . because . . ." and then I'm into discussing it.

Here, the client gives a "yes" response. She indicates she has gotten the therapist's point.

T: That's right, it's tricky.

N: He's demanding. What do I do then?

T: Well, as I said, it is how to respond to that in a way that delegitimizes his unreasonableness, because it needs to be for his own benefit, in a way that just cuts it short, no discussion, it's not worth discussing and, also, where it doesn't lead to further polemics, that is, doesn't get his back up.

N: That's the problem.

T: I'd say a part of it may depend on your willingness to be a bit arbitrary for his sake, because arbitrariness is a way of cutting short things, like, "Go fight City Hall." I'm not saying to say that but just everyday arbitrariness.

Despite the client's apparent readiness to take a different tack, the therapist is still being noncommittal and probably unnecessarily cautious.

N: So I just have to be firm in the . . ." I can't handle this, I can't deal, I can't answer your problem; you are going to have to do this. That's it!"

T: Well, it would have to be something that is just unarguable, no point.

N: I haven't found one of those.

T: Well, if you don't mind the onus, since you've said, looking back, there are a number of things I've done, a lot of things I've done that I don't think have been for the best. . . .

N: Of course.

T: Okay. So to that extent, it would be quite true, you could say that you haven't been as good a mother as you would have liked.

N: Uh huh.

T: And that if you don't mind the onus, you might be willing to say "that's wrong." That after talking with me, you've come to realize that you haven't been "as good a mother as I had hoped."

N: And?

T: Period. Then, when he calls and says, "I want you to take care of this," you can say, "No, I won't. If I were a better mother, I would."

The therapist has finally decided to be more specific judging from the client's attempts to formulate some specific plan. As the reader can see, the therapist hasn't simply come out with, "Here's what to say . . ." but has built a logical sequence of thoughts, each resting on the previous one. This is rather usual for us, since it gives the therapist a chance to back away if the client is not giving "yes" responses at each step. Here, Nancy responds with "Of course." and "Uh huh.")

(Long pause)

N: How interesting! *(Laughs)* This is so good because I would have come at it from the other side: "I am being a good mother now, by not solving all your . . ." and I would have gone into this long dissertation making me look okay because I wasn't doing what I *knew* I shouldn't be doing. That's wonderful!

This is a very encouraging "yes" response. Quite often, when the client is intrigued by a suggestion, one can be fairly certain the client will carry it out. In her final statement, "That's wonderful," the therapist avoids a one-up stance by making a one-down comment, in this case, "Well, keep your fingers crossed." This is intended to imply that the suggestion might not work at all and, therefore, might not be such a brilliant piece of work. Avoiding a one-up stance allows the therapist to take a flexible position regarding a suggestion: it will either work and thus maintain or increase his or her credibility or it won't work, something the therapist will have already entertained and, in that way, protect his credibility. Also, we prefer that the client not feel she is a passive and helpless puppet fortunate enough to have encountered a master puppeteer but is an active participant in the resolution of the problem.

N: Oh, it may not always work, but it certainly . . . it will stop him for a while.

SUMMARY

In all, eight sessions were spent. Bob was seen twice more (one of them a split session with his mother); the rest of the sessions were with Nancy. The sessions with Bob confirmed our initial impression that he was the less strategic person with whom to work. He remained quite passive in his participation. The work with Nancy pursued the strategy begun in the second session with her, mainly to get her to depart from her customary attempts to have Bob accept her "No" by trying to convince him of the legitimacy of that "No." As a way of departing from that, the therapist reinforced the suggestion that she limit the explanation of her "No" to simply reflecting that she was a "bad mother." By the seventh session, she reported she had taken an opportunity to implement this suggestion, with surprisingly gratifying results: Bob had asked her for the use of her car and she replied she wouldn't do it. When he asked her, "Why not?" she replied that if she were a better mother she would agree but that she wasn't that good a mother. Bob had just shrugged his shoulders, said "Okay," and walked away without any further fuss. By the eighth session she said that there had been some remarkable changes in his mood and his behavior. He seemed happier and had volunteered to help her with the care of the home, As a final comment on his change, she reported on his recent confrontation with police investigating a disturbance. Bob was polite to them and the police wound up apologizing for inconveniencing him.

   Since we offer clients 10 sessions in the Brief Therapy Center, the therapist suggested that the remaining 2 sessions be "kept in the bank to be drawn on if and when the need should arise." Nancy was agreeable to this arrangement.

FOLLOW-UP

As is also our practice, we do a telephone follow-up 3 months after the last appointment. Nancy said that her concern about Bob's violence and his demandingness at home was much less. He had gotten a job as a landscaper and had taken up surfing for recreation. There had been no further treatment. Bob reported that he was better able to control his temper and that his relationship with his mother was much improved. He added that he was no longer depressed and that he had not sought any additional treatment.

EDITORS' QUESTIONS

Q: Your approach can be categorized as "minimalist" in that you focus immediately on creating a small change that will interdict some aspect of the interactional cycle in which the problem is embedded. The solution—oriented models have also been described as "minimalist," although they emphasize "exceptions to the problem" rather than the problem itself. What do you see as the advantages of one approach over the other?

A: We agree that both our approach and that of de Shazer (1985, 1988), as the leader of "solution-focused" therapy, can be considered "minimalistic," not only in seeking a small initial change that will lead on to more but also in seeking theoretical simplicity—though it should equally be emphasized that applying either of these orientations in practice may be far from simple. Beyond that we do not see these two approaches as opposed or contradictory. De Shazer was in contact with and influenced by the work of MRI at least from 1972, when he took one of our early brief therapy workshops, and our approaches have much in common. However, we focus primarily on attempted solutions that do not work and maintain the problem, but with some attention to noting and promoting actions that have worked; de Shazer and his followers, in our view, have the inverse emphasis. The two are complementary.

Q: On what basis do you make the decision about who in the family provides the greatest leverage for change? What are your criteria for determining who is the "customer"? By talking initially with only one family member on the phone, aren't you vulnerable to getting a skewed perspective on the motivations of other family members?

A: Our primary criterion in deciding whom we will work with in treatment is, "Who is most concerned to make change in the problem situation?" That is, who is most ready not only to voice a complaint but to take some action about it. A second criterion may be, "Who has the most power to effect change?" This is most significant in child-centered problems; parents have much more power than a child—although they may not recognize this.

In initially talking to only one family member, by telephone or in person, there is, of course, a possibility—in fact, a certainty—of getting an incomplete or biased account of the problem situation. But there are also several important factors that minimize the likelihood of being seriously misled. First, our inquiries always focus on getting specific, concrete descriptive information about the problem—who says what, who does what? Such information is much more reliable than general statements. Second, we usually inquire whether anyone other than the initial complainant is significantly involved in either the occurrence of the problem or attempts to resolve it; if so, we usually arrange to meet with that person or persons also. Finally, accumulating experience in talking, either conjointly or separately, with the various persons involved in a problem leads to the increasing ability to evaluate and interpret the partial accounts of persons seen alone.

Q: In your interview there is no mention of the father. What factors in treatment might have led you to ask about the father's role/involvement, etc., and to consider this person in your treatment planning?

A: We routinely ask clients what help or advice about the problem they may be receiving from anyone else, and if it appears that another person is significantly involved, we will often meet with that person or persons also. In this case, neither the identified patient nor his mother indicated that the divorced father was much involved.

Q: What do you see as some of the advantages of using a "complaint-based" approach in contrast to one that uses a predefined set of diagnostic criteria?

A: To answer this large and basic question fully would require at least another article, but some main points may be reemphasized here. We do not believe that there is only one correct or "normal" way for every individual or every family to think and act. Accordingly, in each case, rather than trying to fit people into a predetermined system of categories, we want to know, as clearly and specifically as possible, what is seen as the main problem by the specific client(s) involved, how this is seen as a problem, and what would be seen as a satisfactory resolution. These are the matters that matter to our clients, and for which they are paying us—as their agents—for professional help.

Q: What do you do when you are left with a client who is not a "customer" (e.g., someone referred to you by the courts)? Do you have some strategies for transforming a "visitor" into a "customer"? In what situations would you agree to meet with several family members at once?

A: There are two different situations involving clients who come to treatment under duress. When someone comes because of pressure from a family member (or possibly from a friend), we attempt to see and work with the more concerned other person, as we did in the case presented here. If a client comes under legal duress, this is not usually a feasible course. Then we first take steps to define ourselves as separate from the referring authority, and not necessarily in agreement with its views of the client and the problem. After this, it is possible to inquire if the client himself sees any problem that it might be useful to work on. As a last resort, it may be suggested that there is one evident problem— that the client is under duress from an authority—and ways of handling this might be worth discussing. But unless something the *client* perceives as a problem can be established initially, therapy is apt to be only a futile effort.

Q: When the therapist says, "That's because the reasonableness doesn't work" (p. 312), in response to the mother's question, isn't he presenting a linear formulation (i.e., giving an explanation of *why* something is not working)? How does this fit with the idea that the MRI model is based on a circular (nonlinear) notion of causality?

A: The therapist is not really giving an explanation so much as pointing out, "Here is another example of your attempted solution— reasonableness—not working, not producing the effect you desire." Like most people, clients see causation as linear, and we see it as circular, but we do not think it necessary to teach our clients a new general view. If we can just get them to handle the problem behavior differently in specific ways, there will be different responses, and the vicious circle will be broken.

Q: The intervention is a clever and useful one. Did you think about, and reject, other alternative interventions? Could you tell us what they were and why you chose not to use them? In a similar vein, is it often a matter of trial and error to come up with the "right" intervention, which really ends up working? Are there particular principles or guidelines you use to find or develop such an intervention?

A: In this particular case, we did not entertain any different intervention with the mother. It seemed clear enough that she needed to depart from attempting to have her son acknowledge the legitimacy of her "No," and from experience with similar cases, this can often be done most quickly and easily by having the parent take the position of

"I'm a bad parent." How we motivate the particular parent to adopt that depends on the individual parent. In this case, as in many cases, we will first try by labeling their attempts as "being reasonable with someone who is being unreasonable." In this case it was sufficient so we did not need to look further. In many cases, there is some trial and error, but these different options and trials mainly have to do with finding ways of *motivating* the client to take an action or of designing appropriate actions depending on acceptability to the client, opportunity for implementing them, convenience, and the like. We do not think in terms of "the right" intervention; there are usually many ways of achieving the same goal—the interdiction of the client's attempted solution—and we assume that when an intervention is successful, it is likely that one or more other suggestions and ways of promoting them could also have worked. The basic guideline, of course, is what tack do we want the client to abandon in favor of an alternative behavior that is more likely to be effective.

Q: Would you describe what was happening in treatment sessions 3 through 6, the period after the strategy was suggested and before the mother implemented it? What factors prevented this treatment from being even more efficient (i.e., requiring fewer sessions)?

A: Much of the time during those sessions was still spent with Bob in an attempt to develop more active participation despite our appraisal that he was not a complainant. It is probable that if we had not started with him, we would not have invested the further time as we did. In any case, since this was atypical, we do not feel that additional detail about our efforts with Bob would add to the reader's understanding of what we do, more typically, in our treatment approach. Obviously, if we had proceeded more as usual—started with the mother—we would have been able to save time. We probably would have seen her son only once and also had more continuity in monitoring her compliance with suggestions and their relative success. In any case, saving two or three sessions seems hardly consequential when so much treatment is still measured in terms of years.

Q: What is the average number of sessions that people are seen in treatment? How often do people come back for "booster sessions" after completing the original treatment?

A: Our average number of sessions in the Brief Therapy Center is about 6½.

When we see a case for less than our maximum of 10 sessions, we often, but not always, will tell the client that the remaining sessions are "in the bank," as we did in this case. This primarily is done as a measure of reassurance—you are not completely abandoned and on your own, you can call on us if need be. But given such reassurance, the need seems to arise very rarely—perhaps in only about 1% of our cases.

Q: How long is your average treatment session? If people have 10 sessions in which to work, can these be divided into half or quarter sessions?

A: Our usual treatment session is 1 hour. We do not divide our sessions into smaller units, but from time to time we will stop a session short of the hour, with the patient's acquiescence, especially when we feel an important intervention has been made and we do not want to dilute it by further talk.

Q: How did you become a brief therapist?

WEAKLAND: Not surprisingly, when colleagues discover that I began professional life as a chemical engineer, I am often asked, "How did you become a family therapist particularly interested in brief therapy?" This is not an easy question to answer briefly; only a few turning points can be mentioned.

I spent 6 years in research, development, and plant design as an engineer. I decided to get out of this field when, at last working for a highly competent and well-organized engineering firm, it became increasingly apparent to me that my daily work was like working on an assembly line—technical, but highly specialized and repetitive.

So I returned to graduate school to study sociology and anthropology; I had become interested in the social sciences and psychology through reading plus curiously observing behavior in the organizations in which I had been working. Several years later, I was invited by Gregory Bateson, my first teacher of anthropology, to work with him on some research on communication for which he had just received funding and I accepted.

This communication research covered a wide range, but after a while the work began to focus on studying the communication of schizophrenic patients in the Palo Alto VA Hospital where the project offices were located. Since we were always concerned with the context as well as the content of communication, it was only a next step to begin interviewing patients together with their family members. This, plus the influence of Don Jackson, who had joined us as a consultant on schizophrenia, led to attempts to do therapy with these families. This became one of the main origins of the whole family therapy movement.

At about the same time, Jay Haley and I became interested in hypnosis and began periodic visits to Phoenix to talk with Milton Erickson to discuss hypnosis and also his work with schizophrenic patients. During these meetings it became clear that Erickson often worked quite briefly, and that his work usually involved active behavioral intervention.

As I continued working in family therapy at MRI, which Jackson founded, I was pleased to see that family therapy was developing and spreading. I was not pleased, however, when I began to see articles appear with statements like, "After only a year of family therapy, the nature of the family's problem was becoming clear." After all, work with families had originally been seen (like psychoanalysis) as an effective, and therefore brief, approach to resolving problems, so when Richard Fisch proposed that a small group of us at MRI get together and experiment with keeping treatment brief by focusing on the main presenting problem and very active intervention, I was glad to join with him, and I have not regretted it over 20 some years.

In summation, my story is, "One thing leads to another."

FISCH: I would say it began, if there can be such a thing as a beginning, when I was an undergraduate, majoring in premed. I had the good fortune of taking a couple of classes in sociology from a creative and exciting instructor and I found it appealing to think of people's behavior in terms of social organization and culture. In choosing my psychiatric residency, I think this played a factor in selecting a Sullivanian institute rather than a strict Freudian one. However, much of the training was still Freudian and I recall feeling impatient at the mystification of the therapy process.

When I started working, mostly analytically, it became increasingly uncomfortable to spend much of my day sitting behind a couch while my patients talked into the air and I finally asked my patients if they would be more comfortable sitting up. That "simple" procedural change, of course, changes one's therapy; one is inclined to be more active. This, I think, contributed to a next step, a curiosity about husbands who set up appointments for their wives and then accompany them to the appointment even though most of these wives were capable of driving.

My curiosity led me to ask the spouses if it would be all right if I saw them together. I was struck by the fact that in most cases, the husband seemed more discomfited by the wife's problem than his wife was. Without realizing it, this started putting me on the path of looking at things from an interactional rather than from an intrapsychic explanation. From this, I found myself taking another step by taking some training in family therapy at MRI. This was in 1960, and at that time, family therapy was a very new and exciting approach. At the same time, it gave me an opportunity to get to know some of the people at MRI. Among them was Jay Haley.

At that time, Haley had just written *Strategies of Psychotherapy* (Haley, 1963), and while I was intrigued by his ideas, I still regarded them as too superficial compared with the "real" and "deep" psychodynamic therapy I was still accustomed to using. However, one day I was presented with a patient who spoke almost no English and, in desperation, I mechanically applied the techniques Haley had used in an analogous case. The fact that it worked and quickly (a couple of weeks) put me another step away from my psychoanalytic background and on the path to a problem-solving approach. My therapy became a melange of psychodynamic and family therapy, but when I got stuck, I resorted to a problem-oriented—"prescribing the symptom"—approach, and enough of the time it got the therapy unstuck and the problem resolved. Without planning it, I began to use it more and more, even if I weren't stuck. Then I learned that Haley had gotten some of his inspiration from Milton Erickson and so, in the early 1960s, I took a couple of workshops with Erickson.

This interest in his work, plus the intrigue I found in the rapid changes that can occur in a case when approached in a problem-solving way, led to the next and probably most important step, the formation of the Brief Therapy Center in 1967, a project allowing me, John Weakland, Paul Watzlawick, and, later, many others to research more and more refined ways of shortening treatment and putting what we were doing into some comprehensive order. That was some 24 years ago, and I hope that I, we, continue to evolve into whatever paths it can take us.

REFERENCES

de Shazer, S. (1985). *Keys to solution in brief therapy*. New York: W. W. Norton.

de Shazer, S. (1988). *Clues: Investigating solutions in brief therapy*. New York: W. W. Norton.

Fisch, R., Weakland, J. H., & Segal, L. (1982). *The tactics of change: Doing therapy briefly*. San Francisco: Jossey-Bass.

Haley, J. (1963). *Strategies of psychotherapy*. New York: Grune & Stratton.

Watzlawick, P., Weakland, J. H., & Fisch, R. (1974). *Change: Principles of problem formation and problem resolution*. New York: W. W. Norton.

Weakland, J. H., Fisch, R., Watzlawick, P., & Bodin, A. H. (1974). Brief therapy: Focused problem resolution. *Family Process*, *13*, 141–168.

The Black Sheep of the Family: A Structural Approach to Brief Therapy

HARRY J. APONTE

Structural family therapy (SFT) is not, per se, either a long-term or a brief approach to therapy. However, it does lend itself to short-term work because the model works (1) in the "here and now," (2) through direct, positive action, and (3) for palpable outcomes. The therapeutic process is inherently organized around achieving specific goals (Aponte, 1974) whether short or long term. For brief therapy, the structural model treats the issue of today as the end goal of therapy. For longer-term therapy, today's goal becomes the stepping-stone to the goal of tomorrow as outcome builds on outcome. However, in either case structural family therapy is more than a technical pursuit of the solution of a problem.

THE PRINCIPLES OF STRUCTURAL THERAPY

At the heart of it, SFT balances a focus on results with an emphasis on process. It employs techniques for the resolution of specific problems while calling on the therapist to relate actively to the transactional process of the family (Minuchin & Fishman, 1981). The therapist works both with the process between family and therapist (Aponte, 1982) and with relationships among family members.

Fundamentally, proponents of SFT think of a problem for therapy as standing on the legs of relationships in a social system. The structural patterns of those relationships are the undergirding of the problem. Change the transactional patterns and you alter the outcome—fix the relationship and you solve the problem (Minuchin, 1974). In addition, within the ecology of relationships (Aponte, 1976) are individuals with their own personal emotional makeups, whose behaviors shape relationships. The interactive processes in these relationships then influence the emotions and behavior of the individual in a continuous circular dynamic. Relationships depend on individuals. Individuals depend on relationships. Change either and you affect the other.

Each family system has its characteristic patterns of relationships. However, these patterns are highly complex and never reveal their many intricacies in the transactions around any single issue. Particular issues will draw out people and their interactions in particular ways. The fullest and truest access to an individual's psychology and a family's relational structure is through seeing people in action around a specific issue (i.e., in the enactment of their transactions). All the components of the issue are present in the enactment—the people, their psychology, their relationships, and the social contexts (Aponte, 1990). Seeing people functioning in the actual experience of an issue gives the truest diagnostic picture of the people and their problem. Intervening with them in action has the greatest potential of disrupting and revamping old, unproductive patterns. The intensity of the drama of the here-and-now experience accesses the emotional life of families in a way that facilitates understanding and promotes change at its deepest levels.

A therapist's role vis-à-vis the enactment of a problem is to observe and work with the family's transactions from two vantage points: outside the system or within the action. The therapist directs family members on their interactions from *outside* the encounter if he or she believes that they can respond to confrontations, suggestions, or instructions. However, when the therapist feels that the family needs more active help, he or she will join in the enactment, becoming a player in the interaction. The therapist, thereby, lends his or her person to the family's efforts from *within* the family's transactions to begin solving the problem in the experience of the moment (Aponte, 1981). In either case, the therapist is actively engaged.

BRIEF STRUCTURAL THERAPY

The immediacy of the enactment of a family's problems is the focal point for brief work in SFT. This enactment is a reliving before the therapist of the family problem. That moment's transactional experience joins content with process as people relate to each other around the issue as they do outside therapy. The forces that make for the problem at home come into play in therapy at the moment of the enactment. The therapist can see, feel, and touch the family's experience. This makes it possible for the therapist to create a new experience now, altering some of the basic forces in the system that shape the old transactional pattern. When this relevant, immediate, and intense experience is felt as a solution by a family, the family reorganizes around the new reality.

In order to work with a family in the enactment, a structural therapist does the following:

1. Looks for the enactment to spontaneously develop, or for the opportunity to instigate its actuation in his or her presence;
2. Then, intervenes in the pattern of the transaction as it unfolds through clarification, suggestions, or directions from outside family members' interactions; or
3. Intervenes by participating as an actor in the drama of their enactment in ways that will alter the course of the experience in the session.

A family begins to experience palpable change around their issue—now.

There is an existential quality (Yalom, 1980) to this perspective that examines the life of people through the spotlight of their current experience. The assumption is that the dynamics relevant to the current problem live in the enactment. While past history is acknowledged as shedding light on dynamics that drive a family's life today, the therapist looks for how those forces are shaping family members' actual experience of life now. A therapist targets the residuals of the past in a family's experience of the moment.

A family is emotionally vulnerable in an enactment, which contains all the danger and risk its members know at home when they confront their problems. Any intervention by a therapist that is to have a deep and lasting impact must reach all corners of the family's pathology and potential—and that is done through the living experience of the enactment.

The Method

For brief therapy, a therapist first engages with a family around the enactment, then tries to disrupt (unbalance) the family's accustomed approach to the issue, and, finally, looks for a *positive* way to create a new experience for them around the issue. Particularly for short-term work, family members must get in touch with their ability to solve their problems as they enter the pit of their distress. The therapist uses the distress to help them confront the futility of old patterns and old solutions, then uses the experience of their potential to give them hope and mobilize their resources for new solutions.

Work with the enactment mimics the session, which in turn mimics the entire course of therapy especially in brief therapy. Just as the therapist sets goals for intervening in the enactment that fit the session, he or she has goals for the session that fit with the overall goals of the therapy. Achieving the goal of the enactment builds toward the goal of the session, which culminates in the goal of the therapy. With the powerful mounting effect of these pyramiding goals, change builds on change, resulting in an early outcome.

The momentum of change builds from enactment to enactment and session to session for the whole of therapy. In the course of this process, the therapist aims to do the following:

1. Join with the family members—gaining their trust—so that they will allow the therapist to be actively engaged with the family at both an emotional and a behavioral level, sharing in the experience of their struggle—now.
2. Define the therapeutic goal with the family in terms that can be glimpsed in the current session and achieved in the length of time treatment is to last.
3. Formulate the intervention of the moment in experiential terms—behavior and affect—that relate directly to a family's experience in the session.
4. Block their dysfunctional transaction in the enactment in a way that also incorporates a positive outlook to the family problem.
5. Leave the family with momentum toward change based on having had an emotionally positive and practically successful experience.

Brief therapy depends on generating and maintaining positive momentum throughout the therapeutic process toward palpable goals.

CASE ILLUSTRATION

All the elements of a structural approach to brief therapy are illustrated in the following edited session of a consultation with a family that was about to reenter therapy after a pause in therapy. The family had been in treatment for some time with a series of therapists. The family was reapplying for treatment by order of the courts as a condition of probation for Pam, the 17-year-old, who had been charged with burglary. The family's future therapist requested the consultation. The therapist observed but did not participate in the consultation.

Initially, the consultant sat in the empty seat left free in the middle of the family seating. From right to left family members were seated as follows: Pam, the self-proclaimed black sheep, who had been having school problems and was abusing drugs and alcohol; Betty, 42, the mother, who was depressed and angry over the family situation; and Bev, 15, who had a past history of enuresis and encopresis. Then the consultant. On his right sat Ben, 45, the peripheral parent who had himself abused alcohol and had been hospitalized on several occasions for depression. Finally, on the extreme left sat Penny, 14, the shy one, who had for a time in the past been pulling out her eyebrows. Mother, reportedly, was protective of Bev and Penny. Burt, 18, who was mother's special ally in disciplining the girls, refused to attend the session. Between the parents, mother felt father was a harsh disciplinarian, while he believed she undermined his authority in the home.

This presession information led the consultant to hypothesize that, for whatever reason, Pam was being singled out as the bad one in the family. She was later to confirm this hypothesis when she described herself as the black sheep of the family. The consultant tentatively set the goal of beginning to get Pam out of her "bad" role, in the consultation.

The First Session

After introductions, the consultant talked with the family about the absent son, Burt. He wondered aloud whether Burt was afraid to join the session lest his problems, too, become public. The consultant began immediately to suggest that others in the family, aside from Pam, also had problems. He then moved to engage the apparently peripheral parent, the father, around setting a family focus for the consultation and, ultimately, for the therapy that was to follow.

Consultant: What are you trying to change?

Father: Well, I'd like to see, you know, everybody more cooperative with each other.

C: Who?

F: The kids, mostly.

C: Which ones?

F: At this point—it changes, you know, from month to month, week to week. But, I'd say the last month or so between the three girls. There's a constant friction about, you know, going into each other's rooms, taking the other one's possessions, borrowing the other one's clothes. . . . That makes me very upset. . . . It seems like the sibling rivalry is so intense—that it's like they hate each other and this makes me feel real bad.

C: That's sad.

F: Yeah. It is sad. It bothers me.

C: I was just thinking—trying to put myself in your shoes—I think I would—I'd feel like I failed somehow if my kids just couldn't stand each other or couldn't have a little kindness and caring for one another . . .

F: I think you hit the nail on the head. I couldn't have said it better myself. . . . Maybe we're doing wrong. . . . I always feel guilty coming out of most of these sessions . . . like I've done something terrible. I really have a lot of guilt associated with this thing. . . . [then he added] There's been an awful lot of conflict between my wife and I—you know, how this is to be effective—how, how—

C: How to stop this bickering among the kids?

F: Yeah. Yeah. There's a great deal of difference. At times it's been a bone of contention—more than a bone of contention!

C: What is it that you're trying to do to solve the problem?

F: Gee, it's hard to verbalize.

The father suggested the goal of creating harmony among the girls. As the consultant talked at one level about goal setting, at another he was beginning to work on the structure of relationships within the family. Because the father appeared peripheral, the consultant wanted to join him. The consultant picked up on his feeling of failure and guilt. In the process he learned about the tension between Ben and Betty. He speculated to himself that the division between the parents was behind Pam's being scapegoated. The consultant then invited the parents to enact their disagreements in his presence, living out rather than describing their differences over handling conflicts between the children.

C: Well, where do you two stand on that, Betty and Ben? . . . Do you agree on every aspect of who should be doing what?

Mother: Yes, yes.

F: No way.

M: (*giggle*) All right.

. . .

C: What is the best one [example] to talk about? Is it the shoes or . . . dishes?

*The parents quickly got into disagreeing about what would best exemplify the kids'
bickering. But then, as the tension between the parents rose, Pam began rocking in her
chair. She finally burst in with the answer.*

Pam: It's neither.

M: It's neither?

. . .

P: It doesn't really have to do with the dishes or the shoes. It's nobody
can agree on anything. Nobody shares anything. Everybody constantly fights.

. . .

*Pam drew attention away from the parents and diffused their struggle. If Pam had been
trying to save her parents by getting herself into trouble, the consultant would attempt to
convert her negative solution into something positive.*

C: Okay Pam. I'm going to let you, in a way, run this interview right
now. I'll tell you how. People are fighting in your family a lot. Okay?
And they're fighting about a lot of different things. I'm looking for
something that's specific; something that's important to you.

P: All right.

. . .

Okay. This is what really gets me. This gets me. It's like—I feel
like—kind of like the black sheep of the family, right?

C: Umhm!

P: Like everybody's good. Everybody does their—goes to school,
right? Does everything good. Does their homework and—and it has
to do with a lot of little things that get the fights started, but—what
it is, is mostly, I'm in the wrong. Like somebody, like somebody,
either one of my parents, will stick up for my sisters when they
don't even know who started it, what's going on or anything. And
like, my mother will be the first one up—screaming and yelling at
me, and then my father will come up screaming and yelling at me
and I—like—like I'll try—I'll be trying to tell him, you know,
what's going on and nobody's listening to me and—it's like they get
off the hook and I'm stuck and I'm pissed and—

C: These two [her sisters] get off the hook?

P: Yeah.

. . .

And I blow up. Like I have a tendency to blow up. I try to hold back, but it hurts me so much to be called all different things and get accused for all different things that I just swear at them and I say, "I hate you! I don't want anything to do with you!" And I just slam my door. And then I feel like—I'm sitting there all by myself and it's five against one and it's so hard. I mean, in school, even in school one day I couldn't take it—really bad. I just cried right in the middle of class. And I never do that. Like I keep my emotions in a lot and just couldn't take it.

C: Now, when you say five against one, you're including your brother?

P: Yeah. He's one of the worst.

C: Okay. Go ahead.

P: And I don't know. I just want like a fair chance. I mean, like, I'm not the only one that's a little brat in the house.

C: Okay. I'm trying to find a way of—I want you to win right now. Okay?

P: That sounds good.

C: I don't know if I can help you to win because I suspect that you're doing a lot of things to screw up.

P: Yeah.

C: Okay. And that you're making it hard for people to get on your side.

P: Yeah.

. . .

C: At the same time, I have no doubt, Pam, that you're right and that there are plenty of times when your point of view is correct—

P: Yes.

C: And nobody listens to you.

P: Yeah.

C: Because they're so busy fighting you from all the other problems. So, I'm not going to give you—say that you're right all the time, but I do want you to win now. I want you to help me to help you win. Okay? If you could? Is there something specific about which you're fighting with your parents right now or your sisters—or all of them right now? Is there something specific that you can think of that perhaps I could be on your side about? . . .

The consultant was trying to set up the enactment and invited Pam to name the issue. He promised to help her experience a success if she would work with him.

P: So, you just want me to think of something right off the top of my head?

C: If you can.

P: I've got something.

C: Okay. Go ahead.

P: Okay. Like—I got a record collection. . . . Okay? And I don't have a record player. . . . The only record player that works in the house is in my sisters' room. All right?

. . .

And usually after school. Like, I'm usually the first one home and my brother's asleep and I go in there, and I put the earphones on and just listen to some tunes for a while. You know? And when I'm done, I'll take my records out and put them back into the covers— like I take really good care of them. I take care of all my things because they mean something. Every little thing I have in my room means something to me, personally. So I take care of it and then, like maybe I'll go out that night and I'll come back and I'll go in my room and it's dumped upside down. This is missing and that's gone and this is tipped over and my records will be in her room [Bev's room, which she shares with Penny] scattered all over the place. Like the record will be out of the cover and in with her records, underneath and everything—getting scratched and everything—and I get really mad, you know, and I'll say, "Stay out of my room. How many times have I told you?" . . . And she'll come up and start yelling, "You go in my room all the time. You go through my stuff. Why can't I go in your room and do that—do the same?"

Bev: You know, you dump ashes and your clothes and garbage in my room and you don't clean it up. And I saw a couple of ashes up in my room. You know, when you leave your cigarette with the ashes still on and don't bring an ashtray, my room smells like smoke. I mean there is a garbage bag for trash in there.

With just a few words, Bev attempted to maneuver Pam back into the role of the black sheep. At this point, the consultant encouraged Pam to solve the record problem directly with her sisters. As the family enactment began, the consultant removed himself from between the girls and had them sit together.

P: No. I go into your room just to listen to my records and I smoke cigarettes. Okay—I'll bring my ashtray and put them out. And I'll take my records and leave, and that's all I'll touch because that's all I touch anyway. All right? But if you're going to go in my room, ask me what you want.

B: That means you would have to ask me if you can use my stereo.

P: Ask me what you want. Don't just go into my room and take it and go through my things. I'll go in and get it for you. If I'm not there, wait—

B: Well, you don't wait for me to get home.

P: Well, that's because you go upstairs in your room and want to do your homework and you make a big screaming fit out of it.

B: I don't go up there all the time at first when I get home.

P: (*Turning to the consultant in desperation*) Too many difficulties. I don't know what else to say.

C: Well, fight a little harder. Or get some help. Get someone to side with you, then.

M: Can I put in my two cents in on this? Just one thing—(*to Pam*) a lack of consideration on your part that you weren't thinking about. Remember the day Bev had a day off from school? And she did not have to get up in the morning. You did go into her room and turn the stereo on without the earphones. She was trying to sleep and she had a day off. She had a right to sleep. You turned the stereo on blasting loud.

P: No, it wasn't. No, it wasn't.

M: I heard it all the way downstairs. You woke her up. If you had gone in there and plugged the earphones in so you can't hear anything, it would have been all right, but you made her upset and angry at you. And, it was an inconsiderate thing on your part . . .

The enactment was revealing family patterns. Betty reflexively backed Bev, not Pam, and Pam was back on the defensive. The consultant handled it by inviting mother out of the girls' negotiations. He then redirected Pam to talk with Penny about her problems. Penny was more amenable to sharing the stereo. With his support, Pam succeeded in reaching an agreement with her youngest sister. Suddenly without mother, Bev felt isolated as Pam and Penny got together. To get back in with them, Bev quickly made concessions, and all three girls reached a consensus. The consultant then moved to the next stage of the session.

C: (*to Pam*) You kind of won . . . [but] you know . . . when you leave here and you go back home, it's going to be pretty much the way it was.

P: It usually happens?

C: Yeah. And I'm just going to take a guess and say your parents have something to do with why it's not going to work.

P: I can kind of see it, but I don't know what it's about.

C: Somehow, I feel that if your parents work together, that they should be able to help the three of you work this kind of thing out. Look what just happened. You three just worked this thing out very nicely.

P: Yeah.

C: And, I can't help but believe that your parents should be able to help the three of you do that [at home] . . .

P: Yeah.

. . .

C: Okay. Why don't you check out with them, and find out whether they're going to back you on this one. You've got a partial victory. You can't win without that.

P: (*to Betty*) Mom?

M: I've heard all the rules and I think they're very clear and I think Penny and Bev and you have an excellent arrangement. Why haven't you been able to do this before? It's what I've been trying to get you to do.

C: (*to Pam*) You see what just happened? . . .

P: Yes.

C: She just made you wrong.

M: I did?

F: She what?

. . .

C: (*to Pam*) You know what your mother said to you? She didn't say, "Pam, you did a good job."

P: She said "Why didn't you—try to do it before."

C: "Why didn't you do it before? What was wrong with you [that you did not do this] before?" . . . So you end up losing.

. . .

M: Oh! The clouds have just opened. I haven't looked at it that way.

. . .

During the subsequent discussion among Betty, Pam, and the consultant, Ben had trouble breaking in. He would finally no longer brook further delay.

F: Can I say one thing? I've waited long enough.

P: (*laughter*) Go ahead.

M: Wow!

F: (*to Pam*) There's a secret ingredient in this agreement that I can see is a pitfall already. . . . You [Bev] spend an awful lot of time in your room doing homework and listening to records. And, Pam gets the balance of the time [to play her records] and I see nothing, but frustration . . . you [Pam] might be boxed out of that room by the agreement itself.

. . .

P: Hold it. First of all, I'm the first one home. Okay? I go upstairs and listen to the records and at 3:00 [when Bev arrives from school] I watch my soap opera. So —

C: Pam, you're right. Again.

P: I love it!

(*General laughter*)

C: . . . you know what your father did? Takes off on another situation . . . a legitimate issue, but it has nothing to do with what you worked out. That would have to be another conversation. . . . Now what you want to know, I assume, is—is your father going to back you on what you worked out or not?

P: Yeah! Yeah! Dad?

F: All right. The wording was, if they're not in their room. Right? Okay. I missed that.

. . .

C: (*to Pam*) I don't know if we accomplished anything at all except to make you feel that you won for 1 hour of your life. All right?

P: Thank you.

C: Your welcome.

P: It made me feel good.

C: I'm glad it makes you feel good. It makes me feel good too because I know how unhappy you were at the beginning when you were talking about how you were feeling everybody was against you.

P: I almost cried.

C: I know you almost cried and I think that if you are feeling that people are against you, you're going to be angry all the time and . . . you're going to do things to hurt other people. And one way . . . is by hurting yourself . . . I hope you can treat you differently so that will change. . . .

P: I am trying.

C: . . . Now, I'm saying this to you . . . it's not going to work like I said. . . . You're going back out tonight or tomorrow and you're going to mess yourself up. Okay? And they're [your parents] going to mess this whole thing up. What you're going to need is . . . a therapist I think to sit down and talk to you and to say to you, "Grow up, Pam."

. . .

At the same time, I hope somebody will sit down with all of you and help them [your parents] to learn how to back you up when it's right . . . and how to come down hard on you when you're doing things that deserve for you to get into trouble . . . I don't think you're going to do this completely by yourself.

P: No way. That's what I've been saying for a while. I can't do it myself.

C: Good.

M: I can see something that you pointed out about my not saying it was great the way she had Bev and Penny solve the problem. . . . It was a matter of language.

. . .

C: Betty, I know your feelings are there [for Pam], but the two of you [parents], you're so accustomed to fighting with Pam . . . you get a habit of thinking negatively.

F: I want to say one thing and I want to say it very sincerely. This is the first time that I've been with a therapist . . . where I have been found to be wrong and [have been] pointed out and not come away hostile or feeling bad about myself, and I thank you.

C: You're welcome.

Ben: . . . You made me feel good . . .

Betty: It opens your mind.

With that, the consultant ended the session, and said his good-byes to the family.

DISCUSSION

In this interview, the family had a new experience, an experience of change. Pam, the black sheep of the family, was recast as a competant family member. Father's goal of harmony among the girls was experienced in the session. The accustomed loyalties in the sibling subsystem shifted and Pam was included with Bev and Penny. All three girls were able to share in Pam's success because they reached agreement without their parents' help.

The parents were able to appreciate Pam's effectiveness in this experience and found they could support her without being disloyal to the other children. Although the parents were faced with their negative attitude about Pam, they too, as a couple, were made to share in Pam's success. They had a role in supporting Pam and the agreement, and as such could see themselves as good parents. They will need help with their relationship, but for the moment Pam was out of the loop of their marital struggles.

Finally, the paradoxical suggestion that the therapeutic gains made during the session would not last was intended to protect the family against the shock of the real world outside where they would soon face their old foibles. It was intended to protect the experience, as a precious seed that would need nurturing, not to be thrown out with the storm of the next family fight. In summary, the family had the experience of success where they had always experienced failure. They now left with reason to hope they could work together toward a successful solution to an old problem.

FOLLOW-UP

This interview took place as part of a workshop over 10 years ago. It was a one-time intervention. The family followed up by entering therapy. However, rather remarkably, as the author was considering using the interview for this chapter, the family contacted the therapist to whom they had been referred at the time of the workshop and asked about seeing the videotape of the original consultation. They explained that the experience had made such a difference in their lives that they would like to see it again as a family.

This author called Betty [mother], and she reported that she and Ben are doing well together. They are "joined at the hip" and are playing golf together and preparing for retirement in Florida where they have bought a home. Pam, a part-time hairdresser, has been married for 5 years and has an 18-month-old child. She made a turnabout in the year after the consultation. Bev is divorced with a child, and living at home with her parents while she completes college. She is in her last year. Peggy, the shy one, is now an outgoing young woman soon to be married. Burt, who had not participated in the consult and had been mother's enforcer with the younger children, became a policeman!

EDITORS' QUESTIONS

Q: Since your goal is to create an immediate shift in the family dynamics, it is important that you achieve maximal leverage for creating change. What strategies do you use to join with family members in order to be trusted, respected, and given permission to intervene in the way you do?

A: In this model, families must feel understood, cared about and safe—*now*. This calls for connecting with them from the very first moment of contact. The therapist must be personally open to making the therapeutic encounter a real experience for them, built around where they are at that moment with their life struggle. Then, the therapist assumes leadership and direction of the session in a way that not only feels relevant to their concerns but also conveys the therapist's emotional and technical ability to handle productively their personal turmoil. This all translates into the therapist's being personally present and active from the start, shaping the context and the relationship for therapy.

Q: Why do you allow Pam to divert you from your initial focus on the parents? It seems like Pam's typical role is to draw attention to herself and detour conflicts away from the parental relationship. How did you decide to move to empower Pam and retreat from your original focus? What do you mean when you say, "If Pam had been trying to save her parents by getting into trouble, the consultant would attempt to convert her negative solution into something positive"?

A: This is an important and difficult question to answer. I could have completely blocked Pam's intrusion, but that would have meant braking the momentum she sparked at that juncture. The parents were not supplying it. I wanted the family enveloped as quickly as possible in an enactment that would generate intensity from the heat of their struggle. What better way than to have Pam thrust before everyone what most bothered her and to have her sisters join in? However, since this was not just a diagnostic exercise, I wanted to cast Pam in a good light rather than a bad light. Pam was accustomed to detouring parental conflict by being a troublemaker. I would have her remove herself and her sisters from her parents' troubles by solving their own problems under Pam's leadership. I would convert the momentum of Pam's usual negative intrusion to a positive transaction.

Q: You met with the family even though one member was absent. What if only the parents and Pam had come to this appointment? Would you have seen them anyway and what is your basic stance about who needs to be present for treatment?

A: I prefer to have everyone at the first session but will try working with whomever comes. Had I only Pam and her parents, I would have focused much more on the parents and their relationship, in order to take the heat off Pam. In the actual session, we had the other girls to share the spotlight. However, if the members of a family who are present cannot solve a problem without the missing parties, I will either hold out for the rest of the family or adjust our goals to what those present can achieve by themselves.

Q: How did you know that you could join with Pam in being "successful," while maintaining your alliance with the parents? I would imagine that some parents in that situation would get upset by such a therapeutic maneuver. The mother says, "Oh! The clouds have just opened. I haven't looked at it that way." A terrific acceptance of a new frame of reference. What if she had said, "You keep trying to defend her [Pam]. She is just a terrible kid and is making my life miserable. You can say this stuff because you don't live with her."

A: There was no way to "know" the parents would accept Pam's being "successful," but there was reason to believe they would if the other kids and the parents, themselves, could be part of that success. From the beginning, these parents came across as wanting to be "good" parents who had their kids' well-being at heart. Mother's problem was that she felt she had to choose between Pam and the child she instinctively recognized as the more vulnerable one, Bev. She chose to put the pressure on the "stronger" one, Pam, not because she wanted to hurt her but because she felt Pam could take it. Had the mother felt otherwise, we would have had a different interview. I might have put more energy into getting the parents to own and deal with their difficulty cooperating with each other, as well as have worked more on having the kids' experience and articulate satisfaction with what *they* had achieved with each other, leaving little room for the parents to criticize Pam.

Q: Had you continued to see this family beyond the initial consultation, how would you have planned future sessions? How often would you schedule appointments? Would you meet with the family on a weekly basis or intermittently (e.g., every 2–3 weeks)? How would you know that it was time to terminate treatment?

A: The shorter I wanted the treatment to be, the longer would I make the sessions, such as 2-hour-long interviews, and the more frequent. Greater intensity creates more momentum for immediate change. Our goals would determine the intensity and length of treatment. If the goal had been only to put Pam in a more positive position within the family and keep her out of the loop of the parents' troubles, we could have achieved it pretty quickly with the start we had. However, to have dealt fully with the parents' issues, with the problems Bev and Peggy were manifesting, and with the poor self-image Pam had internalized, we would have needed a longer-term effort. Nonetheless, even with longer-term work, we would plan it in modules focused on specific goals. We would try to create a therapeutic context, relationship, and momentum for each of our goals, adjusting these factors to our goals as our objectives evolved during the course of treatment.

Q: Since you use the family's *enactment* of their usual patterns and process as a basis for both assessment and intervention, how would you handle a family whose members have a history of being verbally and, on occasion, physically abusive with one another?

A: First of all, the therapist must always have control of creating the context for therapy, that is, the parameters for interaction in the session. Second, an enactment does not have to literally contain all the behaviors seen at home. It does need to include the essential *dynamics* of the relationships that underlie the problem. The dynamics behind a family's physical fight can be fully present in a verbal argument, or even in their tense jockeying to control a session. It is up to the therapist to decide on the context in which to intervene in this family struggle.

Q: Do you ever use homework assignments or tasks in your therapy? And if so, what kinds of assignments do you find most useful in working with families?

A: I use homework assignments to maintain and build on the momentum of the work done in the clinical session. Some families carry home their own momentum and need little coaching about following up at home. However, most need some help to know what to do and not do to protect the gains of a session and to further the work they started. In this model, the most useful assignments grow out of what happened in the session. They feed off the momentum of the session and carry the family right into the next clinical contact. Properly done, these home assignments intensify the therapy and shorten it.

Q: Since the consultation you presented took place over 10 years ago, I wonder how you might have approached this family differently today. How has your approach evolved over the years?

A: I do not doubt that I would be different with the family today because I am ten years older, but how, I cannot say. However, from a technical standpoint, I do not know that I would approach the family much differently in a brief therapeutic encounter. Nevertheless, I do believe that my longer-term work has changed because I am including more family-of-origin work in my therapy, and am also more consciously and consistently working through my relationships with families in therapy. Not that I was unaware of the use of myself with Pam's family. Although I encouraged Pam to negotiate with her sisters on her own, I knew that I had assumed a very central position within the family in the way I supported Pam's leadership in the session, and related to the whole family as good folk, whatever their foibles (Aponte, in press). I am well aware that these parents must have had a history that I would have had to tap to inform my therapy with them over the long haul. There was also enough emotional vulnerability throughout this family that I would have had to use myself to provide much personal support and safety through the therapeutic relationship.

Q: How did you become a brief therapist?

A: My original training in psychotherapy was psychoanalytic. I spent 8 years at the Menninger Clinic in Topeka, Kansas. However, I was wanting to get back to my roots on the East Coast to work with poor minority families. The Philadelphia Child Guidance Clinic gave me that opportunity. It was the late 1960s. Much of the field was still being shaped by the "war on poverty" and the newly born community mental health movement. Minuchin and his colleagues had just come out with *Families of the Slums*.

Structural family therapy was taking its character from the work with the poor. This therapy necessarily had to be outcome oriented, reality based, and action (vs. talk) directed. It resulted in a relatively brief mode of therapy. Its practitioners learned to be focused and active and to work intensively for palpable results. With time, we discovered that it got results not only with the poor but with families from all socioeconomic levels.

The structural model has become part of the core of my clinical perspective, although it has needed broadening to address more completely the range of problems we encounter in therapy. It has needed to be more deeply rooted in an ecological perspective to account systematically for the societal context of families. It has needed family-of-origin work to understand the family roots of current family functioning. And, it has needed a more deliberate and systematic approach to the use of the self in therapy to humanize SFT's therapeutic process and to maximize the use of the person of the therapist in SFT's here-and-now interventions in family enactments.

REFERENCES

Aponte, H. J. (1974). Organizing treatment around the family's problems and their structural bases. *The Psychiatric Quarterly, 48*, 209–222.

Aponte, H. J. (1976). The family-school interview: An eco-structural approach. *Family Process, 15*, 303–311.

Aponte, H. J. (1981). Structural family therapy. In A. S. Gurman & D. P. Kniskern (Eds.), *Handbook of family therapy* (pp. 310–360). New York: Brunner/Mazel.

Aponte, H. J. (1982). The person of therapist: The cornerstone of therapy. *The Family Therapy NetWorker, 6*, 19–21, 46.

Aponte, H. J. (1990). "Too many bosses": An eco-structural intervention with a family and its community. *Journal of Strategic and Systemic Therapies, 9*, 49–63.

Aponte, H. J. (in press). Training the person of therapist in structural family therapy. *Journal of Marital and Family Therapy.*

Minuchin, S. (1974). *Families & family therapy.* Cambridge, MA: Harvard University Press.

Minuchin, S., & Fishman, H. C. (1981). *Family therapy techniques.* Cambridge, MA: Harvard University Press.

Yalom, E. D. (1980). *Existential psychotherapy.* New York: Basic Books.

CONCLUSION

Last Words
on First Sessions

SIMON H. BUDMAN
STEVEN FRIEDMAN
MICHAEL F. HOYT

As we have seen, the initial session of brief treatment is a critical one. Although the clinicians who have delineated their models and shared their work in this volume have certain similarities in their approaches, there are also major differences. Some of the therapists describe their approach as making extensive use of homework assignments (Friedman, Chapter 13), while others never do so (Butler, Strupp, & Binder, Chapter 5). Some take the client's request at face value (Weakland & Fisch, Chapter 14) while others often look "beyond" the immediate request (Budman & Gurman, Chapter 6). Whereas some of the models described espouse time limits of one kind or another (Butler, Strupp, & Binder, Chapter 5; Hoyt, Rosenbaum, & Talmon, Chapter 4; Weakland & Fisch, Chapter 14) others operate with no specific guidelines regarding time other than that the time be used as efficiently and effectively as possible (Budman & Gurman, Chapter 6; Friedman, Chapter 13; Gurman, Chapter 9). With so many differences, an uninformed onlooker observing these models of brief treatment in practice might be hard pressed to know what makes them comparable.

Although it may not be readily apparent, all the brief treatment models presented in this volume, as well as other models not described here, share a number of common ingredients.[1] Various authors (Budman & Gurman, 1988; Friedman & Fanger, 1991; Hoyt & Austad, 1992; Wells & Phelps, 1990) have attempted to synthesize the "universal elements" shared by the majority of brief therapies. The most frequently cited generic components of brief treatment are:

1. *Rapid and generally positive working alliance between therapist and patient.* Therapy may proceed most directly and effectively when the patient and therapist form a "customer" relationship (de Shazer, 1985; Berg & Miller, 1992); that is, the patient recognizes the centrality of his or her role in solving the problem that led him or her to therapy. Other patients may recognize that there is a problem but believe that the solution lies with someone else's changing or may see no problem and seek no solution (de Shazer refers to these respective types as "complainants" and "visitors"). These patients need to be recognized as such and worked with differently or first converted to "customers."[2]

2. *Focality, the clear specification of achievable treatment goals.* Whatever model(s) and intervention approach(es) the therapist takes, first-session interviewing involves a constructivistic search (recognized or not) for applicable data. The patient's "presentation" may lead to a focus, and the therapist's "focus" (or lens) may lead to perceiving certain data. A workable focus is negotiated.[3]

3. *Clear definition of patient and therapist responsibilities*, with the therapist being prudently active and authoritative while assisting the patient in a constructive direction (sometimes including "homework" and behavioral tasks outside the session) (see Levy & Shelton, 1990).[4]

4. *Expectation of change, the belief that improvement is within the patient's (immediate) grasp.* Hope and optimism are fostered, which help engenders the motivation to make changes. This heartening influence occurs through various means: the therapist's professional manner, his or her providing understanding and a rationale for improvement, the recommendation of a relatively brief length of treatment suggesting the (often self-fulfilling) belief that work can be accomplished in a timely manner, discussion of various positive outcomes in a relatively problem-free future, and the rapid introduction of novelty (discussed below) and recognition of already occurring change.

5. *Here-and-now orientation*, the primary focus being on current life situations and patterns in thinking, feeling, and behaving—and their alternatives—rather than extensive reviewing of the "past" or "origins" of problems.

6. *Time sensitivity*, an awareness that life is limited and a concomitant awareness that all problems cannot be solved at once, that other things may have to occur first, and that "life is the great teacher" (Rosenbaum, Hoyt, & Talmon, 1990), and that pieces of therapy may be done on an intermittent or serial basis (Cummings, 1991; Budman, 1990).

Most brief therapists, regardless of orientation, also strive to accomplish certain tasks in the first meeting:

1. Establish rapport.
2. Define purpose of meeting, orient and instruct patient on how to use therapy.
3. Establish an opportunity for the patient to express thoughts, feelings, and behaviors.
4. Assess the patient's problems, strengths, motivations, expectations, and goals.
5. Evaluate possible psychiatric complaints when indicated, including biological factors, suicide/homicide risk, and alcohol/drug abuse when appropriate.
6. Mutually formulate a treatment focus.
7. Make initial treatment interventions and assess their effects.
8. Suggest "homework" or other tasks.
9. Define treatment parameters (such as who will attend sessions and estimating length of therapy or at least implying time sensitivity by suggesting "only as long as needed").
10. Make future appointments as needed.
11. Handle fees and payments.

THE RAPID INTRODUCTION OF NOVELTY

We believe that besides those elements already described, a striking universal component of all the brief therapies explicated in this volume is that *there is an emphasis on the rapid introduction of a novel set of thoughts, interpretations, and/or tasks.* This introduction of novelty occurs quite early in the therapy—often in the very first visit. In one way or another, every model of psychotherapeutic treatment—long or short, continuous or intermittent—strives to help the patient *do, think,* and/or *feel* differently than before the therapy began. The active ingredients of the therapy are all aimed at helping change occur in one or more of these areas. In treatment that is short term or time effective, such change must be initiated quite rapidly. Writing from varied viewpoints, the authors of the preceding chapters have indicated what they do early on to rapidly introduce such a change process.

If the therapist has an extended period within which to operate, he or she can allow much time to expire in the treatment *before* introducing a novel perspective. Rather than adding anything new over the course of early conversations with the patient, the therapist might commence an extended period of assessment, data gathering, and relationship building during which he or she essentially remains relatively noncommittal concerning formulations, interpretations, treatment plan, goals, and/or structure. The brief, time-effective therapist, on the other hand, regardless of his or her theoretical persuasion, quickly attempts to introduce to the patient a novel way of viewing the problem(s) and/or acting in the face of the presenting difficulties or concerns. The patient quickly begins to experience a healthier way of "viewing and doing" (O'Hanlon & Weiner-Davis, 1988).[5]

"Newness" introduced by the brief therapist must be different enough from the ways in which the patient has been trying to address the problem. The brief therapist's interventions, however, cannot be so totally at variance with the patient's ideas about the world or him or herself that they are rejected as shocking, impossible, or undesirable. [An exception to this statement would occur when the therapist is engaging in the use of paradoxical interventions (Fay, 1978). Under these circumstances the novelty comes from the new perspectives, actions, and/or feelings that are elicited through the patient's *rejection* of an intervention.]

THE IMPORTANCE OF NOVELTY

The client is often "stuck" and caught up in a cyclical pattern of "repeating sameness." Remembering the adage, "If we don't change direction we'll wind up where we are heading" (Hoyt, 1990), it is the therapist's job to disrupt these repeating cycles by introducing a novel perspective or by setting the stage for the client to be receptive to information in his or her natural environment that will open up options for change. As we have seen, a major element in the work of effective brief therapists is the introduction of new ideas into the early encounters with the client. This not only activates and arouses the client's interest but disorients the client in a positive way and creates perturbations in the client's prior assumptions and established sets. Whatever the length of treatment, the often touted "corrective emotional experience" (Alexander & French, 1946/1976; Marmor, 1986) results when the patient's habitual and self-limiting *modus operandi* are disconfirmed and disengaged by the advent of new information.

Bateson (1972) defines "information" as "a difference which makes a difference" (p. 453) and research reported by Lanzetta (1970) finds that "active information acquisition and processing is more probable under conditions of heightened uncertainty" (p. 144). What are the implications of these ideas for doing effective brief treatment? First, they suggest that for therapy to be effective, the clinician must present ideas in such a way that the client is activated to notice something new or different, second, by "heightening uncertainty" (i.e., introducing ideas in a novel manner), the client is more likely to integrate this information into his or her already established schemata or sets.

Early experiments in the psychology of learning (see Woodworth & Schlossberg, 1954) demonstrated how rigid sets or patterns in problem solving impeded the development of new problem-solving strategies. The more the subject becomes immersed in a fixed set, the less able he or she is to think creatively and maintain a perspective on alternative routes to a successful outcome. Such "tunnel vision" is common among clients who present for treatment. It then becomes the task of therapy to creatively evoke and facilitate the generation of alternative options for understanding and action.

Milton Erickson (e.g., see Haley, 1973; Rosen, 1982) was a master at both activating the client and creating a context in which new ideas would be received, processed and acted upon. In one case (see Rosen, 1982, pp. 152–154), Erickson treated an 8-year-old girl who "hates herself" because of the freckles that cover her face. Notice how, in the excerpt to follow, Erickson effectively activates the client's attention and then presents a novel frame in which a perceived deficit is turned into an asset and becomes the point of departure for a successful therapeutic outcome.

Erickson tells the story this way:

> I sat at my desk . . . the girl came in and stood in the doorway, her fists clenched, her jaw jutting out, glowering at me and ready for a fight. As she stood there, I looked at her and said, "You're a thief! You steal!" She said that she was not a thief and did not steal . . . "Oh, yes you're a thief. You steal things. I even know what you stole. I even have proof that you stole." The girl was thoroughly angry with me. I said, "I'll tell you where you were and what you stole. You were standing at the kitchen table. You were reaching up to the cookie jar, containing cinnamon cookies, cinnamon buns, cinnamon rolls—and you spilled some cinnamon on your face. You're a Cinnamon Face." (Rosen, 1982, p. 153)

Erickson knew from the mother that one of the child's favorite things to eat was cinnamon rolls. This was the beginning of a change process in which the child began to take pride in her new name, "Cinnamon Face."

From birth, we are "programmed" to search for differences in the environment (e.g., Friedman, 1975; Haith, 1980). Neurophysiological studies (e.g., Hubel & Weisel, 1962) have demonstrated that organisms are "wired" to detect change and difference. A significant body of research (e.g., Berlyne, 1960; Hunt, 1965) has also repeatedly confirmed the idea that we are more receptive to input when the information offered is slightly different from our expectations. However, when information is too different, too discrepant, or too incongruous, humans (as well as other animals) react in an avoidant manner (e.g., Carpenter, Tecce, Stechler, & Friedman, 1970; Fiske & Maddi, 1961; Hebb, 1946). By offering ideas that are slightly incongruent with the level of expectation of the client, the possibility is increased that the input offered will be assimilated and integrated into existing cognitions.

Along these lines, Andersen (1987), who has developed the idea of the reflecting team in clinical intervention, recommends that therapy teams present ideas in ways that offer the family something new or different in terms of meanings and understandings, yet not so different to be rejected out of hand. Andersen has found that presenting input to the family that is very discrepant from their established views has a "disorganizing effect on the system" that is not therapeutic. In their chapter on single-session therapy, Hoyt and his colleagues (Chapter 4, this volume) similarly recommend encouraging only a small step, one that can set positive changes into motion but which is close enough to the families so as not to be so challenging to the existing system or to set off untoward "resistance."

According to Friedman and Fanger (1991): "Part of the therapist's job is to enlarge client's perceptions of options and to create a context in which the client can experience increased variety. . . . [The therapist's goal is to] . . . help clients get past the rigid mind-sets they have developed" (p. 17).

By providing either a context for the generation of new ideas in the therapy encounter itself or assigning homework tasks outside the therapy room that provide feedback, the clinician can create a context in which change becomes more probable. "Learning is more efficient if a certain degree of change [from] the familiar . . . is periodically introduced" (Welker, 1961, p. 203). By engaging the client in a dialogue in which novel ideas are presented, the probability is increased that the client will begin to perceive new options and develop alternative understandings that will then lead to new pathways for action. The use of "reframing" (Bandler & Grinder, 1982), "pivot chords" (Rosenbaum, 1990), and "positive connotation" (Selvini-Palazolli, Boscolo, Cecchin, & Prata, 1978) can all function to provide freshness and expansion beyond the familiar.

THE IMPACT OF NOVELTY IN BRIEF THERAPY

The brief and time-effective therapists who have written chapters for this book appear to us to be highly skilled in rapidly introducing novel possibilities to the patient that allow him or her to modify or interrupt repetitive solutions that have not worked in the past. All the therapists introduce a new element, novelty, or change in the direction of therapeutic movement. Some do this with an explanation or interpretation, some giving instructions or directions, some by offering a new kind of relating. In all cases, something new happens; more of the same does not produce change.

In treating a woman with a phobia of bees, for example, Andreas (Chapter 2, this volume) waits only a few moments before requesting that she literally see her problem from a different, fresh perspective— the projection booth of a movie theater, watching herself on a screen. The therapist in Chapter 4 (Hoyt et al., this volume) suggests to the patient that he [the patient] engage in a dialogue with his father right there and then and that the therapist will play the patient's role while the patient plays his father. The therapist in Chapter 6 (Budman and Gurman, this volume) offers the patient the opportunity to immediately do something different and begin to change by not drinking. Further, he helps her recognize her own developmental imperative to change associated with the impending arrival of her 30th birthday. Friedman, Chapter 13 (this volume), indicates to the family the new idea that they are *already* changing and that they can change even more by catching their son doing something good. In Chapter 5 (Butler, et al., this volume) a patient who expects rejection instead encounters a therapist who demonstrates an abiding interest

In Table 16.1, we list some of the ways in which the various chapter authors introduce a novel idea or task in the beginning session of the treatment process.

VERY LAST WORDS ON FIRST SESSIONS

The brief therapist who is attempting to help his or her patients use treatment in the most productive, time-effective manner possible is advised to pay special heed to the opening phases of therapy. Although there are widely varied possibilities for the proficient practice of such treatment, the successful clinician "hits the ground running." It is unlikely that treatment that fails to quickly set a tone of active, dynamic intervention and change will lead to celeritous, positive outcomes.

At the most basic level, doing effective brief psychotherapy requires that the therapist adopt a specific attitude, posture, and set of expectations about change. As Friedman and Fanger (1991) point out, "The therapist thinks about the psychotherapy process, not as . . . reconstructive surgery, but as an attempt to catalyze the client or client

TABLE 16.1 Novelty in the Initial Session of Brief and Time-Effective Therapy

Author(s) and approach	Initial problem	Novel element introduced	How achieved
Andreas & Andreas (NLP)	1. Phobia 2. Posttraumatic stress	1. Phobic person is taught to view self with bees from a new perspective 2. Change focus from injured victim to capable and effective intervenor	1. Imagery exercise, seeing self on screen 2. Imagery exercise
Ellis (RET)	Panic attacks	Patient is helped to see that he need not always be perfect; "musturbating" is unnecessary	Rational discussion with the patient appealing to his intelligence and ability to cognitively modify irrational aspects of his behavior
Hoyt, Rosenbaum, & Talmon (SST)	Stressed by pressures from boss	Imagines self as powerfully standing up to his father (and boss)	Role-playing exercise with therapist
Butler, Strupp, & Binder (TLDP)	Depression (devalued image of self and others)	Patient feels valued and cared for	Therapist listens carefully, doesn't require patient to accommodate to him; gives extra sessions
Budman & Gurman (IDE)	Panic attacks	Therapist assists patient in recognizing that *she* wishes to change and is developmentally ready to do so; he also aids her in realizing that she can make an immediate change by stopping drinking and substance abuse	Therapist passes the patient's "test"; he does so by being accepting, but clear and firm with her
Turner (CBT)	Overdose and depression, relationship problems	Patient's feelings and capabilities are validated; hope for positive future renewed	Therapist treats the patient respectfully, offers support and instructions to help the patient find her own direction

TABLE 16.1 (continued)

Author(s) and approach	Initial problem	Novel element introduced	How achieved
Yapko (Ericksonian)	Difficulty deciding whether to stay married or not	Patient renews her confidence in her reasoning and decision making	Therapist reframes indecision and "dissociation," guides/ clarifies thinking and indicates resources
Gurman (IMT)	"Communication turmoil in our relationship"	Reframes problem from one of communication to one of intimacy	Persistently pursues and hones in on unresolved attachment issues; challenges couples distancing maneuvers
Johnson & Greenberg (EFT)	Wife angry, resentful at husband for making family move; wife feeling depressed, lonely, unsupported; husband sees problem as wife's irritability and lack of commitment to the relationship; "power struggle"	In first few minutes of session, therapist confronts couple with the discrepancy between their outward appearance and their stated problem; therapist then hones in on w's "loss of control" over her life	Therapist pushes each spouse to share painful and previously unresolved affects with the other while supporting their ability to do this
Baucom, Epstein, & Carels (CBT)	Couple rarely have sex	Therapist introduces idea that each member of the couple comes from "different backgrounds in terms of how negative feelings are handled"	Therapist expands focus of couple from sexual area to broader relationship issues that impact on the sexual problem
Davidson & Lax (Reflecting Team)	Wife's concerns about couple's sexual relationship; "no sex for a long time"	Therapists have a conversation in the presence of the couple; allow the couple to eavesdrop on their ideas	Therapists provide reflections about ongoing process in a nonjudgmental way that opens up options

(continued)

TABLE 16.1 (continued)

Author(s) and approach	Initial problem	Novel element introduced	How achieved
Friedman (Solution Oriented)	9-year-old boy, aggressive, poor impulse control, poor self-esteem; school performance below potential	Therapist quickly refocuses family on points of positive change in son's behavior and gets them to provide a picture of life without the problem; therapist also indirectly deals with father's drinking problem by framing interventions as for the son's benefit	Therapist asks the "miracle question" early in the interview refocusing families' attention on goals for change; also sends family letters that amplify family strengths and provide a revised picture of the family's ability to overcome obstacles
Weakland & Fisch (MRI Approach)	Young adult son is demanding and uncooperative; mother is looking for a way to help her change this behavior	Therapist rapidly recommends that mother respond to son's unreasonable demands by saying to him, "I haven't been as good a mother as I had hoped"	Direct recommendation that mother no longer approach the problem in the manner she had been previously; that is, indicating that it would probably not work to argue with son, cajole or persuade him to act better; mother encouraged to take a "one-down" position in gaining the upper hand.
Aponte (Structural)	17-year-old girl involved in burglary and seen for treatment as condition or probation	Therapist immediately presents his view to the family that he would also feel like a failure if "my kids just couldn't stand one another . . ."; empowers the IP to "win" in her efforts to deal with other family members	Therapist takes empathic position to parents' plight; actively encourages identified patient to get other family members "on her side"; pushes customary family interactions beyond their usual limits

system to use his (or their) resources to . . . reach a well-specified goal" (p. 39). By maintaining a set of expectations that favor optimism about change, by quickly establishing rapport and focus, by providing feedback that is slightly unfamiliar, unexpected, or novel, and by activating the client to take action, the stage is set for time-effective therapy.

NOTES

1. There are also more general features that brief treatments share with all effective psychotherapies, as described by Frank in *Persuasion and Healing*:

1. Emotional arousal.
2. An intense emotionally charged confiding relationship with a healing person.
3. Expectation of help because of the therapist's personal qualities and social status as healer.
4. Each approach has a theory, a rationale or a "myth," that makes sense of the person's trouble and how to get relief from it.
5. Provision of new information to the patient about problems and solutions.
6. Enhanced sense of self-effectiveness as a result of some successful experiences.

2. Looked at from a somewhat different perspective (Prochaska, 1991; Prochaska & DiClemente, 1984), we can recognize the importance of the patient's stage of change: Is the patient in the precontemplation, contemplation, action, or maintenance stage? What needs to occur before desired changes can be made?

3. It is interesting to remember that the word "fact" comes from Latin roots meaning "do or to make" (as in *factory* or *manufacturing*). First (and subsequent) sessions involve the cocreation of a "reality" that yields a useful explanation of where the patient is stuck and what is needed to get unstuck. The constructivist argument was well made by the three baseball umpires contesting their acumen: The first one declared, "I call 'em as I see 'em." The second responded: "I call 'em as they are." To which the third replied: "They ain't nothing until I call 'em."

4. Fully appreciating patients' strengths and capacities for self-determination enhances their inchoate sense of autonomy and personal empowerment. As the titles of a number of useful books have it: *The Power Is in the Patient* (Goulding & Goulding, 1978), and *The Answer Within* (Lankton & Lankton, 1983), so *In Search of Solutions* (O'Hanlon & Weiner-Davis, 1988), we explore *The Frontier of Brief Psychotherapy* (Malan, 1976) and the *Theory and Practice of Brief Therapy* (Budman & Gurman, 1988), while considering *Uncommon Therapy* (Haley, 1973) and welcoming *Keys to Solutions in Brief Therapy* (de Shazer, 1985)

that may produce *Expanding Therapeutic Possibilities* (Friedman & Fanger, 1991) and yield valuable results, perhaps even in *Single-Session Therapy* (Talmon, 1990). The effective brief therapist often functions more as a facilitator or "midwife" than as someone who "makes" change occur.

5. As a corollary to this distinction, it also seems that therapists' beliefs about specific mechanisms of change are often different in longer and shorter treatments. Longer treatments generally emphasize recapitulation and stability. ("He's been through so much trauma that he needs me as a stable object in his life.") The implication here is that one important aspect of what will lead to change is *predictable* in the therapeutic relationship. In contrast, shorter and time-effective intermittent treatments appear to emphasize the rapid introduction of novel thoughts, actions, and emotions.

REFERENCES

Alexander, F., & French, T. M. (1976) *Psychoanalytic therapy*. Lincoln, NB: University of Nebraska Press. (Original work published 1946)

Andersen, T. (1987). The reflecting team: Dialogue and metadialogue in clinical work. *Family Process, 26*, 415–428.

Bandler, R., & Grinder, J. (1982). *Reframing*. Moab, UT: Real People Press.

Bateson, G. (1972). *Steps to an ecology of mind*. New York: Ballantine Books.

Berg, I. K., & Miller, S. D. (1992). *Working with the problem drinker: A solution-oriented approach*. New York: W. W. Norton.

Berlyne, D. E. (1960). *Conflict arousal and curiosity*. New York: McGraw-Hill.

Budman, S. H. (1990). The myth of termination in brief therapy: It ain't over til it's over. In S. K. Zeig & S. G. Gilligan (Eds.), *Brief therapy: Myths, methods, and metaphors* (pp. 206–218). New York: Brunner/Mazel.

Budman, S. H., & Gurman, A. S. (1988). *Theory and practice of brief therapy*. New York: Guilford Press.

Carpenter, G., Tecce, J., Stechler, G., & Friedman, S. (1970). Differential visual behavior to human and humanoid faces in early infancy. *Merrill-Palmer Quarterly, 16*, 91–108.

Cummings, N. A. (1991). Intermittent therapy throughout the life cycle. In C. S. Austad & W. H. Berman (Eds.), *Psychotherapy in managed health care: The optimal use of and resources* (pp. 35–45). Washington, DC: American Psychological Assocation.

de Shazer, S. (1985). *Keys to solution in brief therapy*. New York: W. W. Norton.

Fay, A. (1978). *Making things better by making them worse*. New York: Hawthorn Books.

Fiske, D. W., & Maddi, S. R. (Eds). (1961). *Functions of varied experience*. Homewood, IL: Dorsey Press.

Frank, J. D. (1974). *Persuasion and healing*. New York: Schocken Books.

Friedman, S. (1975). Infant habituation. Process, problems and possibilities. In N. Ellis (Ed.), *Aberrant development in infancy: Human and animal studies* (pp. 217–239). Hillsdale, NJ: Erlbaum Associates.

Friedman, S., & Fanger, M. T. (1991). *Expanding therapeutic possibilities: Getting results in brief psychotherapy*. New York: Lexington Books/Macmillan.

Goulding, R. L., & Goulding, M. M. (1978). *The Power is in the patient*. San Francisco: Transactional Analysis Press.

Haith, M. (1980). *Rules that babies look by: The organization of newborn visual activity*. Hillsdale, NJ: Erlbaum Associates.

Haley, J. (1973). *Uncommon therapy: The psychiatric techniques of Milton H. Erickson, M.D.* New York: W. W. Norton.

Hebb, D. D. (1946). On the nature of fear. *Psychological Review, 53*, 259–276.

Hoyt, M. F. (1990). On time in brief therapy. In R. A. Wells & V. J. Giannetti (Eds.), *Handbook of the brief psychotherapies* (pp. 115–143). New York: Plenum Press.

Hoyt, M. F., & Austad, C. S. (1992). Psychotherapy in a staff-model Health Maintenance Organization: Providing and assuring quality in the future. *Psychotherapy, 29*, 119–129.

Hubel, D., & Weisel, T. (1962). Receptive fields, binocular interaction, and functional architecture of the cat's visual cortex. *Journal of Physiology, 160*, 106–154.

Hunt, J. M. (1965). Intrinsic motivation and its role in psychological development. In D. Levine (Ed.), *Nebraska symposium of motivation* (Vol. 13). Lincoln, NB: University of Nebraska Press.

Lankton, S., & Lankton, C. (1983). *The answer within: A clinical framework of Ericksonian hypnotherapy*. New York: Brunner/Mazel.

Lanzetta, J. T. (1970). The motivational properties of uncertainty. In H. I. Day, D. E. Berlyne, & D. E. Hunt (Eds.), *Intrinsic motivation: A new direction in education* (pp. 134–147). Toronto: Holt, Rinehart & Winston.

Levy, R. L., & Shelton, J. L. (1990). Tasks in brief therapy. In R. A. Wells & V. J. Giannetti (Eds.), *Handbook of the Brief Psychotherapies* (pp. 145–163). New York: Plenum Press.

Malan, D. H. (1976). *The Frontier of brief psychotherapy*. New York: Plenum Press.

Marmor, J. (1986). The corrective emotional experience revisited. *International Journal of Short-Term Psychotherapy, 1*, 43–47.

O'Hanlon, W. H., & Weiner-Davis, M. (1988). *In search of solutions: A new direction in psychotherapy*. New York: W. W. Norton.

Prochaska, J. O. (1991). Prescribing to the stage and level of phobic patients. *Psychotherapy, 28*, 463–468.

Prochaska, J. O., & DiClemente, C. C. (1984). Transtheoretical therapy: Toward a more integrative model of change. *Psychotherapy: Theory, Research and Practice, 19*, 276–288.

Rosen, S. (1982). *My voice will go with you: The teaching tales of Milton H. Erickson*. New York: W. W. Norton.

Rosenbaum, R. (1990). Strategic psychotherapy. In R. A. Wells & V. J. Giannetti (Eds.), *Handbook of the brief psychotherapies* (pp. 351–403). New York: Plenum Press.

Rosenbaum, R., Hoyt, M. F., & Talmon, M. (1990). The challenge of single-session therapies: Creating pivotal moments. In R. A. Wells & L. J. Giannetti (Eds.), *Handbook of the brief psychotherapies* (pp. 165–189). New York: Plenum Press.

Selvini-Palazolli, M., Boscolo, L., Cecchin, G., & Prata, G. (1978). *Paradox and counterparadox*. New York: Jason Aronson.

Talmon, M. (1990). *Single-session therapy: Maximizing the effect of the first (and often only) therapeutic encounter*. San Francisco: Jossey-Bass.

Welker, W. I. (1961). An analysis of exploratory and play behavior in animals. In D. W. Fiske & S. R. Maddi (Eds.), *Functions of varied experience* (pp. 175–226). Homewood, IL: Dorsey Press.

Wells, R. A., & Phelps, P. A. (1990). The brief psychotherapies: A selective overview. In R. A. Wells & V. J. Giannetti (Eds.), *Handbook of the brief psychotherapies* (pp. 3–26). New York: Plenum Press.

Woodworth, R. S., & Schlossberg, H. (1954). *Experimental psychology*. New York: Holt, Rinehart & Winston.

Index

Abandonment by father, single-session
  therapy for, 70–73
ABC theory of human disturbance, 36–37,
  48, 56
Abuse. *See specific types of abuse*
Accident, anxiety responses to, 24–25
Acts of Others, 99–100
Acts of Others Toward Self, 88
Acts of Self, 88, 99
Acts of Self Toward Self. *See* Introject
Adolescent(s)
  adopted, 142, 147
  cognitive–behavioral therapy case
    illustration, 140–150
  MRI approach and, 318–319
  structural family therapy case and, 327–
    336
Adoption, 142, 147
Affection, in couple's relationship history,
  231–232, 234
Agoraphobia, 23–24
Alcohol abuse
  active, during therapy, 300
  I-D-E therapy for, 119–126
  motivation for change and, 129
  rational–emotive therapy and, 55
  as reaction to tacit schema, 149
  sobriety as focus for interview and,
    289–290
  stress and, 296
  structural family therapy case and,
    327–336
Alcoholics Anonymous (AA), 120,
  128
Andreas, Connirae, 14–35, 352
Andreas, Steve, 14–35, 352
Anticipation, value of, 176
Antidepressants, 106. *See also*
  Pharmacotherapy
Anxiety
  about anxiety, 41
  interpersonal patterns and, 87
  "musts" and, 41–43

responses to, 24–25, 43–48
self-perception and, 149–150
Aponte, Harry J., 324–342, 354
Assessment
  of communication, 238–239
  in emotionally focused couples therapy,
    219
  psychodynamic techniques of, 138
Associated memory, 15
Assumptions, 283
Attachment theory, emotionally focused
    couples therapy and, 206
Auditory modality, 18
Automatic response, changing, 27–28
Autonomy, 11, 64, 90
Avoidant personality case, 91–99
Awareness, of self-defeating patterns, 88

Bauman, Donald H., 225–253, 353
Beck Depression Inventory, 102, 140, 144
Bee phobia, neurolinguistic programming
    for, 16–24, 351
Behavioral change, in couple therapy, 187
Behavioral marital therapies. *See also*
    Cognitive–behavioral marital therapy
  vs. cognitive–behavioral marital therapy,
    248–249
Biasing judgments, 137
Binder, Jeffrey L., 87–109, 352
Blame, 98
Bonding theory, emotionally focused
    couples therapy and, 205, 206
Brief therapy. *See also specific therapeutic
    approaches*
  definition of, 111
  general features of, 355
  universal elements of, 345–346
Budman, Simon H., 3–5, 9–13, 111–133,
  352
Butler, Steven F., 87–109, 352

Carels, Robert, 225–253, 353
Catastrophizing, 137

CBT. *See* Cognitive–behavioral therapy (CBT)
Ceremonies, 67
Change process. *See also* Therapeutic change
  attitudes about, 112
  integrative marital therapy and, 188
  pivot chord for, 66
  seeding, in single-session psychotherapy, 65
Client. *See* Patient
Closeness/distance issue, 191–194, 211–212, 217
CMP. *See* Cyclic maladaptive pattern (CMP)
Cocaine abuse patients, single-session psychotherapy and, 80
Cognition
  as active process, 136
  behavior and, 12
  influencing marital problems, 227–228
Cognitive–behavioral marital therapy, 184, 250–251
  assessment phase, 249
  behavioral interactions and, 225
  case illustration, 228–248
  categories of interest for, 227
  cognitive restructuring in, 227–228
  conceptualization of couple, 239–243, 248
  contributing factors, understanding of, 251
  course of treatment, 252
  current relationship discord and, 247
  educational, skill-building approach, 226–227
  first session, 230–239
  follow-up, 246–247
  goals, negotiation of, 250
  historical factors and, 247–248
  individual factors and, 247
  internal processes and, 225
  lack of collaborative relationship and, 249–250
  length of sessions, 252
  relationship factors and, 247
  social exchange theory and, 226
  social learning theory and, 226
  spacing of sessions, 252
  success, evaluation of, 252
  termination of treatment, 252
  theoretical bases of, 226
  treatment plan, 244–246
  types of couples and, 250–251
  vs. behavioral marital therapies, 248–249
Cognitive–behavioral therapy (CBT)
  basic assumptions of, 135–136

case illustration, 140–150
classical framework of, 137
collaboration in, 136
dynamic framework of, 138
family sessions and, 152
first session, 140–150
follow-up, 150
goal of, 136
initial session in, 139–140
number of sessions, 148, 151–152
origins of, 135
rational–emotive therapy. *See* Rational–emotive therapy
for resistant patient, 150–151
role of therapist in, 136
technical intervention in, 139
treatment failures and, 152–153
Cognitive distortions, 137
Cognitive therapy. *See also specific cognitive approaches*
  focus of, 156
  multidimensional dissociative model and, 175
Cognitive triad, 144
  domains of, 137
Collaboration, in cognitive–behavioral therapy, 136
Commitment, intimacy and, 196
Communication
  assessment of, 238–239
  constructive, instruction for, 249
  problems of, 188–195, 227
Communication behavior, 227
Community mental health services
  single-session psychotherapy and, 79
  time-limited dynamic psychotherapy and, 105
Comprehension, of NLP procedures by patient, 33–34
Conflict handling, history of, 232
Confrontation, managing assertively, 176
Conscious cognition, vs. unconscious cognition, 138
Constructing solutions approach, 185
  active alcohol abuse during therapy and, 300
  assumptions for, 283–285
  case illustration, 285–299
    first session, 286–295
    second session, 295–297
    third session, 298–299
  development of narratives, 299
  leaving room to gather thoughts, 293–294, 301
  letter-writing method and, 294–295, 297–298, 299–300
  "macho man," involvement in therapy, 301–302

maintaining focus, 301
"miracle question" and, 300–301
number of sessions, 303
using capacities and strengths of client, 282–283
vs. traditional family therapy models, 302–303
Constructivist philosophy, 284
Control, 95, 147, 164
consequences and, 170–171
feeling of, for accident scene, 25–27
loss of, resentment toward, 211
in marital relationship, 211–212
Control Mastery Theory, I-D-E model and, 113–115, 121, 128
Coping skills, enhancement of, 63
Core Conflictual Relationship Theme analysis, 138
Corrective emotional experience, 102, 103
Cotherapy team, in reflecting process, 184
Countertransference, 88, 104, 151
Couple therapy, 183–185. See also specific approaches for
brief treatment for, 186
termination of, 186
Course of treatment, for neurolinguistic programming, 30–31
Criticism, 225
Cure
concept of, 63
interpersonal–developmental–existential model and, 112
Cyclic maladaptive pattern (CMP), 99–100
categories of, 88–89, 92
definition of, 88, 104
experiencing different outcome of, 100–102
patient understanding of, 102
reenactment of, 103

Davidson, Judy, 255–279, 353
Deep breathing exercises, 44
Defense mechanisms
maladaptive, therapist's personal reactions to, 87
in time-limited dynamic psychotherapy, 89–90
Denial, 129
Dependent personality, time-limited dynamic psychotherapy case, 91–99
Depending on others, 216
Depression
adolescent, cognitive–behavioral therapy case illustration, 140–150
interpersonal patterns and, 87
musts and, 48
Desire, turning into a "must," 41–43

Developed resource, 168
Developmental focus, for interpersonal–developmental–existential therapy, 117
Developmental issues, integrative marital therapy and, 200
Diary, drug and alcohol, 128
Dichotomous thinking, 137
Discipline, 292–293
Disqualifying the positive, 137
Dissociated memory, 15
Dissociation, 160–162
reframing from negative to positive, 163
types of, 156–157
value of, 163–164
Divorce, decision, 165–168
Drug abuse. See Substance abuse
cognitive–behavioral therapy case illustration, 140–150
Drug and alcohol diary, 128
Drugs. See Pharmacotherapy
Dyadic Adjustment Scale (DAS), 210, 218–219, 221
Dynamic–cognitive–behavioral therapy (D-CBT), 138

EFT. See Emotionally focused couples therapy (EFT)
Ellis, Albert, 36–57, 352
Emotional engagement, marital satisfaction and, 204
Emotionally focused couples therapy (EFT)
appropriateness of, 219–220
assessment sessions, 219
attachment theory and, 206, 207
bonding theory and, 205, 206
case illustration, 209–210
first session, 210–218
follow-up, 218–219
central focus of, 206
change strategies for, 207–209
clinical issues in, 209
content of, 207
contraindications, 210, 222
criteria for longer-term basis, 221
Dyadic Adjustment Scale and, 218–219, 221
focus of, 204–205
goal of, 205
homework assignments and tasks for, 222
impact of problem on relationship and, 221
improvement or change in, 220–221
indications for, 219–220, 221–222
main tasks for therapist, 208
number of sessions for, 220
positions and patterns, 209
present process and, 209

Emotionally focused couples therapy (EFT)
  (*continued*)
  primary emotion and, 209
  redefinition of relationship in, 205
  referrals from, 219–220
  spacing of sessions, 220
  steps in, 208
  termination of treatment, 220–221
  theoretical perspectives, 206–207
  therapist role, 205
Emotionally focused therapy, 184
Emotional reasoning, 137
Emotions. *See* Feelings
Empowerment, 170
Enactment, in structural family therapy,
  326–327, 331–333
Encouragement, in single-session
  psychotherapy, 63
Epstein, Norman, 225–253, 353
Exclusion therapy, 129
Expectations of Others, 93–94, 99
Expectations of Others' Reactions, 88
Experience
  of different outcome, in therapeutic
    relationship, 88
  modalities of, 14
Explicit level, vs. tacit level, 138
Externalization of voices, 139
Extramarital affair, 91–92

Family members, as active partners in
  therapy, 284
Family system, characteristic patterns of
  relationships in, 325
Family therapy, 183–185. *See also specific*
    approaches for
  brief treatment for, 186
  couples therapy in, 261
  I-D-E model and, 132
  political domain of, 132
  as science, 303
  vs. individual therapy, 132
  wellness model of, 283
"Fascism" factor, 152
Father, abandonment by, 70–73
Feedforward mechanisms, 138, 151
Feeling Good: The New Mood Therapy, Burns,
  140, 148
Feelings
  discussion of, 97
  expression of, 206, 269
  interventions for, 244–246
  management of, 147
  negative
    directed toward therapist, 98
    expression of, 242–243
    handling of, 232–233

of others, tolerance for, 269
  primary source of, 207
  underlying, interpretation by therapist,
    214–215
First session, 3–5, 351, 355
  asking questions and, 257–259
  for cognitive–behavioral marital therapy,
    230–239
  for cognitive–behavioral therapy, 139–150
  for constructing solutions approach,
    286–295
  differences in, 345
  early interactional change and, 5
  format for, 256–257
  for integrative marital therapy, 188–195
  for interpersonal–developmental–
    existential (I-D-E) model, 116–126
  for interpersonal–developmental–
    existential therapy, 116–126
  for neurolinguistic programming, 16–22
  patients' requests during, 4–5
  for rational–emotive therapy, 39–52
  reflecting process in. *See* Reflection
    process
  return rate for, 61, 74–75
  for single-session psychotherapy, 68–74
  theoretical perspectives of, 255
  for time-limited dynamic psychotherapy,
    91–92
  tone and direction of therapy and, 9
Fisch, Richard, 306–323, 354
Focal psychotherapy, 112. *See also specific*
    time-limited therapies
Focus, 9
  in brief therapy, 346
  developmental, 117
  for integrative marital therapy, 188
  on relational strengths, 236–238
Follow-up, 10
  for emotionally focused couples therapy,
    218–219
  for neurolinguistic programming, 28
  for neurolinguistic programming case
    illustration, 22–24
  for rational–emotive therapy case
    illustration, 52–53
  for single-session psychotherapy, 74
  for single-session therapy, 74
Framing, 159. *See also* Reframing
  of introject, 97
  of "new beginning", 286–287
Friedman, Steven, 3–5, 9–13, 282–304,
  354
Frustration tolerance, low, 53

General Systems Theory, integrative
  marital therapy and, 187

Gestalt-type exercises, 67
Global Assessment Scale (GAS), 102
Global Severity Index of the Symptom
    Checklist 90–Revised, 102
Goals
    of cognitive–behavioral therapy, 136
    of emotionally focused couples therapy,
        205
    first session
        in multidimensional dissociative
            therapy, 158–159
        in rational–emotive therapy, 39
        for therapist, 336–347
    negotiation of, 250, 283
    in single-session psychotherapy, 76–77
    turning into "musts," 41–43
Greenberg, Leslie S., 204–223, 353
Grief, neurolinguistic programming and, 32
Growth, facilitation of, 63
Gurman, Alan S., 111–133, 186–203, 352,
    353

Habitual responses, swish pattern and, 29
Health Maintenance Organization (HMO),
    therapy for, 68, 78, 105
Here-and-now orientation, 346
History
    of idea to come to therapy, as focus of
        interview, 261–264
    patient view of, 130
    of relationship, 230–236
History taking
    for I-D-E approach, 130
    in time-limited dynamic psychotherapy,
        91
HMO therapy, 68, 78, 105
Homework assignments
    for cognitive–behavioral therapy, 146,
        148, 151
    for emotionally focused couples therapy,
        222
    for integrative marital therapy, 200–201
    for structural family therapy, 340–341
    for time-limited dynamic psychotherapy,
        105–106
How to Stubbornly Refuse to Make Yourself
    Miserable About Anything—Yes,
    Anything, 49, 53
Hoyt, Michael F., 3–5, 9–13, 59–84, 352
Humor
    constructivism and, 284
    integrative marital therapy and, 199–200
    in reflection process for couple/family
        therapy, 278
Hypnosis
    contradictions for, 179
    formal vs. informal, 175

indications for, 175
multidimensional dissociative model
    and, 157–158
role in multidimensional dissociative
    model, 174–175

Iatrogenic resistance, 76
I-D-E model. See Interpersonal–
    developmental–existential (I-D-E)
    model
Imagery, 67
Improvement, interpersonal–developmental–
    existential model and, 112
IMT. See Integrative marital therapy (IMT)
Incest, psychological sequelae of, 130
Incest survivor(s)
    I-D-E approach case, 116–126
    intermittent, time-sensitive approach
        and, 130–131
    longer-term individual therapy for, 221
    therapeutic events in healing, 131
Individual change, in couple therapy, 187
Individual therapy. See also specific
        approaches for
    approaches for, 9–13
    vs. family therapy, 132
Individuation process, 149
Information
    definition of, 348
    different, acceptance of, 349–350
Information gathering methods
    for neurolinguistic programming, 31–32
    for single-session therapy, 65–66
Initial interview or session. See First
        session
Insurance coverage, as time limit for
        therapy, 90
Integrative marital therapy (IMT)
    aims of, 187
    assessment in, 198–199
    basic premises of, 187
    case illustration
        first session, 188–195
        second session, 195–196
        third session, 196
    change process in, 202
    contraindications for, 198
    course of therapy, 195–197
    developmental issues and, 200
    evolution of, 197–198
    first session
        aims of, 188
        prior information for, 199
    General Systems Theory and, 187
    humor and, 199–200
    integrative nature of, 197–198
    negotiation of treatment contract, 201

Integrative marital therapy (IMT)
    (*continued*)
  number of sessions, 195
  object relations theory and, 187
  principles guiding therapist, 187
  social learning theory and, 187
  techniques for, 187
  termination of, 201
  time-limit for treatment, 201
Interaction process, in Emotionally
    Focused Couples Therapy, 205
Interminability, 177
Intermittency of sessions, 11, 177–178
Interpersonal assumptions, underlying,
    detection of, 93
Interpersonal–development–existential
    (I-D-E) model, 11–12
  alcohol, 127
  case illustration, 116–126
  Control Mastery Theory and, 121, 128
  course of treatment, 126–127
  current motivation for therapy, 116,
    123–126
  essential elements of, 112
  focal areas, 112–113, 114
  follow-up, 127
  session summary, 123
  therapeutic relationship and, 114–115
  time-effective, 11–112
  time sensitivity of, 111
Interpersonal or dynamic focus, 99
Interpersonal patterns, maladaptive, 87
Interpersonal problems, as therapy focus, 186
Interpersonal psychodynamic model, 11
Interpersonal relationships, in dynamic–
    cognitive–behavioral therapy, 138
Interpersonal therapy, focus of, 156
Interruption of client, 266
Interview room, leaving, to gather
    thoughts, 293–294, 301
Intimacy
  avoidance of, 90
  commitment and, 196
  discomfort with, 241, 243
  interventions for, 244
  nonsexual, 245
Intrapersonal potential, 168–169
Introject, 97, 100
Irrational beliefs, 37, 49, 56

Johnson, Susan M., 204–223, 353

Kinesthetic modality, 18

Labels, 160–162, 165
Language, possibility-oriented perspective
    of, 284

Lax, William D., 255–279, 353
Learning, cognition and, 136
Length of session, for single-session
    therapy, 66
Length of treatment, for rational–emotive
    therapy, 54
Letter-writing method
  benefits of, 299–300
  to emphasize session, 294–295, 297–298
Linguistic style, of family, 284
Listening position, 259, 269

Major depression and dysthymia, time-
    limited dynamic psychotherapy case,
    91–99
Marital conflict/distress
  attributes of, 228
  breaking of relational "rules" and, 187
  escalation of dysfunction, 225
  experiences of distressed spouses and,
    225
  multidimensional dissociative model
    case, 159–174
  nature of, 204
Marital relationship
  ambivalence toward, 165–167
  current strengths and concerns, 236–238
  history of, 230–236
Marital satisfaction, noncommunicative
  behavior and, 227
Marital therapy. *See also specific therapeutic
    approaches*
  I-D-E model and, 132
Medications. *See* Pharmacotherapy
Memory, racall modes, 15
Mental Research Institute brief therapy,
    185
  alternative interventions and, 319–320
  booster sessions and, 320–321
  case illustration, 309–317
    first session, 311–313
    follow-up, 316–317
    second session, 313–316
  complaint-based approach, advantages
    of, 318
  constructing solutions approach and,
    302
  focus on presenting complaint, 307
  general aspects, 307–308
  involvement of others, 318
  length of treatment session, 321
  leverage for change, customer for, 317–
    318
  minimalist approach, 317
  motivation and, 320
  nonlinear causality and, 319
  number of sessions, 320–321

problem definition, 308
problem resolution and, 307
progression of sessions, 320
psychodynamic approach and, 306
speaking client's language and, 309
transforming visitor into customer, 318–319
Metaphor, 284
Methadone, 143
Milan Associates, 274
Millon Clinical Multiaxial inventory, 48, 53
"Miracle" question, 287–288, 300–301
Mirror, one-way, 259, 272, 277
Modalities of experience, 14
Motivation, 31
    for change in substance abusing
        patients, 129
    current, for therapy, 116, 123–126
    multidimensional dissociative model
        and, 177
    rational-emotive therapy and, 54
Multidimensional dissociative model, 156–157
    case illustration, 159–174
        first session, 160–173
        follow-up, 173–174
    cognitive therapy and, 175
    course of treatment, 176–177
    first session, goals for, 158–159
    hypnotic framework and, 157–158
    length of sessions, 177
    length of treatment, 176–177
    motivation and, 177
    personality change and, 175–176
    prognosis for, 176–177
    spacing of sessions, 177
    style of functioning and, 175–176
    termination of, 178
    treatment failures, dealing with, 178–179
"Musts," 41–43

Nail-biting habit, swish pattern and, 29
Narrative psychology, 130
Narratives, 130
    development of, 299
    interactions with others and, 275
Negative feelings
    directed toward therapist, 98
    expression of, 242–243
    handling of, 232–233
Negotiation, of goals, 250, 283
Neurolinguistic programming (NLP), 10
    anxiety responses and, 25–26
    brief therapy field and, 14
    case illustration, 16–28
    commonalities in procedures, 23
    contraindications, 32

course of treatment, 30–31
creating new self-image, 25–27
creating panic and, 25
dangers of, 32
distinct differences of, 33–34
nonverbal cues and, 15
for panic response, 24–28
prognosis for, 30–31
psychoactive or psychotropic drugs and,
    32–33
reluctance and, 30
resistance and, 30
skepticism and disbelief of, 21–22
steps in, 15–16
submodality shifts and, 14–15
treatment failures and, 31–32
for vague or unclear problems, 31
wide range of interventions for, 29–30
Neurotic behavior
    model of, 41–43
    panic attacks. See Panic
A New Guide to Rational Living, 49
NLP. See Neurolinguistic programming
    (NLP)
Noncommunication behavior, 227
Nonproductive exchanges, extended, in
    brief therapy, 191
Nonverbal cues, 15, 19, 209
Novelty
    in couple/family approaches, 183
    in first session, 352–354
    impact on brief therapy, 350–351
    importance of, 348–350
    rapid introduction of, 347–348

Object relations theory, integrative marital
    therapy and, 187
Observing position, 270
Obsessive–compulsive disorder, 140
One-down comment, 315
One-session treatment, 10–11
One-up stance, 315
Operant conditioning, 226
Optimism for change
    in brief therapy, 346
    in constructing solutions approach, 283
    in reflecting process, 278–279
Out-of-session tasks, integrative marital
    therapy and, 200–201
Overgeneralization, 137

Panic, 26, 140, 264
    about panic, 41
    creating, 25
    interpersonal–developmental–existential
        therapy for, 116–126
    rational–emotive therapy case, 38–53

Paranoid personality, time-limited dynamic
psychotherapy case, 91–99
Parenting, stress of, 69–70
Parenting responsibilities stress of, 69–70
Passive–aggressive response, 242
Passivity, 95, 172
Patient
relationship with therapist. *See*
Therapist–patient relationship
responsibilities, definition of, in brief
therapy, 346
self-determination capacities, 355–356
tunnel vision of, 349
Patient satisfaction, 5, 67
Patient–therapist relationship
quality of bond in, 91
small talk and, 93
in time-limited dynamic psychotherapy,
87
Patriarchal families, 290–291
Peace-keeping responsibility, 95–96
Perception, enlarging, 350
Perfectionism, 40, 43, 48
Personality change
multidimensional dissociative model
and, 175–176
in time-limited dynamic psychotherapy,
104
Personality disorders, rational-emotive
therapy and, 54
Personalization, 137
Personal narratives. *See* Narratives
Personal potential, 168
Perspective
of couple, on presenting complaint, 243
new, in single-session therapy, 66
Pharmacotherapy
rational–emotive therapy and, 55
with time-limited dynamic
psychotherapy, 106
Phobia
neurolinguistic programming for, 16–24,
32
NLP process definition of, 23
Pivot chord for change, 66
Playfulness, 244–245, 284
Postmodernism, 275–276
Potential imminence, 64
Power struggle, 211
Preferences, 40–41
changing into musts, 48
turning into a "must," 41–43
Pretending, 18
Pretest, of phobic state, 17
Prior information, for integrative marital
therapy, 199
Priorities, clarifying, 160–161

Problematic behavior, ascription of
meaning and, 275
Problem resolution, behavioral change and,
307
Problems
circular view of, 319
conceptualization of, 239–243
cyclic or circular view of, 215–216,
308–309
definition of, 308
interactional view of, 307, 308
inventing, 47
solution as, 308
vague or unclear, 31, 55
Problem solving, in multidimensional
dissociative model, 159–174
Pruning, of personal narrative, 130
Psychoactive or psychotropic drugs,
neurolinguistic programming and, 32–
33
Psychological reactance, 76
Psychometric assessment devices, 140
Psychotherapy
definition of, 156
effective, commonalities of, 12–13
Pursue/withdraw pattern, 196, 205

Question(s)
asking, in first session, 257–259
"miracle," 287–288, 300–301
opening, 286

Rapport, gaining, small talk for, 16–17
Rational–emotive therapy (RET), 10
ABC theory of human disturbance and,
36–37
alcohol abuse and, 55
books, 53
case illustration, 38–53
first session, 39–50
follow-up, 52–53
second session, 50–51
third session, 51–52
changes in, 56
considerations, 56
course of treatment, 54
early development of, 36
frequency of sessions, 54–55
goals for first sessions, 39
length of sessions, 54–55
length of treatment, 54
main therapeutic aspect of, 38
medications for panic disorder and, 55
motivation and, 54
pamphlets, 49, 53
personality disorders and, 54
prognosis, 54

resistant patients and, 54
self-actualization and, 37–38
self-sabotaging and, 37–38
spacing of sessions, 54–55
treatment failures, 56
for vague or unclear problems, 55
Rational Recovery meetings, 128
Readiness
single-session psychotherapy and, 64–65
for therapy, 113
to try a different approach, 314–315
Reality testing, 177
Reauthoring, 113
Recall, modes of, 15
Recording of sessions, 49
Referrals, 128, 159
Reflection process, 184
case illustration, 260–274
first session, 261–271
follow up, 273–274
other sessions, 271–273
comments on, 260
guidelines for, 259–260
humor, 278
Milan Associates and, 274
modification for single practitioner, 277–278
respect and sensitivity toward client, 274–275
sharing of thoughts and ideas, 278
theoretical framework for, 255–256
Refocusing, 213
Reframing, 129, 159
advantages of, 312
of dissociation from negative to positive, 163
of hurtful feelings, 171
in single-session therapy, 66
Relational developmental dysynchrony, 189
Relaxation exercises, 44
Reluctance, neurolinguistic programming and, 30
Repetition, in rational–emotive therapy, 49–50
Reprocessing, 218
Resistance
to cognitive–behavioral therapy, 150–151
identification, in couple therapy, 186
to neurolinguistic programming, 30
problems outside therapy and, 87
to rational–emotive therapy, 54
to substance abuse issues, 128
to therapeutic interventions, 226
to time-limited dynamic psychotherapy, 104
to treatment termination, 90

Respect
for family's original request, 283
for family system and resources, 283
Restatement, before time-out, 67
Return for second visit, 74–75
Right, as relative term, 171
Rigidity, 161
Rituals, 67
Role playing
for cognitive–behavioral therapy, 151
impact of novelty and, 351
in single-session therapy, 67, 72–73
Role Relationship Model analysis, 138, 149
Romance, in couple's relationship history, 231–232
Rosenbaum, Robert, 59–84, 352

Scapegoating, 301
Schema, 137, 149
School adjustment case, 285–299
Science, family therapy as, 303
Secondary gain, agoraphobia and, 24
Selectivity, 164
Self-actualization, 37
Self-defeating feelings, 37
Self-defeating patterns, awareness of, 88
Self-destructive behavior, 97
Self hating, 43
Self-help report forms, 48–49
Self-image, creating new, 25–27
Self-mastery, 67
Self-perception, 149–150
Self-sabotaging, 37–38
Sensate focus exercises, 244
Sentiment override, 228
Separation, marital, 165
Separation–individuation, time and, 90
Sessions. See also specific therapeutic approaches
first. See First session
one, importance of, 69
recording of, 49
Sex, initiation of, 241–242, 245–246
"Sex scrabble," 245
Sexual abuse
I-D-E approach and, 126–127
reflection process and, 261–274
Sexual anxiety, 46–47
Sexual problem case, cognitive–behavioral marital therapy for, 230–247
SFT. See Structural family therapy (SFT)
Should statements, 137
Single-session psychotherapy, 10–11
advantages of, 80–81
assumptions of, 80
attitudes for, 61–62

Single-session psychotherapy (*continued*)
case illustration, 68–74
first session, 68–74
follow-up, 74
clinical guidelines for, 65–68
contraindications, 62–63, 70, 80
differences in, 75–76
eclectic nature of, 75–76
ending, and leaving open door for
future change, 67–68, 73–74
failures and, 76–77
feedback, final, 67
format, adherence to, 76
fundamental eclecticism and, 63–65
goals in, 76–77
indications for, 62
induction and preparation for, 65
last-minute issues, 67
long-term benefits, 60
making a living at, 81
new perspective and, 63
patient complaints and, 78
patient population for, 78–79
patient power or autonomy and, 64
readiness and, 64–65
resistant patients and, 79–80
second session, need for, 76–77
steps in, 75
success of, 60–61
theoretical perspectives, 59–60
therapist–patient relationship and, 64
training new clinicians and, 77–78
Skepticism, of neurolinguistic
programming, 21–22
Small talk, important messages in, 93
Sobriety, as focus for interview, 289–290
Social exchange theory, cognitive–
behavioral marital therapy and, 226
Social learning theory
central concepts in, 226
cognitive–behavioral marital therapy
and, 226
integrative marital therapy and, 187
Softening, definition of, 218
Solution suggestions, making precipitously,
313–314
Solving Emotional Problems, 53
Spouse abuse, 189–190
allowance of, 98
resignation to, 92
risk for, 96
State-specific learning, drugs and, 32–33
Strengths, patient, looking for, 66–67
Stress
reactions to, 43–45
relief, single-session psychotherapy for,
68–74

Structural family therapy (SFT), 185
brief, 324, 325–326
method of, 326–327
case illustration, 327–336
converting negative solution into
positive, 338–339
dynamics for enactment, 340
evolution of approach, 341
follow-up, 337–338
homework assignments and tasks, 340–
341
number of sessions, 340
planning for future sessions and, 339–
340
presence of all family members and, 339
principles of, 324–325
termination of treatment, 340
therapist role in, 326
trust and respect of therapist and, 338
viewpoint for, 339
Strupp, Hans H., 87–109, 352
Stuttering, 292
Style of functioning, multidimensional
dissociative model and, 175–176
Submodalities, 14–15
Substance abuse, 129. *See also* Alcohol
abuse
in family, I-D-E therapy for, 119–126
hard-line position on, 121–122
as reaction to tacit schema, 149
single-session psychotherapy and, 80
willingness to reframe, 129
Suicidal patient(s)
case illustration, cognitive–behavioral
therapy, 140–150
single-session psychotherapy and, 80
Swish pattern, 29

Tacit level, vs. explicit level, 138
Tacit schema, 149
Talking, help and, 69
Talking position, 259
Talmon, Moshe, 59–84, 352
Taping of therapy sessions, 159
Tasks, out-of-session. *See* Homework
assignments
Team approach, in reflection process, 261–
274
Termination
of cognitive–behavioral marital therapy, 252
of cognitive–behavioral therapy, 140
of couple therapy, 186
of emotionally focused couples therapy,
220–221
of integrative marital therapy, 201
of multidimensional dissociative therapy,
178

of structural family therapy, 340
of time-limited therapy, 102
of treatment, resistance to, 90
Therapeutic alliance. *See also* Therapist–
    patient relationship
active monitoring of, 89–90
in brief therapy, 346
deterrents to, 87
endangerment, prevention of, 199–200
for single-session therapy, 65
working, 69, 87, 346
Therapeutic approaches. *See also specific*
    approaches
commonalities of, 156
underlying structure of, 156
Therapeutic change. *See also* Change
    process
in couple therapy, 187
essence of, 103
expectation of, in brief therapy, 346
occurence in I-D-E model, 131–132
optimism for, therapst's role in, 278 279
in short vs. long therapy, 356
in time-limited dynamic psychotherapy,
    88
in time-limited therapy, 100–102
Therapeutic conversation, halting of, 276
Therapeutic experience, 67
Therapeutic relationship. *See* Therapist–
    patient relationship
Therapeutic uncertainty, 302–303
Therapist(s)
checking observations, 20–21
confidence, success of single-session
    therapy and, 60–61
goals for first session, 346–347
for individual approaches, 132
long-term vs. short-term, dominant
    values of, 113
noncommittal statements of, 311–314
as participant–observer, 11
responsibilities in brief therapy, 346
in time-limited dynamic psychotherapy, 89
willingness to help, 69
Therapist–patient relationship. *See also*
    Therapeutic alliance
expectations for, 94
halting of therapeutic conversation, 276
I-D-E model and, 114–115
lateral position of, 256, 258, 276–277
positive, 10
premature or out-of-context references
    to, 92
promotion of adaptive experience, 103.
    See also Corrective emotional
    experience
in single-session psychotherapy, 64

Time-effective brief treatment, pivotal
    values of, 112–113
Time-limited dynamic psychotherapy
    (TLDP)
assessment of outcome, 100–102
case illustration, 90–99
    first session, 91–92
    second session, 92
    third session, 92–99
course of, 104–105
development of, 87
differentiation from other therapies,
    103–104
homework and, 105–106
indications for, 106
interpersonal focus in, 99, 102
length of treatment, rationale for, 105
personality change and, 104
potential contribution of, 89
principles of, 104
procedures of, 104
prognosis for, 104–105
role of time limits in, 89–90
style of function of patient and, 104
subtle reactions and, 93, 109
success and, 108
technical interventions of, 88–89
treatment failures, 106
Time-out, 67
Time sensitivity
of brief therapy, 346
of I-D-E model, 111
TLDP. *See* Time-limited dynamic
    psychotherapy (TLDP)
Training clinicians, in single-session
    psychotherapy, 77–78
Transference, 78, 149
definition of, 87
entanglement of therapist, 151
well-timed, 67
Treatment failures
in congitive–behavioral therapy, 152–
    153
in multidimensional dissociative therapy,
    178–179
neurolinguistic programming and, 31–32
in rational–emotive therapy, 56
in single-session psychotherapy, 76–77
in time-limited dynamic psychotherapy,
    106
Treatment focus. *See* Focus
Triple-column strategy, 139
Trust, 338
Turner, Ralph M., 135–153, 352

Ultrabrief therapy. *See* Single-session
    psychotherapy

Ultrabrief therapy (Single-session therapy),
    10–11
Unconditionally Accepting Yourself and Others,
    53
Unconscious cognition, vs. conscious
    cognition, 138

Vague or unclear problems
    neurolinguistic programming and,
        31
    rational–emotive therapy and, 55
Verbal abuse/aggression case, 310–317
Visualization, 18–19
Vulnerability, perceived, 235, 243

Want–fear duality, in relationships, 96–97
Weakland, John, 306–322, 354
Willingness
    of patient, 129, 294
    of therapist, 69
Workaholic, 31
Work-related stress, 69
Wrong, as relative term, 171

Xanax, 141, 144

Yapko, Michael, 156–179, 352

"Zooming in", 25, 27–28